A HISTORY OF
PREVENTIVE MEDICINE

A HISTORY OF
PREVENTIVE MEDICINE

By

HARRY WAIN, B.S., M.D., M.S.P.H.

Diplomate, American Board of Preventive Medicine

Fellow, American College of Preventive Medicine

Fellow, American Public Health Association

Fellow, Royal Society of Health, London, England

Instructor, Preventive Medicine, Ohio State University

Health Commissioner, Mansfield-Richland County, Ohio

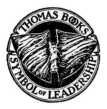

CHARLES C THOMAS · PUBLISHER
Springfield · Illinois · U.S.A.

Published and Distributed Throughout the World by
CHARLES C THOMAS · PUBLISHER
Bᴀɴɴᴇʀsᴛoɴᴇ Hoᴜsᴇ
301-327 East Lawrence Avenue, Springfield, Illinois, U.S.A.
Nᴀᴛᴄʜᴇᴢ Pʟᴀɴᴛᴀᴛɪoɴ Hoᴜsᴇ
735 North Atlantic Boulevard, Fort Lauderdale, Florida, U.S.A.

© *1970, by* CHARLES C THOMAS · PUBLISHER
Library of Congress Catalog Card Number: 77-97539

With THOMAS BOOKS *careful attention is given to all details of manufacturing and design. It is the Publisher's desire to present books that are satisfactory as to their physical qualities and artistic possibilities and appropriate for their particular use.* THOMAS BOOKS *will be true to those laws of quality that assure a good name and good will.*

Printed in the United States of America
H-15

To
My Grandchildren
May They, And All Mankind Know
That

**"AN OUNCE OF PREVENTION
IS WORTH A POUND OF CURE"**

PREFACE

ONCE UPON A TIME, and not so very long ago, the world was a very unsafe place in which to live. Periodically plague, pestilence, pandemics and epidemics swept across the world like great disastrous tidal waves, leaving behind them a terrible toll of death, disease and human misery.

The human race has more than once been threatened with extinction because of plague and pestilence. Disastrous outbreaks of disease frequently brought about the mass migrations of early peoples, often changed national customs and greatly influenced religious development. Practically every great war of history has been accompanied by epidemics of disease that greatly influenced the outcome. Battles and campaigns were as often won or lost by plague and pestilence as by the brains of the generals or the might of the armies. The scourge of disease has frequently shaped the course of history and brought about far reaching changes in the destinies of peoples and nations.

In times past, mankind's thinking was negative as far as disease prevention was concerned, and most of his efforts were centered upon curative medicine. Diseases and epidemics were considerd as inevitable visitations of providence, and civilization was content to take action to try to protect itself only when disease actually occurred.

Until comparatively recent times there was very little that mankind knew or could do to prevent death and disease, except to resort to prayer and flee in terror before the numerous plagues and epidemics that occurred. The concept of disease prevention was unthought of, and scientific knowledge as to the cause and prevention of disease was unknown.

Progress was painfully slow over the centuries and preventive medicine as a true scientific discipline was not born until after Pasteur's great discoveries of the nineteenth century. Thus freedom from the fearful epidemics of the past and the control of contagion are relatively recent accomplishments. Although scientific preventive medicine and effective public health practice is of recent birth, its roots extend far back into antiquity.

The aim of this book is to present the historical progress of preventive medicine from its earliest beginnings up to relatively modern times. It portrays the fascinating story of the pestilence-ridden centuries of the past and tells the tale of the many talented "pioneers of prevention" who contributed so significantly to our progress. Since preventive medicine grew out of, and developed along with, mankind's social, medical and scientific advancement, the book includes pertinent historical accounts of these advances.

In order to keep the book readable and of a reasonable size, only the most interesting and important historical events are presented. The historical progress of preventive medicine is carried through the nineteenth century and on into the early twentieth century.

Because preventive medicine moved forward so rapidly during the twentieth century and because it is difficult to have a proper perspective of contemporary contributions, the book draws to a conclusion at this period of time. Hence, events occurring beyond the early twentieth century are dealt with briefly or not at all.

The book has taken over ten years to write, and a great deal of painstaking reading and research has gone into its preparation. Every effort has been made to insure historical accuracy and at the same time to write in an interesting fashion so as to maintain the reader's interest.

CONTENTS

                                      Page

Preface vii

Chapter

1. IN THE BEGINNING 3
2. MOSES AND THE HEBRAIC HEALTH CODE 7
3. HEALTH IN THE GOLDEN AGE OF GREECE 12
4. THE ROMANS—PIONEERS OF PUBLIC SANITATION 17
5. DARKNESS OVER EUROPE AND THE LIGHT IN THE EAST 29
6. PILGRIMS AND CRUSADERS 35
7. THE SCHOOL OF SALERNO AND SENSIBLE LIVING 41
8. THEY SHALL CRY, "UNCLEAN" 49
9. THE PLAGUE 54
10. OTHER MEDIEVAL EPIDEMICS AND DISEASES 64
11. THE RENAISSANCE AND THE REBIRTH OF MEDICINE 74
12. SYPHILIS—SCOURGE OF THE RENAISSANCE AND A NEW
    CONCEPT OF CONTAGION 86
13. THE SCIENTIFIC AND MEDICAL ADVANCES OF THE
    SEVENTEENTH CENTURY 100
14. VAN LEEUWENHOEK'S TINY LITTLE BEASTIES AND THE
    INVISIBLE WORLD OF THE MICROSCOPISTS 115
15. THE BOOKKEEPING OF LIFE AND THE BIRTH OF VITAL STATISTICS 121
16. PLAGUE—FIRE—PEOPLE AND PROGRESS 126
17. THE EIGHTEENTH CENTURY 132
18. THE STORY OF SMALLPOX AND THE BIRTH OF PREVENTIVE
    MEDICINE 167
19. THE CONQUEST OF SCURVY AND THE ADVANCE OF NAVAL
    AND MILITARY HYGIENE 196
20. LATE EIGHTEENTH AND EARLY NINETEENTH CENTURY:
    FOUNDATION STONES FOR MODERN PUBLIC HEALTH AND
    PREVENTIVE MEDICINE 205

Chapter	Page
21. THE LADY WITH THE LAMP	213
22. DOCTORS! WASH YOUR HANDS	220
23. PASTEUR AND THE BIRTH OF BACTERIOLOGY	227
24. THE GOLDEN AGE OF MEDICAL DISCOVERY	243
25. MILK-BORNE DISEASES	250
26. THE WATER-BORNE AND FECAL DISCHARGE DISEASES	264
27. CHOLERA AND TYPHOID	281
28. BITING BUGS, THE HISTORY OF ARTHROPOD-BORNE DISEASE	290
29. LICE, FLEAS AND DDT	301
30. WINGED DEATH, THE STORY OF MALARIA AND YELLOW FEVER	308
31. THE GREAT WHITE PLAGUE	324
32. GONORRHEA—CRIPPLER OF MEN, WRECKER OF WOMEN AND BLINDER OF BABIES	341
33. DIPHTHERIA—KILLER OF CHILDREN	353
34. POLIO PREVENTION	359
35. THE DEFICIENCY DISEASES	368
36. RECENT PROGRESS AND PROMISE FOR THE FUTURE	381
Bibliography	392
Name Index	397
Subject Index	404

A HISTORY OF
PREVENTIVE MEDICINE

Chapter 1

IN THE BEGINNING

PRIMITIVE MAN and all early civilizations regarded the visitation of disease either as the work of evil spirits or as a manifestation of anger upon the part of the gods. Early mankind's attempts to prevent or cure disease consisted of rites and incantations to ward off or to drive out the evil spirits, or of attempts to propitiate and appease the anger of the gods through sacrificial offerings, rites and prayers.

Historically, it is known that some of the primitive peoples did make sporadic attempts to protect and preserve their health. From bitter experience they learned that it would help to preserve their lives if they kept their surroundings clean. They also recognized that certain diseases were contagious or catching. Through trial and error, they developed some basic empiric rules of sanitation, health and hygiene.

The story of health and mankind's fight against death and disease begins with the dawn of history. History began on the broad plain between the Tigris and the Euphrates Rivers called Mesopotamia.

Historians and archeologists tell us that here was developed an early civilization known as the Sumerian. Excavations have shown us that the ancient Sumerians possessed some knowledge of the rudiments of sanitation. Evidence has been found that some of the ancient Sumerian houses possessed well-laid drains and cesspools.

The successors to the Sumerians were the Chaldeans, Assyrians and Babylonians. These ancient peoples showed some advance in the knowledge of sanitation. It is known that they brought public water supplies to their villages and cities over long distances in open channels.

They also constructed drains and sewers, and excavations have revealed houses that had well-laid bathroom floors, and latrines that were built into recesses of the wall, along with drains carrying off the effluent.

[3]

The healers or physicians of these people were priests whose methods of cure most often consisted of the exorcism of the demons of disease. Specific demons were considered to preside over special parts of the body and to cause special complaints.

The Babylonian priest-physicians, along with their chants and incantations, had a certain amount of inquisitiveness concerning the anatomy of the human body. They placed great emphasis upon the liver, believing that knowledge as to the state of health or disease was reflected in the shape of this organ. The priests studied and used the livers of sheep and provided themselves with little clay models of this organ, which they presented to the gods as votive offerings. Later they made models of other organs and portions of the anatomy, which were offered to the various deities, along with prayers imploring the gods to restore them to health.

That the Babylonians developed an extensive medico-surgical lore and practice is shown by the fact that the famous Code of Hammurabi, which was written in 2,000 B.C. and which is our earliest compilation of laws, contained severe penalties for medical malpractice.

They practiced a crude form of surgery, treating fractures and injuries, lancing abscesses and trephining the skull to release the demons of disease that possessed the patient. Archeologists have found Babylonian tablets which mentioned over three hundred drugs used in the medical practice of that ancient civilization. Included were plants, trees, herbs, roots, seeds, juices and mineral substances.

Amulets were worn for prophylactic protection and grotesque masks were fashioned to terrorize and drive off the demons of disease. Especial precautions were used to ward off the vicious "southwest wind" whose terrible, hot breath produced an agonizing fever which could consume both man and beast. This particular demon was represented as a frightful-looking, dog-bodied eagle with lion's paws. Clay and metal images of him were placed over every door and window, so that when he tried to enter a house he would be frightened off by seeing his own terrifying image.

It is of great interest to note that the Babylonians, in vague anticipation of preventive medicine and the germ theory, believed that insects spread and caused disease. They directly blamed Baal-Zebub, the god of flies, gnats and all other insects, for disease and ill health. A Babylonian court physician named Arad-Nana advised his master Assurbanipal to "Beware of flies and shun lice in the interest of good health."

The Babylonians also exhibited some tendency toward quarantine and isolation because they knew that where many men were dying, others too would soon fall ill and die.

The Egyptians had a well-developed medical system which was under the complete and exclusive control of their priests. Diseases were commonly considered to be caused by incurring the anger of the gods, usually by transgressions of the ritual laws.

Numerous gods guided the destinies of the ancient Egyptians. One of the most popular and powerful was Ra, the sun god, who was depicted as having the head of a falcon. Thoth, who had the head of an ibis, was the god of wisdom. Imhotep, a priest-physician who lived about 3,000 B.C., had been considered such a great physician by the Egyptians that he grew in stature with the years until he acquired divinity and became the god who presided over the medical scene. Sekhem was the god who protected mothers in childbirth, and the "Eye of Horus" was considered to be all-powerful. According to legend, as a child the god Horus lost an eye in battle with Seth, the demon of evil. In desperation his mother Isis promptly called upon Thoth, the god of wisdom, for help. Using his great wisdom, Thoth restored the eye along with its power of vision. This led the Egyptians, who from time immemorial suffered from trachoma and other eye afflictions, to revere the Eye of Horus as a sacred symbol capable of protecting the vision and healing the eyes. In time the magic powers of the Eye of Horus were expanded so that this symbol came to be used as a prophylactic charm for protecting health in general, for warding off all diseases, and for guarding against all manner of evil.

Egyptian theology interfered with objective medicine because of the restrictions against profaning the body. This was based upon the assumption that the body must be carefully preserved until the time of resurrection. Thus while they developed embalming into a fine art, they learned little of anatomy.

Egypt can be considered as the birthplace of medical science. However, knowledge of Egyptian medicine was unknown and clothed in mystery until the Ebers Papyrus was discovered in Thebes in 1872. In this famous historical document which dates from 1550 B.C., over seven hundred drugs are mentioned. Some of these such as opium, olive oil and saffron are still in use today. However, the Egyptians also used many malodorous and unesthetic substances which were applied with the idea that they would render the affected part so objectionable that the evil spirits producing the disease would leave.

The Egyptians performed much surgery; they lanced abscesses, sutured lacerations, manipulated dislocations, splinted fractures, amputated, excised tumors, operated for cataracts, and opened the bladder for removal of stones.

The Egyptians had some concept of preventive medicine and practiced a definite hygienic regimen. They had specific rules on the cleanliness of women, and sexual intercourse was forbidden during the menstrual period. Parturient women were declared unclean for forty days. They practiced circumcision as a hygienic rite as far back as 4,000 B.C., and the Jews probably acquired this ritual from them.

They worshipped the scarabaeus or dung beetle because of its scavenging powers and its symbolic contribution to cleanliness of the environment.

The Egyptians were admonished to keep their houses clean and bathe frequently, and great value was placed upon a pure water supply.

Undoubtedly the individual and public hygiene practiced by the Egyptians influenced the ancient Hebrews. The Bible tells us in Acts 7:22 that Moses was "learned in all the wisdom of the Egyptians."

Chapter 2

MOSES AND THE HEBRAIC HEALTH CODE

THE ANCIENT HEBREWS were probably the first people in the world to disbelieve the primitive superstitious concept that diseases were caused by evil spirits and demons. They believed that disease was an expression of the divine wrath of Jehovah and that surcease from suffering was to be brought about only by prayers, fasting and observance of the moral law.

The Bible, which is the classic of ancient records concerning disease, places greater emphasis upon the prevention of disease than upon the treatment of bodily ailments. In Exodus 15:26 we read, "If thou wilt diligently hearken to the voice of the Lord thy God, and wilt do that which is right in his sight, and wilt give ear to his commandments, and keep all his statutes, I will put none of these diseases upon thee, which I have brought upon the Egyptians; for I am the Lord that healeth thee."

The Bible clearly shows that the ancient Hebrews were the pioneers of public health and hygiene. By incorporating Egyptian hygienic thought and behavior along with their own experience and thinking, they promulgated the world's first hygienic code. This code dealt with a wide variety of personal and community responsibilities, including the introduction of a full day of rest after every six days of labor. It also dealt with cleanliness of the body, protection against the spread of contagious diseases, the isolation of lepers, the disinfection of dwellings following illness, the sanitation of camp sites, the disposal of excreta and refuse, the protection of the water and food supply, and the hygiene of sex and maternity.

Because the people of the Children of Israel were becoming more and mightier than the Egyptians, Pharaoh became fearful and commanded that every newborn male Israelite be slain. In defiance of Pharaoh's cruel edict Moses was saved from death by his mother.

Hidden in the bulrushes and watched over by his sister, the infant Moses was found and adopted by Pharaoh's daughter.

Raised as a Royal Prince of Egypt, Moses acquired the administrative, legal and medical wisdom of Pharaoh's priests and politicians. Moses was thus uniquely qualified and gifted to become the great law-giver and leader of his people. He united the Hebrew tribes into a confederacy and ushered in their national life.

"Then the Lord said unto Moses, Go in unto Pharaoh, and tell him, Thus saith the Lord God of the Hebrews, Let my people go" (Exodus 9:1). But Pharaoh's heart was hardened and he would not let the people go. Then the Lord laid his hand upon Egypt and the river was turned into blood, the frogs were sent, the dust was turned into lice, there was a plague of flies, a murain of beasts, a plague of boils and blains, the hail, a plague of locusts, and of darkness. But still Pharaoh's heart was hardened and then in Exodus 12:29 we read, "And it came to pass, that at midnight the Lord smote all of the first born in the land of Egypt, from the first born to Pharaoh that sat on his throne unto the first born of the captive that was in the dungeon, and all the first born of cattle."

Then Pharaoh (Exodus 12:31) "Called for Moses and Aaron by night and said, Rise up, and get you forth from among my people, both ye and the Children of Israel; and go."

"And the Children of Israel journeyed from Ram-eses to Suc-coth, about six hundred thousand on foot that were men, beside children. And a mixed multitude went also with them" (Exodus 12:37-38). Thus Moses in about 1300 to 1200 b.c. led his people out of the land of bondage into the wilderness, where they wandered for forty years.

Moses faced the responsibility of guiding and governing the people of Israel, ministering to their religious needs and keeping them steadfast in their faith. In addition he had the tremendous task of protecting and preserving the health of an entire nation on the move.

In order to protect the health of the Children of Israel, Moses gave to them, and thus to the world, mankind's first effective system of sanitation, health and hygiene. These rules are part of the Mosaic law and are set forth in the Bible in the Books of Leviticus, Numbers and Deuteronomy.

To get the people of Israel to obey the Commands of God, Moses told them that, "The Lord will take away from thee all sickness" (Deut. 7:15). On the other hand he admonished his people that if the commandments were not kept "The Lord will smite thee with the botch* of Egypt and with the emerods†, and with the scab, and with the itch, whereof thou canst not be healed" (Deut. 20:27; 28:27).

To insure basic sanitation in their camps and to properly dispose of human body wastes the ancient Hebrews were adjured as follows: "Thou shalt have a place also without the camp, whither thou shalt go forth abroad: And thou shalt have a paddle upon thy weapon; and it shall be, when thou wilt ease thyself abroad, thou shalt dig therewith, and shalt turn back and cover that which cometh from thee" (Deut. 23:12-13). It is interesting to note that the sanitary practice of the burial of human body wastes is as sound a rule of public health today as it was in 1,200 B.C.

The ancient Hebrews had a keen understanding of the contagiousness and communicability of certain diseases. They were perhaps the first to recognize that the chain of infection could be broken by keeping the sick away from the well. This is best illustrated by the following passage from Leviticus (13:45-46), "And the leper in whom the plague is, his clothes shall be rent, and his head bare, and he shall put a covering upon his upper lip, and shall cry, unclean, unclean. All the days wherein the plague shall be in him he shall be defiled; he is unclean; he shall dwell alone; without the camp shall his habitation be."

Moses had practical ideas about the isolation of the sick, and he set forth regulations for the control of contagion, along with explicit directions for supervision by the priests.

For example, the thirteenth and fourteenth chapters of Leviticus are given over to the diagnosis and recognition of leprosy, and the rites and sacrifices to be used in cleansing the leper, his garments and his dwelling.

In the fifteenth chapter of the Book of Leviticus we find a clear-cut description of venereal disease and the laws designed to prevent

---

* Botch: a large ulcerous affliction of boils (smallpox? bubonic plague?)
† Emerods: Hemorrhoids (possibly rectal and intestinal diseases, such as typhoid, dysentery, cholera, etc.)

its spread. Gonorrhea was no mysterious affliction to Moses: he knew it well, as can be seen from the following extracts from Leviticus 15: ". . . And the Lord spoke unto Moses and to Aaron, saying: Speak unto the Children of Israel, and say unto them: When any man has an issue running out of his flesh, because of his issue he is unclean. . . . 4: Every Bed, whereon he lieth that hath the issue is unclean; and every thing, whereon he sitteth, shall be unclean. . . . 9: And what saddle soever he rideth upon that hath the issue shall be unclean. . . . 13: And when he that hath an issue is cleansed of his issue, then he shall number for himself seven days for his cleansing, and wash his clothes, and bathe his flesh in running water, and shall be clean. . . . 32: This is the law of him that hath an issue, and of him whose seed goeth from him, and is defiled therewith. . . . 33: And of her that is sick of her flowers and of him that hath an issue, of the man, of the woman, and of him that lieth with her that is unclean."

There are numerous other references in the Bible to venereal plagues and disease, all of which probably were gonorrheal in nature. However, the descriptions are not as accurate or clear as those in Leviticus. In the twenty-fifth chapter of the Book of Numbers is recorded the plague of Baal Peor, which states, "And Israel abode in Shittim and the people began to commit whoredom with the daughters of Moab." This debauchery resulted in a venereal epidemic among the Children of Israel.

Moses, great and stern leader that he was, took drastic action to save his people. He instructed the judges of Israel to slay every one of his men who led this corrupt life with the Moabite women, and we read in Numbers 25:8 "So the plague was stayed from the Children of Israel."

The Hebrews were among the first peoples of the world to protect their individual and community health by nutritional precepts, dietary rules and sanitary food practices. The eleventh chapter of Leviticus tells the people of Israel what beasts may and may not be eaten. All creeping and loathsome creatures such as the snake, the lizard, the weasel, the mole and the mouse are forbidden. Unappetizing, readily spoilable and possibly poisonous sea foods are eliminated from the diet as shown by the following quotation from Leviticus (11:10) "And all that have not fins and scales in the seas, and in the rivers, of all that move in the waters, and of any living thing which is in the waters they shall be an abomination unto you."

The well-known prohibition against eating pork and the less-known one against rabbit have direct public health implications even today, because these foods can and do cause trichinosis and tularemia.

The Hebrew dietary laws and practices were later amplified and expanded in the Talmud. This is a book of Jewish civil and religious laws which had its beginning about the time of Ezra in about 538 B.C. The word "Kosher," which is now part of our modern language, is a Hebrew word meaning clean, and is applied by the Jews to articles of food, particularly meat, that have been prepared in a manner conforming to the pronouncements laid down in the Talmud. This book also recommends moderation in eating and the use of a variety of foodstuffs. It sets forth the merits of fasting, as can be seen by the following quotation. "The best cure for a bad dream is a day's fasting." The Hebraic dietary laws are still observed by Orthodox Jews the world over.

One has but to read the Bible carefully and thoughtfully to conclude that the wisdom expressed therein regarding health, hygiene and sanitation forms the basic groundwork of today's public health rules. As one closes the book he must realize that these biblical rules on health and hygiene were far in advance of, and superior to, any which then existed in the world. Many of these hygienic precepts have been little improved upon to this day, and are as worth following now as when they were first promulgated.

Chapter 3

HEALTH IN THE GOLDEN AGE OF GREECE

SOMEWHAT LATER than the Hebrews in the history of western civilization, the foundations of medicine were laid in Greece. While the beginnings of Greek medicine date back beyond recorded history, it emerged upon the world scene in about 500 B.C. as a curious mixture of mythology and rationality known as the "Cult of Asclepius."

Asclepius is first mentioned in Greek literature in the Iliad where he is represented as an aristocratic tribal leader, famous as a priest-physician, and possessed of superior medical knowledge and skill. Over the centuries the stature of Asclepius continued to grow until, in about 525 B.C. he emerged as the legendary Greek god of medicine.

In the ancient Greek mythology Asclepius was the son of the god Apollo and the nymph Coronis. He possessed curative powers beyond mortal ability and was so proficient in the art of healing that Pluto accused him of decreasing the number of souls in Hades. This accusation, along with the jealousy that his great popularity aroused among the other gods, caused Zeus to destroy him with a thunderbolt.

After his death he not only became an object of worship, but was considered the father of all physicians and the founder of the healing cult of Asclepius. He was represented as a heroic bearded figure who always carried in his hand the symbolic caduceus.

To this day the caduceus is used as the symbol or insignia of medicine. It is now usually represented as a staff or wand with wings, around which twin serpents are entwined. The true caduceus or "staff of Asclepius" consisted of a wand around which a single serpent was entwined. The serpent was used as a sacred symbol of healing because, according to Greek mythology, it was a serpent that brought to Asclepius a special herb possessed of great healing powers. Serpents were also considered as symbols of healing because they shed their skins, and this was looked upon as a process of renewal and healing.

Greek legend also endowed Asclepius with two lovely daughters, Hygeia and Panacea. Hygeia was the gracious Greek goddess of health from whom is descended our term and science of hygiene. His other daughter, Panacea, had "all-healing" powers and is remembered in modern medicine by the term "panacea" which is applied to any "cure-all" drug.

The priest-physicians of the cult of Asclepius endeavored to heal the sick by a fusion of superstitious rites and practical means. They erected "temples of healing" in honor of Asclepius which were dedicated to his worship.

These "Asclepieia" consisted of a group of buildings and courtyards, located, with an eye to beauty and health, among a grove of trees and close to a spring, stream, or by the sea. Centrally placed of course, was the beautifully ornate temple reserved for prayer and worship. The second most important building was the "Abaton," where the sick pilgrims could retire to be visited and cured by the god of health while they slept. The remaining buildings consisted of hostels, baths and gymnasiums.

The Asclepieia were staffed by a large corps of priests, helpers, choirboys and musicians, while sacred serpents and other animals roamed the grounds. Diet, rest, exercise, massage, baths and heliotherapy were all employed to help cure the sick.

Not only did the sick and ailing come to the Temples of Asclepius, but these health centers were also visited in large numbers by the healthy. They came to pray for continued well-being while they relaxed and enjoyed the healthful environment.

Despite the popularity of the Asclepian cults, Greek medicine made a decisive change from these magico-religious practices, to a rational naturalistic type of healing. The priest-physicians gave way to the philosopher-physicians, and a little later a separate professional class of physicians came into being. These Greek physicians were skilled craftsmen, apprentice-trained and bound to their masters by an oath which reflected the high ethical standards of the profession.

Empedocles (490-430 B.C.), a Greek philosopher-physician, originated the doctrine that the human body is made up of four elements; earth, air, fire and water, and that the imbalance of these elements within the body causes disease. This was called the humoral theory of pathology, and unfortunately it influenced medical thinking for many centuries, until the Middle Ages. The acceptance of this fallacious theory of disease causation made attempts at preventive medicine well-nigh futile.

However, Empedocles did have some concepts of disease prevention, and he is sometimes referred to as the "First Sanitarian." He once altered a mountain so that the north wind blew the plague away from his native city of Agrigentum. He also diverted a river and drained a marsh near the neighboring city of Salinus and thus freed the town of a pestilence.

The greatest of Greek physicians was Hippocrates, who became known as the "Father of Medicine," and whose name, for more than 2,000 years, has been symbolic of the beauty, dignity and high ethical ideals of medicine.

Very little is known about Hippocrates' personal life. He was born about 460 B. C. on the little island of Cos in the Aegean Sea, the second of seven sons of a physician named Heracleides. According to tradition, Hippocrates began studying medicine at the Asclepieion of Cos, later studying at Cnidus, Thasos and Thessaly. He is also said to have studied in Egypt, Lydia and Scythia. He traveled widely, while practicing his profession, collecting ideas and visiting many foreign countries, as well as many cities in Greece. He achieved great renown during his lifetime and is said to have died in 361 B.C. at the age of ninety-nine.

Hippocrates dissociated himself from Greek magic and supernaturalism. He gave no recognition to the emblematic symbol of healing, the staff of Asclepius or caduceus. His fame grew out of the fact that he studied and described the symptoms of many diseases with such great clarity that these diseases can be recognized today. He concerned himself primarily with prognosis and treatment of the patient as a whole. All treatment was intended primarily to assist nature. Diet was of primary importance in both health and disease. He employed few drugs and used them only when diet failed. Surgery was applied only for injuries, and when diet and drugs were of no avail.

A number of treatises have come down to us under the name of Hippocrates. It is quite certain that not all of these were written by him, but that some are the works of later physician-authors. However all of these writings are collectively known as the "Corpus

Hippocraticum." They consist of a number of treatises variously titled: on the heart, on articulations, on fractures, on injuries of the head, etc. He also wrote a separate treatise on epilepsy, which was entitled "The Sacred Disease." Among his better-known works are his "Aphorisms" and the famous "Oath of Hippocrates."

Hippocrates accurately described most of the common diseases of mankind and named many of them. His writings laid the foundations of medicine and separated it from religion and philosophy.

Among his works are three on sanitation and hygiene, one of which is entitled "On Airs, Waters and Places." Hippocrates predicted a pestilence in Attica from the direction of the prevailing winds from a nearby outbreak of disease. It may have been that the epidemic was malaria and its spread was due to mosquitoes that were carried on the wings of the wind.

While the Greeks greatly advanced the healing arts, and Hippocrates is considered the Father of Medicine, little stress was placed upon preventive medicine, and Greek laws and customs did not emphasize the protection of the public health.

The really great contribution of the Greeks to hygiene was not so much the advancement of medicine as it was the development of a marvelous system of personal hygiene. Their ideal was to attain a sound mind in a sound body. They were pioneers in the fields of personal hygiene and physical education. There was universal physical training for boys aimed at the harmonious development of all their physical faculties in order to attain physical perfection and a body beautiful. The system was founded upon daily exercise from earliest youth to ripe manhood under the supervision of experienced and practical leaders. The youths of ancient Greece spent much of their time in gymnastic exercises, running, jumping, discus throwing, javelin casting, boxing and, above all, wrestling. When they reached the age of eighteen they devoted two years to the study of arms and military maneuvers and had to undergo a rigid physical examination every ten days. The system not only dealt with exercises and athletics, but combined all parts of hygiene into a unified whole. It stressed the preservation of health and care of the body by bathing and massage, proper rest and sleep, and set forth regulations as to diet and sexual life.

While military supremacy and world conquest was the principle aim of the Greeks, they did realize that to attain this end, physical fitness and good health were essential. The pursuit of personal hygiene in Greece reached a perfection never achieved anywhere else in the world before or since. The influence of the Greeks on athletics and physical fitness is felt to this day, and we have our Olympic games and our Marathon contests.

The glory of Greece culminated in the career of Alexander the Great who died in 323 B.C. at the age of thirty-three from an infectious disease. The decline of the power and civilization of Greece received a decided impetus from disease. There is reliable historical evidence that malaria was introduced into Greece from Africa in about the fourth century B.C. From then on the marvelous physiques of the Grecian Society began to deteriorate from the ravages of this disease.

Hippocrates described a remittant fever, accompanied by an enlarged spleen which occurred among persons living near marshes. He deduced a connection between this disease and the nearby swamps, a connection which, it is known today, was due to the anopheles mosquitoes which carried the malarial parasites. Thus the course of history and civilization was altered by disease.

Chapter 4

THE ROMANS
PIONEERS OF PUBLIC SANITATION

W HILE GRECIAN CULTURE AND CIVILIZATION was declining, there was developing on the Latin peninsula a new and mighty nation. Driven by the twin desires of wealth and world conquest, the rising power of Rome eventually put an end to all the lesser empires of the world. Through military might and the continuous conquest of new territories Rome became the undisputed "Mistress of the World."

Roman medicine had existed only in a primitive and unorganized way prior to the creation and expansion of the Empire. Because the Roman leaders had a patrician contempt for all the practical and manual arts, they considered medicine as essentially a menial craft, fit only for slaves or foreigners to practice.

Greek medical knowledge had become concentrated in the great library at Alexandria, and when the empire of Alexander the Great crumbled, Grecian medical knowledge began to flow into Rome. With the rise of Rome many of the Alexandrian physicians migrated to that city, while others settled in the newly rising cities on the roads that led to Rome. Thus Roman medicine was borrowed from the Greeks and was in the hands of foreign physicians. While the thriving prosperity of the expanding Roman empire attracted many skillful and learned Greek and Alexandrian physicians, it also attracted the rascals, self-seekers and charlatans.

The Romans accepted and absorbed all of the practical methods of Greek medical practice consisting of the familiar "nature-cure" methods of diet, exercise, massage and hydrotherapy. The old Greek methods of establishing a balance between the four humors of the body were persisted in, and blood-letting and purgation were popular forms of treatment. There was an extension of the use and compounding of herbs, potions and drugs. However, Asclepius was still the God

[17]

of Medicine and widespread belief in the powers of the supernatural existed. Quacks flourished everywhere, preying upon the superstitions of the people.

Although medical practice was in the hands of the Greeks, many of the great Roman landlords had the habit of doctoring the members of their own estates. Either they themselves, their womenfolk, or more frequently one of their higher class slaves functioned as the estate's private physician. For the guidance of these "kitchen-closet" practitioners, a Roman aristocrat, Aurelius Cornelius Celsus (25 B.C. to A.D. 50) compiled what was perhaps the world's first "medical advisor or encyclopedia." Celsus was not a physician himself and was apparently completely ignored by the recognized physicians of his day. However, he was deeply interested in medicine and in about 30 A.D. he compiled an outstanding medical work which qualified him as one of the most judicious medical authors of antiquity. This great book was entitled *De Medicina* and was an extensive general medical textbook containing the contemporary medical knowledge of his times. In it is Celsus's classic description of inflammation which even today is familiar to every medical student; redness and swelling with heat and pain (*rubor et tumor, cum calore et dolar*). It is of interest to note that after the invention of printing, this was one of the first medical books ever to be published. It was published in 1478 under the title of *De Re Medicina* and retained its position as a medical text until the middle of the eighteenth century.

The greatest name of Roman medicine, and one that was to influence medical thinking for forty-five generations, was that of Claudius Galen (130-201 A.D.). Galen was born in the Greek city of Pergamon in Asia Minor and was the only child of Nikon, a wealthy architect. Nikon supervised and guided his son's early education, giving him a thorough foundation in philosophy and mathematics. He directed him to attend courses at Pergamon in the four leading philosophic systems of the day so as to instill within him a spirit of impartiality. At the age of seventeen Galen began the study of anatomy which was followed by medical studies at Smyrna, Corinth and Alexandria.

At the age of twenty-eight Galen returned to Pergamon where he was appointed physician to the gladiators. This gave him practical experience in hygiene and medicine, as well as an opportunity to develop his surgical skill and anatomical knowledge from treating the terrible wounds suffered by the gladiatorial contestants.

Four years later, about 167 A.D., Galen departed for Rome, which was then the capital of the world. Through a series of brilliant diagnoses and spectacular cures, he soon achieved such fame and success that he was acclaimed the "Prince of Physicians." This, together with his public lectures, physiologic demonstrations and his writings, so increased his reputation that he was appointed physician to the Emperor Marcus Aurelius and later to his son and successor Commodus.

In addition to being an able surgeon and a shrewd clinician, Galen was a good observer and an excellent scholar. He frequently absented himself from Rome to go on lengthy research and study trips which took him to many lands and added to his vast store of medical knowledge.

He was a scientist as well as a practitioner and through experimentation he made many contributions to anatomy and physiology. He is considered historically to be the father of experimental physiology. While Galen did not dissect humans, he did do animal dissections using monkeys and pigs. He cleared up many basic anatomical problems, giving excellent descriptions of bones and muscles, as well as describing the origin of the blood vessels of the heart, and the nerves of the central nervous system.

Galen's accomplishments were manifold and he was the most prolific of all ancient writers. He is said to have written over five hundred treatises on medicine, logic and ethics. Only eighty-three of these are now acknowledged to be genuine. The origins of some of the remainder are doubtful, and others are obviously spurious. He wrote his medical treatises on anatomy, physiology, pathology, pharmacy, medicine and hygiene.

In the field of pharmacy he is remembered for using extremely complex prescriptions, frequently containing dozens of ingredients. He described and used over five hundred vegetable drugs, and because of this such drugs of natural origin are still called "Galenical preparations." One of his most famous prescriptions is the commonly used cold cream, which formerly was called "ceratum refrigerans Galeni."

For treatment Galen in general followed the Hippocratic tradition, using diet and physiotherapy for many conditions. He recognized cholera, hydrophobia, malaria and tuberculosis as definite disease entities.

While interested in hygiene and preventive medicine, Galen made little or no contributions to this field of medicine. He missed his great opportunity to fight and study plague and pestilence when he left Rome about 167 A.D. While claiming to have left Rome in order to escape assassination at the hands of jealous rivals, the truth probably is that he left because of an epidemic. Apparently Galen was too selfish to expose himself to death when a disastrous pestilence from the East turned Rome into a madhouse and a morgue. He had little to say about this or other epidemics and apparently believed that plague and pestilence were caused by unfavorable meteorological conditions.

It is difficult to decide just how much importance Galen attached to the idea of contagion. He recognized the importance of personal contact in cases of tuberculosis and stated that "it is a matter of experience that those who sleep in the same bed with consumptives fall into consumption and also those who live long with them, eat and drink with them or wear their clothes and linens." However he placed little or no emphasis upon personal contact as a cause of epidemics. He ascribed plague and pestilence to two causes, the first being a pestilential state of the air caused by a great irregularity in the seasons, and the second being a vitiated condition of the human body due to corrupt or defective food.

This Greek physician of Rome stands out as one of the great medical men of antiquity; medicine gained a wealth of ideas, facts and knowledge from him. His encyclopedic writings represented a synthesis of medical thought and knowledge which was solid enough to last for nearly 1,500 years.

Galen was accepted and perpetuated as the highest authority and infallible master on all matters relating to medicine, anatomy and physiology, until his errors were finally challenged by the sixteenth century physicians.

Mankind learns from experience and necessity. Because the Romans always had numerous cases requiring surgical attention they became quite proficient in this field. For centuries the Romans were engaged in almost continuous warfare and even in the short intervals between wars, they engaged in realistic mock battles. For the amusement of the populace they had their fierce and cruel gladiatorial contests. As a result, they always had a large variety of serious wounds and injuries to care for.

The Romans were forced to carry out many major surgical procedures, such as arresting hemorrhages, suturing serious wounds, reducing dislocations, setting fractures and performing amputations. They treated abdominal injuries with confidence and skill, arresting bleeding, replacing extruded viscera, debriding the wound, and suturing the muscles and skin. They became adept in the art of plastic surgery and were even able to restore the famous Roman nose after injury. They discovered the technique of applying ligatures and arrested bleeding by catching up the blood vessels on hooks and twisting them many times in order to close them.

They developed and used many surgical instruments. Celsus described over one hundred different instruments, including forceps, scalpels, trephines and amputation saws. Excavations at Pompeii have uncovered over two hundred different surgical instruments.

Because Rome marched to world power on the strength and efficiency of its military machine, the health and welfare of its soldiers was of prime importance. At first the Romans had no organized system of military medicine and the soldiers had to look after themselves. They were given crude medical supplies and they treated and bound up each other's wounds and injuries.

The inadequacies of this crude system soon made it necessary for the Romans to officially appoint Greek immigrant and slave physicians to care for the soldiers. From this beginning, the organizational and administrative abilities of the Romans soon led them to develop a full scale military medical service. They set up battlefield first aid stations and full scale military hospitals. Regularly appointed physicians were assigned to serve the troops, with as many as four surgeons assigned to care for each 1,000 or 1,500 men. Later these medical and hospital services were extended to also care for the athletes, gladiators and the sick poor.

The Romans were responsible for the establishment of the first state or national medical service the world has ever known. They introduced the first organized hospital system, setting up both military and civilian hospitals. Physicians were appointed by the government to all large towns and rural centers, each being responsible for the care of a certain number of inhabitants. While they were paid by the state and their services were free to the poor, they were extended the privilege of private practice among the wealthy. Their status was similar to that of a civil servant of the higher grade.

These physicians also functioned as health officers, checking on the water supply, the drainage system, the public baths, latrines and brothels. They were charged with eliminating public nuisances and preventing foul odors. They tested the accuracy of weights and measures in the market place, checked on the quality of food for sale, and were empowered to destroy tainted foods.

The outstanding and lasting contributions of the Romans were not in the advancement of curative medicine but were in the field of public health and sanitation. They were the founders of civic hygiene and public sanitation. They gave the world its first practical application of public health by their stupendous feats of public engineering, in the construction of huge aqueducts which brought abundant water supplies to their cities. Their public works also included paved roads and streets, drains and sewers, as well as public baths and latrines.

According to legend Rome was founded in about 753 B.C. by Romulus. The new city was built on the Palatine, which was one of seven hills situated along the banks of the River Tiber and located about fourteen miles from its mouth. Other settlements were made on the neighboring hills and in time these all merged into one city which became known as the "City of the Seven Hills."

The site of early Rome was well supplied with water; springs were abundant and wells could be sunk to find water at no great depth. Rainwater was collected in cisterns and water from the Tiber was used.

The center of activity of ancient Rome was the market and assembly place which was known as the Forum. This lay in a hollow place between the Palatine, the Quirnal, and the Capitoline hills. Because the Forum and other low-lying areas of the city were unpleasantly marshy and wet, the Romans early recognized the need for drains and sewers. Thus the sewers of Rome preceded the public water supply.

The sewers of Rome were begun under the reign of the kings in the sixth century B.C. Rome's Cloaca Maxima, which is the oldest and most famous sewer in the world, was built during the reign of the Emperor Tarquinas Priscus (616-579 B.C.). Sir John Harington in his "The Metamorphosis of Ajax" states that, "This worthie Prince is reported by that excellent historian (Livy), to have made two provisions for his citie, one for warre, the other for peace, both verie commendable: for warre a stone wall about the towne, to defend them from outward invasions; and for peace, a goodly Jakes within the towne, with a vault to convey all the filth into the Tyber, to preserve them from inward infection."

As Rome grew the sewers were continually extended and improved until a vast network of them conveyed the drainage and sewage of the city into the River Tiber. Every ancient Roman street had its lateral drain diminishing in size as the distance from the main sewer increased. These cloacae or sewers were designed and constructed on so grandiose a scale that in certain places a wagon-load of hay could be driven through them with ease. They were so solidly constructed that the mouth of the largest and oldest of them, the Cloaca Maxima, which served as the central collector for all of the others, can still be seen opening into the river. Its semicircular arch is five meters in diameter and is as perfect today as it was in the days of the kings.

To supplement their engineering skill and in order to insure the proper functioning of their sewers and drains, the ancient Romans displayed great imagination by designating a "diety" to take care of the whole messy business. The Goddess Cloacina was the designated "divinity" who presided over the sewers and drains of ancient Rome. Personifying the vapors stemming from the stench of the sewers, her powers were invoked for protection against diseases due to the drains. In prayers and supplications she was euphemistically addressed as "Sweet Cloacina." Pliny relates that the Romans and Sabines when about to engage in battle on account of the rape of the Sabine virgins, lay down their arms and made atonement on the spot where later the temple and statue of Venus Cloacina stood.

As the city grew its springs and wells became inadequate as a source of water and the Romans were forced more and more to use the sewage-polluted waters of the Tiber. As a result of drinking their own sewage they paid a terrific penalty in the form of death and disease. Thus through bitter experience the importance and value of a pure water supply was realized. Roman engineering genius came to the fore and an abundant supply of pure water was brought to the city. The aqueducts of Rome were among the most stupendous and successful engineering feats of the ancient world. In 312 B.C. the first of the great aqueducts was built by the famous censor Appius Claudius, who also built the famous road known as the Appian Way. This aqueduct was eleven miles long with all but three hundred feet of it underground. This and the Anis Vetus, built forty years later, supplied the lower levels of the city. In 140 B.C. the first high-level aqueduct, the fifty-six mile long Marcia, was built by Quintus Marcius Rex to bring water to the top of the Capitoline Hill. Its water was, and still is, particularly good and cold. Three more aqueducts were built during the Republic and at least seven under the Empire, so that ancient Rome was at last supplied by eleven or more aqueducts. Modern Rome is supplied by four aqueducts which are the sources, and occasionally the channels, of as many of the ancient ones.

Sextus Julius Frontinus (A.D. 40-103) a Roman soldier, engineer and author, in his book *De Aquis Urbus Romanae,* gives us an accurate history and description of the water supply of Rome, including the laws relating to its use and maintenance. According to Frontinus, during his time eight aqueducts brought 222,237,060 gallons of water a day into the city of Rome.

The channels of the aqueducts were built of masonry because their pipes were insufficient in size and strength. Cast iron was unknown to the Romans, and bronze would have been too expensive. The aqueducts carried the water by gravity. They were built at a very easy slope and frequently were carried around hills and valleys, although tunnels and bridges were used in some instances. The great arches, so impressive in their ruins, were used for comparatively short distances, and most of the channels were underground.

In the city the water was carried into distributing reservoirs (castella), and from there it ran into the street mains. The water mains were laid down the middle of the streets and from these, lead pipes (fistulae) carried the water into the houses or to the numerous public fountains. These pipes were made of strips of sheet lead with the edges pulled together and soldered at the joining; thus the pipes were pear-shaped rather than round. These pipes were frequently stamped with the names of the owner and user and thus the finding of these pipes in modern times has helped locate the site of the residences of many distinguished Romans.

Vitruvius, one of the great Roman architects and engineers, writing in about 25 to 20 B.C. during the reign of Augustus, laid great stress upon a community's need for a pure and abundant water supply. He also wrote on building in great detail, giving much information about Roman buildings and houses.

The belief that the ancient Romans enjoyed modern plumbing similar to ours and had hot and cold running water at their disposal or that they had flush toilets with water-carried sewage is largely a myth. While water was piped directly into the houses of the wealthy and well-to-do, it never extended above the ground floor, and was not carried into very many rooms of the house. The water was usually piped to a fountain in the peristylium or reception hall of the house and usually a jet was placed in the bath houses. However the majority of the Romans did not have water piped into their homes. Water for household use had to be drawn and carried in from the nearest public fountain in the street. The better classes used slaves as water carriers, while the poor had to carry their own.

While many of the homes of the wealthy and well-to-do had indoor latrines connected directly to the sewers, most of them did not. They had cesspools or used chamber pots or commodes which their servants or slaves emptied into the sewers in the streets.

The Romans had public latrines or toilets located at points along the routes of the sewers. Some of these were quite lavish and ornate and were constructed in a rectangle or semicircle. Water flowed through them in continuous channels and seats were fixed in front of these channels. The seats were of marble and frequently had dolphins sculptured on their backs. Above the seats there were niches in the walls containing statues of various gods and heroes.

These latrines were a curious mixture of delicacy and coarseness. People met there, conversed and visited with each other and even exchanged invitations to dinner with no embarrassment. Even the latrine at the Imperial Palace at Rome had three seats arranged side by side.

The public latrines were public only in the sense that they were open to all who could or would pay the fees charged for their use. Thus the poor, the misers and the slaves did not use the public latrines, but used chamber pots which they emptied in the streets. The more slovenly hurled the contents of their chamber pots out of their windows into the streets below. Many of the Romans used any available facility and with so little regard for public decency that the Emperor Flavius Vespasius was forced to issue an imperial edict against "pissing on the Palace walls."

Although the Romans had laws prohibiting these unsanitary practices, they were extremely difficult to enforce. Accumulations of filth, open latrines, sewage pits and cesspools abounded throughout the city. Despite its marvelous aqueducts and its extensive sewage system, ancient Rome still stunk.

To the Romans of early times bathing was for health and decency only. They washed their arms and legs daily because their manners of dress left these parts exposed. They usually bathed their bodies once a week, bathing at home in a primitive washroom off of the kitchen where they heated the water. Later on bathing assumed great importance to the Romans from a social as well as a health standpoint.

The aristocratic and wealthy Romans fitted out elaborate bathrooms in their houses, having both hot and cold baths and a separate room called the "unctorium" where oils and ointments were rubbed upon their bodies by their slaves.

Public baths were set up for the large masses of Roman citizens. These were operated on a large scale in all parts of Rome and even in the smaller towns and provinces. Many of these public baths were large-scale luxurious establishments which could accommodate from one to three thousand people. All sorts of baths were offered such as plain, hot or cold, douche or plunge. Massage, exercises, games, reading and conversation were all offered to the patrons. The public baths became an important part of the social life of the Romans and can probably best be compared to our present day athletic or health clubs.

The baths were frequently located near hot or mineral springs or in natural spa areas. They were open to all citizens who could pay the fees. By 33 B.C. there were at least one hundred and seventy public baths in Rome and later the city had over eight hundred of them. The Baths of Diocletian, dedicated in 305 A.D., were said to have been the largest and most luxurious ever constructed.

At first the public baths were hygienic, health-giving and relaxing, but as time went on they degenerated and many evils flourished there. Mixed bathing between the sexes and nude athletic games were sanctioned, while under the stately porticos of the bathhouses there were vendors of rich foods, strong drinks and procurers for both sexes. Debauchery, vice and corruption became commonplace and it was said that the baths, wine and women helped to destroy the might of Rome.

While her achievements had been great, the "greatest hours" of Roman power and glory had passed. Luxury, ease, vice and corruption took its toll of the ruling classes while the tremendous numbers of the lower classes and the massive slave population within the empire grew poorer and poorer. The disintegration of Roman power was a gradual process brought about by many complex causes. Although the decline and fall of the Roman Empire is usually attributed to a combination of causes, such as social, religious, political and economic, there was also a medical one.

Despite all of their tremendous accomplishments in the field of public sanitation, the Romans were still helpless before the disastrous depredations of epidemic diseases such as smallpox and bubonic plague. Their abundant supplies of pure water, their extensive systems of sewers and their emphasis upon community cleanliness all helped to restrict and curtail certain types of epidemic diseases. However these advantages were more than offset by other conditions which helped to produce epidemics, such as the concentration of large populations within their cities and their extensive trade activities with all parts of the world. Their constant military activities, with the movements of large forces back and forth throughout the world caused pestilence and epidemics to follow the Roman Eagle and to periodically spread misery and death among the population.

Thus the Roman world from the year one to the days of the final barbarian triumphs was periodically weakened and disorganized by calamitous epidemics which again and again swept through the population during some of their most turbulent political periods.

Tacitus described a plague occurring during the reign of Nero which was so severe "that corpses were in all the houses and the streets were filled with funeral processions." This was probably an outbreak of bubonic plague.

The plague of Antoninus is said to have started in 165 A.D. in the army of Verus while he campaigned in the East. As the army returned homeward it scattered the disease far and wide and finally brought it to Rome. Orosius stated that so many people died that villages, cities and even whole provinces were abandoned and fell in ruins. This epidemic lasted about fourteen years and demoralized social, political and economic life. Dio Casius records that the epidemic broke out again in 189 A.D. and that at its height, caused 2,000 deaths a day in Rome. From descriptions of symptoms it is difficult to fully identify the disease, but most historians feel that it was either an epidemic of smallpox or bubonic plague.

Another epidemic described by Saint Cyprian as occurring in about 250 A.D. was said to have originated in Ethiopia. From here it reached Europe after passing across Egypt. This plague continued in recurring waves for a period of fifteen or sixteen years. Saint Cyprian made many conversions to Christianity by reason of the fear, terror and sadness occasioned by the epidemic. While the descriptions are vague this appears to have been an outbreak of bubonic plague.

In addition to these acute epidemics the enervating and deadly disease of malaria had gained a foothold on the Latin peninsula and found a fertile field in the weakened and decadent population.

Thus the Roman Empire, its strength sapped by disease as well as by poverty and political unrest, was no longer able to withstand the attacks of the Goths, Vandals, Huns and other Barbarians. Rome became untenable. The government was transferred to Constantinople and finally the Western Roman Empire fell in 476 A.D. When the mighty Roman Empire crumbled and fell, culture and knowledge disappeared for a thousand years and darkness descended upon Western civilization.

Chapter 5

DARKNESS OVER EUROPE AND
THE LIGHT IN THE EAST

After the fall of Rome the barbaric hordes from the north put out completely the light of Roman wisdom. The clock of Western Civilization ran backwards and the centuries that followed were appropriately known as the Dark Ages. The history of the Dark Ages is one continuous story of plague, pestilence, poverty, famine and war.

With the passing of Rome, medicine ceased to be a science or even a profession. Medical schools disappeared and the Greek and Roman medical manuscripts were lost or destroyed. For centuries it seemed that Hippocrates and Galen had labored in vain. Mystery and magic returned, and charms, incantations and superstitious rites took the place of rational medical treatment.

Barbarian hygiene and sanitation was as bad as the culture of the uncouth conquerors. The world went from the "Glory of Greece" and the "Splendor of Rome" into an era of dirt, disorder and disease. The sound principles of personal hygiene so well developed during the golden age of Greece were completely disregarded. The early Christians in protest and reaction to the lasciviousness of the Roman baths and the gross immorality of the times placed great emphasis upon asceticism and made neglect of the body holy. The magnificent public sanitation of the Romans was abandoned and such sanitation as existed in Europe during the Dark Ages would have appalled any self-respecting Roman of Caesar's times.

In the country the common people were little better than slaves chained to the land by the feudal lords. While the lords lived in their manor houses with every comfort and luxury that wealth could buy, their serfs lived in dark, damp, one-room huts. These hovels were smoky, drafty and cold in the winter and stifling hot in the summer. They frequently had dirt floors and the roofs were thatched with reeds or rushes. Poorly ventilated, the windows were few and small, with canvas or waxed cloth stretched across the openings. The peasants lived in these hovels with less comfort than the domestic animals they cared for. Overcrowded, poorly nourished and vermin infested, the miserable inhabitants of these unlovely living quarters were easy victims of infection and disease.

Town life for the masses was even more squalid. The walled cities of Western Europe were malodorous, filthy, pestilential places. The people lived in picturesque timbered houses, which were dark, damp and grossly over-crowded. Poorly heated, lighted and ventilated, neither sunshine nor fresh air penetrated the putrid atmosphere of these houses. Down the middle of the unpaved narrow streets, open drains received all sorts of garbage and excrement, sometimes carelessly thrown out of the overhanging upper stories. There were no proper water supplies, no drains or sewers, few baths and fewer lavatories, but there was an abundance of dirt and filth. Adding to the general unpleasantness the public latrines were seldom flushed or cleaned. Poorly constructed and poorly maintained privys and private cesspools abounded throughout the community, adding to the all-prevailing stench of the towns.

As a result of these filthy, unsanitary conditions, plague, pestilence and frightful epidemics took a terrific toll. Life was uncertain and the infant mortality rate rose while the life span declined.

With the rise of Christianity the church attained a position of tremendous influence, power and wealth. The churches, cathedrals and monasteries became the centers of such culture and learning as remained or existed in the Western World. Knowledge was preserved and kept alive in the monasteries, but unfortunately it was copied rather than studied. The monks were more interested in the techniques and artistry of fine writing than in measuring the thoughts they translated. Rigid church dogma suppressed the free-thinking philosophy of the Greeks and Romans, and so the church severed its connections with progressive philosophic and scientific thought. While no genuine progress was made, at least part of the Greek and Roman literature was preserved for later generations.

Medieval Christian teaching emphasized that life on this earth had meaning only as a spiritual preparation for the next, and that heaven alone could confer eternal happiness. It preached that the masses could look for their delivery from misery and sorrow only in the life after death. Because their teachings demanded unquestioning submission to the church and to the feudal lords, any potential genius among the people was suppressed or directed into channels barren of results.

The church brought forward again the earlier beliefs that sickness and disease were punishments that befell mankind because of his sins. Therefore the only thing that he could do to effect a cure was to atone for his sins by fasting and prayers. Because of these beliefs and the fact that the only learned people of the times, the clerics and monks, were forbidden to study or practice medicine, the science of medicine deteriorated. Nothing could be added to anatomical knowledge because the human body was considered divine and anatomical dissection was considered a crime against God and man. Hence the times were sterile and devoid of progress and learning. No significant contributions were made toward the advancement of science, medicine or public health.

However, the belief that good deeds on earth would surely win a heavenly reward brought about the practice of Christian charity. The teachings of Jesus inspired sympathy and compassion for the unfortunate and the down-trodden. Thus, the church considered it a religious duty to aid the sick, the helpless and the homeless. Money collected from the faithful and the fearful was used by the church to establish almshouses, orphanages, and institutions to care for the sick poor.

The medieval monasteries and convents were really self-contained little villages. They were well built, well drained and had good water supplies. Infirmaries and facilities for the care of the sick and the poor were built within their walls. While the medical care given to the patients was elementary, they were given food, warmth, shelter and kindness.

The monks and nuns, not being medically skilled, served more as devoted nurses than as physicians. Thus the monks in these monasteries contributed more to medicine than those who labored as scribes copying manuscripts.

Through their self-sacrifice and devotion to religious duty in offering sanctuary and hospitality to the sick, the poor and the needy, they enriched medicine with Christian ideals of charity and brotherly love. Thus the monasteries and convents of the medieval church served as the forerunners of our present day hospitals.

Even though Europe was engulfed in darkness and Greco-Roman medicine was virtually lost, the light of knowledge had not been completely extinguished. There was "a light in the East" and the Byzantine or Eastern Empire stood as a bulwark against the inroads of the barbarians. It guarded the precious legacy of culture and knowledge which had been left by the ancients.

In 330 A.D. Constantine the Great officially transferred the Roman government to the city of Byzantium on the shores of the Bosphorus and christened it New Rome. Later the city was called Constantinople in his honor. He thus established the Byzantine Empire which was also called the Eastern or Later Roman Empire.

Many Romans moved to the new capital, among them numerous physicians who brought with them their favorite texts and manuscripts. Hence many works of Hippocrates and Galen were safely brought to Constantinople. Thus Greco-Roman medical knowledge was preserved and incorporated into Byzantine medicine.

While medicine itself remained static in the Eastern Empire, the medical manuscripts and texts that had been brought from the west were copied, translated, and preserved. Among the most diligent of the copyists were a heretical sect of Christians known as the Nestorians. This sect followed the teachings of Nestorius whom they considered to be the one true patriarch of Constantinople. Because of their beliefs they were driven out of Constantinople by other Christian sects about 451 A.D. They settled at Djondisapour in Persia and founded a hospital which subsequently developed into a medical school. They translated the works of Hippocrates, Celsus, and Galen into Syriac. For more than 300 years their precious treasures attracted little outside interest.

In this period of time came Mohammed the Prophet and the rise of Arabian power and civilization. The Moslem Arabs swept from Arabia through the Eastern Roman Empire, over Egypt, North Africa, and Spain, and by 737 A.D. they reached the banks of the

Loire in France. With their rise to power the Arabs built up their civilization, culture and knowledge.

All over the Near and Middle East was a desire for knowledge and learning, and the science of medicine was begun again. Thanks to the Nestorians it did not have to start from the beginning. The translations they had made from the Greek into Syriac were now translated into Arabic and the medical knowledge of Greece and Rome came to light again. By the tenth century all the essential Greco-Roman medical writings had been translated and were in use in the cultural centers of the Arabian world at Damascus, Cairo and Baghdad. In the process of translation the Arabians added their own terminology. This gave rise to confusion later when these manuscripts were retranslated back into Latin.

The foremost of Arabian physicians and writers was Rhazes (850-923), who is sometimes referred to as the "Arabic Galen." Abu-Bakr Muhammed ibn Zakvriya or Rhazes was born in the Persian City of Rai and did not become interested in medicine until his thirtieth year. Then while visiting a Baghdad hospital he is said to have become so interested in medicine that he decided to devote the remainder of his life to it. He became so famous as a scholar, practitioner and teacher that he was appointed head of the hospital at Baghdad and court physician to the Caliph. Rhazes is supposed to have written 237 books, of which only 36 have been saved. He was a keen observer and made many practical contributions to medicine, such as introducing mercury compounds as purgatives, and ligatures and sutures made from animal gut. He is said to have been the first to record the reaction of the pupil to light, and is said to have written the first known book on children's diseases. His chief contribution to preventive medicine and his most highly regarded work is his book on smallpox and measles. He was the first to describe these diseases with clinical accuracy and to differentiate and separate them from the confusion which surrounded all of the infectious exanthemata.

Another illustrious light of Arabian medicine was the Persian physician and philosopher known as Avicenna or Ibn Sina (930-1037). He was author of the *Canon,* a huge storehouse of learning in which he codified all of the medical knowledge of his times. This book has been called the greatest medical text ever written and was used in medical schools until the fourteenth and fifteenth centuries. Unfortunately his ranking of surgery as an inferior branch of medicine hindered its progress for many centuries.

Thus while the Western World was in darkness, medicine was not only preserved but made definite progress under the Arabian Moslems.

Chapter 6

PILGRIMS AND CRUSADERS

LESS THAN 200 YEARS after the Prophet Mohammed's death in 632, Islamism had swept across the earth like a wild-wind and had succeeded in conquering one-half of the world. While Islamic power, culture and knowledge were approaching the zenith of prosperity and splendor, Western Europe was in the blackest period of the Dark Ages. Continuous warfare and strife coupled with political and economic chaos produced poverty, famine and pestilence. The fields lay idle and ravaged, while whole villages and burgs were completely or partially abandoned and lay in ruins. Dirt, despair, death and disease were everywhere.

Christianity was not yet fully accepted nor understood by a population still not too far removed from paganism. One set of Christians fought with another, excommunicating each other, and refusing to sanction each other's births and to bury the dead. Each demanded "believe what I believe or die."

As the year 1000 approached there were many who preached the "millennium." Believing in the second coming of Christ, they preached that, "He shall come back on the last stroke of the last hour of the thousand years since his birth." A confusion of cries, prayers and prophecies were heard and believed. There were those who predicted the end of the world, with the righteous ascending to heaven and the wicked descending to everlasting hell. There were others who believed that Christ would descend upon the earth and that peace and paradise would reign forever more.

A type of mass madness descended upon the people as they felt the need to prepare for the "end of the world" or for the "descent of Paradise upon the earth." Large numbers of people went on pilgrimages to the Holy Land to atone for their sins or to be at or near the tomb of Christ when the millennium came.

[35]

The journey to the Holy Land was a dangerous and rigorous one. Of the tens of thousands who set forth on these pilgrimages relatively few ever reached their destination. Thousands died on the road of exhaustion, exposure, hunger, thirst or disease. Others were captured or killed by the Lombards, Greeks or Saracens. Many turned back, broken in spirit and health, before completing their pilgrimage. The pilgrims frequently organized into large bands and sometimes these bands fought each other. More frequently they foraged food, begged or pilfered the countryside. The villages and towns were more afraid of these pilgrim bands in their garb of cassock, cowl and crucifix, than they were of enemy soldiers with their armor and swords. Pilgriming became an excuse for adventurers, pilferers, robbers and degenerates to roam and rob the countryside. The roads of Europe were crowded with rogues, rascals, beggars and cripples, as well as lepers and the insane.

The millennium came and passed and nothing happened. The world neither came to an end, nor had paradise descended to earth. Chaos, disorder, disease, hunger and poverty remained. Religious unrest was everywhere and the Church of Rome and the Church of Constantinople engaged in a bitter fight. Those Christian groups that had preached the millennium were hounded and burned as heretics.

In 1073 the Seljuk Turks had taken Jerusalem, and they laid upon it the heavy hand of intolerance. Returning pilgrims brought back stories of mistreatment and cruelties inflicted by the Moslems on those who journeyed to the Holy Land. Sentiment and emotions mounted, expressing the feeling that it was the duty of the Christian world to free the Holy City from the infidels. Religious leaders preached that it was the duty of every Christian to save the holy places from defamation and desecration.

The Eastern Emperor Alexius appealed to Pope Urban for aid against the Moslem invaders.

At a great church council convoked by Pope Urban II in 1095, it was agreed that the various Christian nations should, at least temporarily, cease waring and fighting among themselves and unite to wrest the Holy Sepulcher from the hands of the infidels and restore it to Christian auspices. So with the blessing of the Pope,

Peter the Hermit preached the First Crusade, calling upon the people to march under the leadership of Christ to Holy Jerusalem and free it from the infidels.

The cry of the Crusader was *"Deus vult"* or God wills it, and the people responded. Behind them were three centuries of hunger, starvation, pestilence, defeats, and deceptions. Being a Holy War the Crusades offered to all who joined complete absolution from all past sins and sure promise of a heavenly reward for the future. In addition there was the immediate and practical opportunity for adventure, romance and riches to be obtained from conquest. Knights and nobles sold their land and belongings, marshalled their men and horses and joined the Crusades. The common people, restless and filled with religious fervor were ready to be freed from the soil and to seek adventure in far off lands.

The army swelled and grew as it advanced; led by the clergy and armoured knights on horseback, they were followed by a vermin-ridden pestilential mob on foot. Poorly planned and poorly equipped, the first crusade was made up of religious warriors from Normandy, France, England, Flanders, Italy and Sicily. They crossed the Bosphorus and followed the route of Alexander the Great until they came to Antioch in 1098. There the Christian army of 300,000 Crusaders beseiged the city for almost a year.

Disease and famine killed so many in so short a time that the dead could not be buried. The pest is said to have killed 100,000 persons during the months of September, October and November. Their cavalry was rendered useless by the death of 5,000 of their 7,000 horses, probably from an outbreak of anthrax.

The city of Antioch was finally captured and the Crusaders marched on to Jerusalem. They were accompanied and harassed by plague and pestilence, an enemy more deadly and potent than the heathen foe. As the sick, weary and dying fell from the ranks and lay down at the side of the road, they were, if fortunate, picked up and cared for by a rear convoy of monks and priests who had organized and formed a crude type of ambulance service. Plague, pestilence, scurvy, and starvation so decimated their ranks that when Jerusalem was finally taken in 1099 only 60,000 of the original 300,000 Crusaders were left.

There were a series of Crusades, extending from 1097 to 1272, all having a sadly similar story. Especially tragic are the accounts of the two Children's Crusades, one of which was begun in France and the other in Germany. In 1212 a French shepherd boy named Stephan had a vision telling him that the Holy Cross could only be redeemed from the hands of the infidels by the pure clean hands of innocent children, that only innocent boys and pure virgins could free the Holy City from the Saracens.

Stephen led the Crusade, aided by some of the clergy. Carrying crosses and candles and chanting hymns, they were impossible to hold back. In a religious frenzy they marched across France, recruiting more and more children, while others fell by the wayside. Poorly equipped and poorly fed, they lived off of the bounty of the countryside.

Begging and stealing, they swarmed across the land while exposure, hunger and disease decimated their ranks in a frightful manner. Finally 30,000 of them reached the shores of the sea and camped at Marseilles. In order to rid the city from this horde of fanatic, unruly and diseased children, as well as the large number of disreputable adult camp followers and hangers-on, two rascally merchants provided seven ships to transport them off across the sea. Two of these rotten boats sank in a storm, losing all aboard. The remaining five ships reached the opposite shore and there through betrayal, were met and captured by the foe, who sold the children into slavery.

In Germany another shepherd boy named Nicholas had a similar vision. He led a somewhat older group composed of young men up to twenty years of age and virgins up to eighteen on another crusade. Approximately 20,000 started on the march across Germany and about 7,000 of them finally reached Genoa, Italy in August of 1212. Here the group split up, some remaining there, others turning back homeward, while many secured passage on ships bound for the Holy Land.

Those who went on to the Holy Land were captured and sold in the slave marts of Asia and Africa. Thousands of the young Crusaders had perished from hunger, cold and disease and those who finally returned home were broken in health and spirit. The maidens who had gone forth as virgins returned as harlots.

The story of the Seven Crusades is not so much one of romance, and chivalry, as it is one of death and disease. The crusaders were more often turned back by epidemics than they were by the armed might of the Saracens. The history of the Crusades reads more like the chronicle of a series of epidemics and plagues, with scurvy and starvation being as deadly as the contagious diseases.

The Crusaders formed a roadway over which many epidemic diseases were introduced into Europe. Prior to these times the medieval lords had stood alone in their petty might, supreme over their estates and serfs. Repelling all intruders, suspicious of strangers and forcing their serfs to remain on the land, they had kept their estates and villages relatively well isolated. This isolation together with the slowness and infrequency of travel had kept epidemic diseases at a relatively low level. However, when the Crusaders opened the way to the East, a living line of communications and travel was formed along which diseases could spread. Smallpox, plague, leprosy, diphtheria and scarlet fever, as well as many other diseases came home with the armies of the Crusaders and when the troops disbanded these diseases were carried into every baronial stronghold and into every medieval city of Europe.

The Crusades placed a great strain upon the charity of the Monks and the various religious orders, who were faced with the problem of helping the pitiful plight of the sick and exhausted Crusaders. Thus the line of travel formed by the Crusaders from Europe to the East was marked here and there by Hospices for the care of the poor and sick. Monasteries with their attendant infirmaries and hospitals grew and expanded to try to meet the urgent needs of the times. New religious and knightly orders, devoted to sheltering and caring for the sick, injured and exhausted Crusaders were formed both in Europe and the Holy Land.

In 1048 the Knights Hospitalers of Saint John had founded a monastery and hospital at Jerusalem to care for the sick pilgrims who had journeyed to the Holy Land. During the Crusades their activities were extended to care for the sick and injured Crusaders.

In 1119 a Knight named Hugh de Payen associated himself with eight other war-weary knights from the Crusades to form an order of "poor fellow soldiers of Christ." They were pledged to protect and help care for the pilgrims and crusaders who had journeyed to the Holy Land. King Baldwin II of Jerusalem gave them a residence near the Temple of Soloman and thus they became known as Templars or Knights of the Temple.

In about the middle of the twelfth century the religious order of Saint Lazarus was founded in Jerusalem for the purpose of caring for sick pilgrims and especially lepers. Later due to the spread of leprosy, branches were established in various parts of Europe.

The Crusades were one of the longest, costliest, bloodiest and cruelest episodes of history. Although the Crusades failed to realize their great ideal these holy wars profoundly influenced European history. They helped destroy feudalism, because large numbers of nobles perished in the Crusades or lost their fortunes and estates and thereby enhanced the power of the kings and the common people. Commercial intercourse was promoted between the East and the West and trade was stimulated. Along with the increase of international trade there was an increased prosperity and a growth of towns and cities all over Europe.

As a result of the Crusades, Europe developed intellectually and culturally by almost three centuries of contact with the more advanced and enlightened culture of the East. European medicine was enriched by contact with the East and some of the long lost Greco-Roman medical knowledge was reintroduced. For example, Salerno, the political capital of southern Italy and Sicily, became famous as a medical center during the eleventh and twelfth centuries. It served as a place of rest and healing for the Crusaders on their way to and from the Holy Land and thus helped introduce Arabian medicine to Western Europe.

Another example of the transmission of Arabian medical knowledge occurred when the merchants of Montpelier in France brought home some Arabian physicians to teach medicine. While there was opposition from the Christian doctors, the lord of the city gave them full freedom to teach. Thus Montpelier became the chief center of medical learning north of the Alps, and was surpassed only by Salerno.

Chapter 7

THE SCHOOL OF SALERNO AND
SENSIBLE LIVING

D<small>URING THE</small> D<small>ARK</small> A<small>GES</small> the dim light of learning continued to burn in an obscure corner of Italy. Near Naples in the tiny seaside town of Salerno, there was established on the smouldering ruins of Greco-Roman medicine Europe's first Christian medical school. In Roman times Salerno, because of its salubrious climate, had been a famous and fashionable health resort. After the fall of Rome it continued to carry on many of the practices and traditions of the ancient world, and served as a meeting ground for people of culture and learning.

The medical school at Salerno came into being in about the year 900. Nobody knows exactly how the school was first established. Some say the school had its origin in the teachings of the nearby monastery of Monte Cassino. This monastery had been founded in 529 by St. Benedict of Nursia upon the site of an old temple of Apollo and operated under the "Rule of St. Benedict" which contained provisions for the care of the sick.

Others say that Salerno's medical school was not a by-product of this great monastery, but that it was founded by Charlemagne. Still another legend and the most commonly accepted one is that the school was founded by four masters or doctors; Elinus, the Jew; Pontus, the Greek; Adale, the Arab; and Salernus, the Latin.

The school was open to men of all nationalities and languages and even to women. The official title of the school was the "Civatas Hippocratica" and the first Salernitan texts were simple compilations of early Roman authors written in miserable Latin. However, through the gradual abandonment of medieval superstitions and by following these texts the Salernitan physicians redirected European medicine back to the sound simplicity of Hippocratic medical thought and therapeutics.

The influence of Arabic medicine was not felt in Europe until the eleventh century when Constantinus Africanus (c. 1020-1087) introduced it at Salerno. Born in Africa, Constantinus had traveled widely in the East, attending various medical schools and especially the one at Baghdad. Upon his return to his native Carthage, charges were brought against him as a magician and he fled to Salerno, where he expounded the teachings of the Arabs and fostered the Latinization of Arabic medical texts. After a period of teaching at Salerno, Constantinus retired to the monastery at Monte Cassino in about 1070 and devoted the remainder of his life to the translations of Arabic, Greek, and Jewish medical texts into Latin.

His familiarity with the medical literature of antiquity as well as Jewish and Arabic medical lore was phenomenal. He became one of the most important medical translators of all times. His translations included the works of Hippocrates and Galen, the Byzantine treatises of Theophilus and Philaretus and the *Perfect Book of the Art of Medicine* by Haly Abbas.

Three other eleventh century physicians who were prominent in the advancement and development of the medical school at Salerno were Gariopontus, Trotula and Alphanus. Gariopontus translated and compiled a handbook of pathology and therapeutics from Greco-Byzantine and Roman authors which achieved great renown. Trotula, a learned matron who was the wife of a physician, compiled a book, *On Diseases of Women*, which contained information on cosmetics and infant care as well as gynecology. Alphanus, the Archbishop of Salerno, who probably had some medical training, either wrote or sponsored several medical works which helped formalize medical education at the School of Salerno.

These books revived a great deal of the long forgotten medical knowledge of the ancients and more importantly they served to introduce the more recent medical advances of the Arabians and the Jews to Salerno. This new knowledge was received with great enthusiasm because these were the first rational medical texts to reach Europe in 500 years. New works on anatomy and surgery based on Constantinus' translations appeared and Salerno's star was in its ascendency.

The medical school at Salerno acquired a wide and revered reputation and became famous throughout Europe. At one time to have studied at Salerno was sufficient to establish the medical reputation of any young physician.

Until the middle of the twelfth century, the methods of teaching and training remained essentially the same as they had been in Roman times; that is, physicians were trained by older physicians on an apprenticeship basis. Salerno was perhaps the first true medical school and the doctors of Salerno were outstanding both as educators and practitioners. They regarded disease as a natural phenomenon and applied common sense treatments to try to effect a cure. They acknowledged surgery as a discipline and were surprisingly skillful. They offered students an extensive curriculum and taught anatomy based on the texts of Galen and Haly Abbas. Because human dissection was forbidden they used pigs for this purpose. Disease was observed and taught at the bedside and students assisted or were present at surgical operations.

Salerno was also the first medical school to urge that people who wanted to practice medicine should be qualified to do so. In 1140 Roger II of Sicily issued the following decree:

> Whosoever will henceforth practice medicine, let him present himself to our officials and judges to be examined by them: but if he presume of his own temerity, let him be imprisoned and all his goods be sold by auction. The object of this is to prevent the subjects of our kingdom incurring peril through the ignorance of physicians.

The School of Salerno gave useful instruction not only in medicine, but in the ethics of medical practice as well. Archimathaeus, a Salernitan professor, in his book *De Adventu Medici* gave such advice, some of which can probably be traced back to Hippocrates and Galen. Later Salernitan and other medieval physicians added to this list; some interesting examples of their combined and assorted advice follows:

> Dress soberly like a clerk and not like a minstrel.
> Keep your fingernails well shaped and clean.
> When called to a patient commend yourself to God.
> Do not walk hastily, which betokens levity, or too slowly which is a sign of faint-heartedness.
> Find out from his messenger as much about the patient as you can

before you arrive. Then if you discover nothing from his pulse or water, you can still astonish him with your knowlege of his condition.

On arrival exchange greetings and ask the friends whether the patient has confessed, for if you bid him to do so after the examination it will frighten him.

Next proceed to feel the pulse, remembering that it may be affected by your arrival or by the thought of the fee you are going to charge.

Tell the patient you will cure him with God's help, but inform the relatives that the case is most grave.

Behave modestly and gravely at all times.

Do not look desirously on the patients wife, daughters or maid servants, or kiss them or fondle their breasts.

Do not talk boastfully, lest you trip on your own words.

Do not disparge your fellow physicians. If you do not know them personally, say you have heard nothing but good of them.

Avoid the company or friendship of laymen. They not only mock doctors, but it is not easy to extract a fee from an intimate.

If you do not wish to take a case pretend to be ill.

If you find the patient dead on your arrival show no surprise but say you knew his case was grave and that he would not recover. This will enhance your professional reputation.

The Crusades had a profound influence upon the development and reorientation of medicine which started at Salerno and spread to the rest of Europe. During the Crusades traffic shuttled through the city between the East and the West and Salerno became a cultural melting pot. Many sick and wounded Crusaders landed there, and stayed for rest and treatment before continuing their journey home across Europe.

Numerous noblemen were among the Crusaders and thus the School of Salerno had a constant flow of famous patients. Perhaps the most famous of these was Robert, Duke of Normandy, the son of William the Conqueror. This Crusading Duke's long absence from home cost him the throne of England and later led to his imprisonment by his usurping brother. However, during his sojurn at Salerno the restoration and maintenance of the Duke's health was of such great concern to the professors of Salerno that they teamed up to write a famous textbook on hygiene. Written in Latin verse, especially for Duke Robert's guidance, this compact book contained such practical health rules as the following:

> The Salerno School doth by these lines impart
> all health to England's King doth advise

> From care his head to keep wrath his heart,
> Drink not much wine sup light and soon arise.

Then follows such excellent advice on the subject of diet:

> A King that cannot rule him his diet,
> Will hardly rule his Realm in piece and quiet.

Little did the professors of Salerno realize that they had produced one of the most famous and popular medical books ever to be written. Known as the *Regimen Sanitatis Salernitum,* this book originally was a collection of 362 verses of practical rules on healthful living. The book counseled moderation in all things and advocated an even, natural way of life. Couched in easy jingles and rhymes which the common man could remember, this book revived long-forgotten concepts of personal hygiene and healthful living. It represented the most significant contribution to preventive medicine and public health made by the School of Salerno.

The *Regimen Sanitatis Salernitum* swept across the Western World and became the most popular book of the Middle Ages next to the Bible. Originally in manuscript form and written in Latin this book was soon translated into all of the common languages of Europe. With the invention of printing in the fifteenth century a large number of relatively inexpensive and popular versions appeared. As time went on later doctors added new verses to each new publication until the original 362 health rules burgeoned into over 3,500 verses.

Thus Salernitan medical wisdom was disseminated to an entire continent and the *Regimen* became the epic guidebook of health and hygiene for all of medieval mankind. Its sage simplicity and practical closeness to daily life left no doubt in the reader's mind as to how to live, what to do and what to avoid. It gave relatively sound advice on sleep, sex, diet, drink and diversion, as well as remedies for such diseases as gout, phlegm and the ague. Its popularity was further insured by the fact that its catchy jingles were so easy to memorize that even the illiterate common masses could commit them to memory.

Quoted here are some of the jingles, poems and advice which were contained in the *Regimen Sanitatis Salernitum*:

> Rise early in the morn and straight remember
> With water cold to wash your hands and eyes.

In gentle fashion reaching every member,
And so refresh your brain when you arise.

From washing after meals two gains arise,
The hands are cleansed and strengthened are the eyes.
If thou in health prolonged wouldst ever stay,
Wash frequently thy hands each passing day.

The healthy man cleans his teeth,
Goes for walks and keeps out of draughts.

If thou to health and vigor wouldst attain
Shun weighty cares—all anger deem profane
From heavy suppers and much wine abstain.

Joy, temperance and repose,
Slam the door on the doctor's nose.

Use three physicians still—first Dr. Quiet,
Then Doctor Merryman and then Doctor Diet.

Great suppers will the stomach's peace impair,
Wouldst lightly rest—curtail thine evening fare.
Nor trivial count it after pompous fare
To rise from table and to take the air.

Shun idle slumber nor delay
The urgent calls of nature to obey.

When moved yourself to nature needs,
Forbear them not, for that much danger breeds.

Some "Don'ts" from the Hortus Sanitas:

Don't read in bed.
Don't drink too much.
Don't love too much.
Don't strain too much.

In addition to these rules of healthful living this long poem embodied the medical teachings of the School of Salerno. It gave specific herbal remedies and treatments for many diseases. Succeeding scholars in later editions added lengthy verses on climate, the four humors, venesection and uroscopy. Such verses provided the medical profession with indispensable precepts and thousands of physicians committed them to memory. Thus the *Regimen* served as a practical handbook of medicine for the physicians of medieval Europe.

This book brought back to Europe a host of Greco-Roman medical ideas. Foremost among these was the "Doctrine of the Four Humors," which became the most powerful concept of medieval medical thinking. Empedocles had laid the foundation 600 years before Christ by teaching that the world consisted of four elements: fire, water, air and earth. Hippocrates and Galen had applied this to man, stating that he was composed of four humors: blood (fire), black bile (water), yellow bile (air), and phlegm (earth). They believed that if the humors were in proper balance man was in good health, but that an upset of the balance of these four humors produced disease.

The Salernitan doctors and later scholars added to this by teaching that the dominant humor determined a person's physical and emotional makeup. For example the Sanguine Person was inclined to be fat, prone to laughter and had hot blood. The Phlegmatic Person was given to sloth and rest while the Choleric Person with yellow bile was violent and fierce, and the Melancholy Man who had black bile was depressed, peevish and passive.

They believed that evacuation of the corrupt or excess humors from the body prevented and cured disease. Hence it was a widespread and popular belief that in order to maintain or regain one's health it was necessary to submit to the three medical procedures of purging, cupping and bleeding. Strange as it may seem these theories held sway until the middle of the nineteenth century when they were finally overthrown by Virchow and his work on cellular pathology.

The *Regimen Sanitatis Salernitum* retained its place as the authoritative "backbone" of medical literature until the time of the Renaissance. There is no record of how many times this remarkable book was reprinted, but it was still being published as late as 1852. It is estimated that approximately 300 editions were issued and that it was translated into all of the known languages of the Western World. Sir John Harington, the godson of Queen Elizabeth, compiled and translated a popular English version in the sixteenth century.

The immense popularity and widespread acceptance of the *Regimen* gave rise to a whole literature on the preservation of health. Popular health books and almanacs flooded medieval Europe soon after the invention of printing. These books dealt with every detail of daily living and gave instructions on how to care for every part of the body. Usually addressed to a person of high rank, these books advised him how to live long and healthfully. Thus health education and personal hygiene were among the most important contributions of the Middle Ages to preventive medicine and public health.

The School of Salerno reached the peak of its prestige in the eleventh and twelfth centuries. With the end of the Crusades in the thirteenth century the routes of trade changed. Salerno which had been the first and foremost center of medical learning slowly declined. However, Salerno had only been the beginning—other centers of learning were founded at Montpelier, Bologna, Paris, and Padua. From 1200 to the end of the Middle Ages the foundation stones for over eighty European universities were laid. By the end of the thirteenth century medical leadership had passed from Salerno to Montpelier. However, Montpelier's fame was relatively short lived for the Black Death in the fourteenth and fifteenth centuries devastated the university, killing off its faculty and students, so that in 1422 only one student was enrolled in the school. This was typical of the times, for the history of the Middle Ages was punctuated with the horror of periodic devastating outbreaks of epidemics, pandemics, plagues and pestilence.

Chapter 8

THEY SHALL CRY, "UNCLEAN"

THE FRENCH PHILOSOPHER Voltaire, commenting cynically on the Crusades said, "Of all that we gained by the Crusades and all of that we have taken, leprosy was the only thing we kept."

The morbid history of leprosy stretches across humanity's trail for untold thousands of years. Ancient records reveal the futile prescriptions of the Egyptians for this affliction. The thirteenth and fourteenth chapters of Leviticus in the Old Testament are given over to the diagnosis and recognition of leprosy, along with the rites and sacrifices to be used in cleansing the leper, his garments and his dwelling. Strict and stern rules were laid down in Leviticus for the enforced isolation of the leper and he was branded as "unclean." The Hebrew word "Zaraath" was applied in the Old Testament to this disease, but undoubtedly it also included a variety of other skin diseases, such as vitiligo, psoriasis, skin cancer and severe ringworm.

Greek records of about 500 B.C. indicate a knowledge of this disease which they called "elephantiasis graecorum." Later Hippocrates referred to this disease, applying to it as well as to a variety of other skin diseases the Greek adjective "lepros," meaning rough or scaly. When the Bible was translated from Hebrew into Greek in about 100 B.C. an attempt was made to find the Greek equivalent of "Zaraath" and the translators decided to use Hippocrates' word lepra. Since then the terms leper and leprosy have been used carrying down through the ages with them a cruel, terrifying and loathsome connotation.

The New Testament also contains references to leprosy and we read in St. Luke 5:12,

> And it came to pass, when he was in a certain city, behold a man full of leprosy; who seeing Jesus fell on his face, and besought him, saying, Lord, if thou wilt thou canst make me clean.

13. And he put forth his hand, and touched him, saying, I will: be thou clean. And immediately the leprosy departed from him. 14. And he charged him to tell no man: but go, and show thyself to the priest, and offer for thy cleansing, according as Moses commanded, for testimony unto them.

While sporadic cases of leprosy had undoubtedly occurred along the Atlantic and Mediterranean coasts of Spain and France even before the Christian era, the disease did not become common in Europe until about the time of the fall of the Roman Empire. In the fifth and sixth centuries its increase in southern and western France aroused serious alarm among the inhabitants. The clergy, concerned for the safety of their flocks and calling to mind the ancient duties of their priesthood, adopted all of the restrictive measures against leprosy contained in the Old Testament. Among the earliest civil restrictions against lepers were those prepared by the Council of Lyons in 583 and the edict promulgated in 644 by Rotharic, King of the Longobardi, which prescribed the strict isolation of lepers.

Leprosy continued to spread widely and soon the outward signs of the disease became terrifyingly familiar to the citizens of medieval Europe. With the thickened skin, the hoarse voice, the many foul-smelling sores that spread and finally rotted, the miserable victims were enough in themselves to produce loathing and hysterical terror. Leprosy was widely disseminated in Europe during the eleventh and twelfth centuries by the returning Crusaders. The social upheaval and the large population movements produced by the Crusades along with poor economic conditions and widespread domestic squalor provided a fertile soil for the rapid spread of leprosy. The disease assumed epidemic proportions and spread at a furious rate throughout Europe and England.

The commonly held view was that such a loathsome disease as leprosy must be the result of sinful behavior. It was thought that the sufferers had probably provoked their condition by dirty habits and sexual license, or even by eating poisonous foods. The moral attitude of the church towards this "unclean" disease gave added weight to these opinions.

The medical opinion of the times held that the disease was spread by personal contact and it was believed that the condition was hopeless, offering no chance for recovery and that "Once a leper, always a leper." Rational and effective treatment for leprosy was nonexistent and this disease was set apart from all others and left exclusively to treatment by divine help and intervention. A common form of treatment which lepers used, was to allow dogs to lick their sores in the futile hope that they thus would be healed. This erroneous belief was based on the passage from the 16th chapter of St. Luke which reads as follows, "And there was a certain beggar named Lazarus, which was laid at his gate, full of sores, and desiring to be fed with the crumbs which fell from the rich man's table; moreover the dogs came and licked his sores."

Both medical and religious opinion held that strict and rigorous isolation and segregation was necessary to control and prevent the spread of leprosy. Therefore every attempt was made to exclude and remove the unfortunate victims as effectively as possible from everyday life.

The church righteously invoked the Biblical restrictions found in Leviticus 13:45-46, which reads as follows: "And the leper in whom the plague is, his clothes shall be rent, and his head bare, and he shall put a covering upon his upper lip, and shall cry, unclean, unclean. All the days wherein the plague shall be in him he shall be defiled, he is unclean: he shall dwell alone; without the camp shall his habitation be."

Strict, detailed and precise regulations governing lepers were enacted. Recognizing the contagiousness of the disease, society forcibly expelled the leper from the community in order to protect its healthy members. Since the disease was incurable the leper became an outcast for life and was socially considered dead long before he recived the merciful release of physical death.

The decision as to who was a leper was given serious consideration; before a person was adjudged a leper he was examined by a special commission. During the early middle ages these commissions consisted of a bishop, several clerics and a person already afflicted with leprosy (because he supposedly had special knowledge of the disease). Later these commissions were expanded to include several prominent physicians and barber surgeons.

The awful finality of excluding a leper from the human community and making him one of "the living dead" was symbolized by an enactment of the funeral service. The leper was clad in a shroud, the solemn mass for the dead was read over him and earth was sprinkled upon him to signify his departure from the living. Then, accompanied by his relatives, friends and neighbors he was conducted by the priest to a designated place outside of the confines of the community. His worldly goods were divided among his rightful heirs and he had to clothe himself in a long black garment and cry out to all who came near, "Unclean, unclean."

Lepers were not permitted to live within the village or city walls, and could not use public fountains or inns. They were not allowed to speak to people and they had to carry and sound a warning rattle, horn or bell. When a leper ventured into the market place he dared only to point with his rod or staff at anything he wished to buy. The leper was a complete social and civil outcast, wandering about the countryside or living by himself in a lonely hut, or in a colony of huts and hovels with other lepers, amid untold squalor and filth. Lepers had to beg for alms to eke out their miserable existence. Groups of them would congregate at the city or village gates and as a traveller would fare forth, this miserable filthy horde would descend upon him crying out for alms. They would threaten to embrace the traveller and in order to escape their loathsome attentions he would cast a handful of copper coins of the lowest denomination as far away from himself as possible. While the miserable lepers scrambled in the dust and dirt to find the coins, the traveller could make his escape.

The general attitude towards lepers was extremely harsh and cruel. For example, Phillip the Fair who ruled France from 1285 to 1314 considered the problem of leprosy and made a concrete suggestion for its control. In effect he said, "Let us collect all of the lepers in one place and burn them. So often as more appear let us also burn them, until the disease is eradicated."

The church was more merciful in its attitude and as a concession to the spiritual welfare of the leper, small windows were built into the walls of the churches, so that the outcast could see, if not share the religious ceremony. However Christian charity and love was not entirely dead and the monastaries of the religious order of Saint Lazarus were set aside as hospitals to care for the ever increasing numbers of lepers.

Both church and government finally provided better care for the lepers and a more practical means of protection for the public. By means of charitable bequests and taxes levied specifically for this purpose, special leper houses and colonies were built. These became known as lazar houses or lazarettos. At one time there were as many as 19,000 such leper houses on the continent and over 200 in England.

Because the disease was so universally feared and loathed a rigorous system for the control of leprosy was developed, including even the most minute details. Isolation was so strict that every possibility was guarded against to prevent direct or indirect contact with lepers, including even their breath. Detailed instructions were given to physicians in order to enable them to diagnose a case and the legal procedures to officially adjudge a person a leper were followed. The lepers were then forcibly isolated in the leper houses or lazarettos. Unfortunately there was one law for the rich and one for the poor. Most wealthy people who contracted the disease were allowed to remain in their own houses, and even if they entered a lazar house, they were permitted to bring with them all of their usual comforts, such as soft bedding, good clothing, special foods and silver tableware. Those who could not pay for such luxuries received the harsh treatment which has always been reserved for the poor.

However in general the isolation and segregation of lepers was quite complete and was enforced without mercy. The continued segregation of lepers for several centuries was successful and it practically eradicated leprosy from Europe. This perhaps, can be regarded as one of the first great victories of preventive medicine. The experience gained in dealing with leprosy influenced medical thought considerably. The concept of contagion, namely, that certain diseases can be spread by direct contact, became firmly fixed in the minds of the medieval physicians.

Another theory advanced for the rather dramatic decline of leprosy is that most of the lepers of Europe, who were segregated in the leper houses, were wiped out by the "Black Death." This great pandemic of bubonic plague struck Europe in 1348 and continued in recurring epidemic waves for several centuries. Undoubtedly the already sick and weakened lepers in their overcrowded lazarettos were easy victims of the plague. Thus the Black Death wiped them out, leaving too few survivors to continue the spread of leprosy.

Chapter 9

THE PLAGUE

IN ANCIENT TIMES when the wrathful gods wanted to strike a punishing blow upon guilty mortals they afflicted them with a plague. Literally this term means a blow and is derived from the Greek word "plege" meaning a blow or stroke. While mankind has been striken by many kinds of plagues and many ailments are said to plague mankind, there is only one true plague, and that is the bubonic plague. While also known as "the Pest," "the Black Death," and "the Black Destroyer," this disease is best known simply as "the Plague."

Plague is probably as ancient as mankind and the antiquity of this dread disease (spread from rats to fleas to man) can logically be assumed from the fact that wherever there were men there were rats, and wherever there were rats plague would occur. Unfortunately, the early historical records of plagues and epidemics were not kept with sufficient accuracy to make diagnosis certain.

One of the earliest records of what was probably an outbreak of plague is recorded in the Bible (I. Samuel, chapters 5 and 6). Here is recorded a great plague among the Philistines which broke out at the seaport town of Achdad and then moved inland to smite 50,070 at Bethshemesh. The Philistines made golden images of their "emerods" and of the mice (rats?) that overran the land in order to stay the pestilence. The "emerods" which are mentioned rather frequently in the Bible are believed by some historians to refer to the ulcerated swellings in the groin known as buboes, which are produced by the plague. The disease of Hezekiah, King of Judah, which is recorded in the Old Testament was probably plague. This was transmitted to the army of Sennacherib, and in Kings 19:35 we read, "And it came to pass that night, that the Angel of the Lord went out and smote in the camp of the Assyrians an hundred forescore and five thousand and when they arose early in the morning, behold, they were all dead corpses."

Over the ensuing centuries plague struck again and again. In the year 68 A.D. plague erupted in Rome, striking down 10,000 people daily at its height. Plague returned again to Rome in the years 79 and 125 A.D. It recurred again in the year 164 and continued to strike in successive waves for the next sixteen years. This outbreak was so severe that it was reported to have exterminated approximately one-half of the population and to have caused even the great physician Galen to flee in terror before it.

The first authentic pandemic of plague began in 542 A.D. at Pelusium in Egypt. This city was an important center of commerce, located on the main trade route between the East and the West. The plague followed the routes of trade across the world and afflicted every country then known between Asia and Ireland. Procopius, a sixth century Roman writer, graphically described the buboes and the black spots on the skin so typically diagnostic of plague. He stated that "at one time the amount of deaths in Constantinople ranged from five to ten thousand each day." He further stated that the plague "spared neither island nor cave nor mountain top where man dwelt. Many homes were left empty and it came to pass that many, from want of relatives, were unburied for several days. At that time it was hard to find anyone at business in Constantinople. Most people met in the street were carrying a corpse. All business had ceased, all craftsmen had deserted their crafts."

After this disastrous pandemic there was a lull, and for approximately eight centuries the civilized world was relatively free from plague.

Coming out of the East and following the routes of trade, the plague returned in the mid-fourteenth century and very nearly annihilated mankind as it swept across the world. No sooner had leprosy passed its zenith and begun to decline in Europe than the even more terrifying and deadlier bubonic plague spread its black robe of pestilence over the Western World. Riding with hurricane speed across the heavens, the dark horseman of the plague scattered death. Spreading the darkness of death over the land, he spared neither field nor farm, village nor city, palace nor hovel.

Originating in the hinterlands of Central Asia from a reservoir of infection existing among the wild rodents of the steppes, the plague spread rapidly westward. By the spring of 1346 it had reached the shores of the Black Sea, from which it was carried on shipboard to Constantinople, Genoa, and Venice. Invading Europe early in 1348 it spread inland attacking Florence, northern Italy and Avignon by April, and reaching Valencia and Barcelona by May. It took approximately three years for this huge pandemic wave of plague to wash over Europe, with secondary waves following at intervals until about 1388.

As widespread sickness and death struck with shocking suddenness, mass madness, hysteria and panic ensued. No living person on earth was free from fear, for none knew when it would be his turn to be smitten. The doomed, living among the dead and dying, responded variously with prayer and hope, fear and despair, wild flight, riot or debauchery. Civilization disintegrated and humanity was abandoned. The sick and dying lay unattended, and sudden agonized death occurred in the houses, fields and streets. The fields lay idle and abandoned, while the villages and cities were left empty and all trade ceased. The land was literally covered with dead bodies in every stage of putrefaction, and the stench of decaying human flesh was everywhere. There were not enough living left to bury the dead. The graveyards were overcrowded and bodies had to be buried in pits or burned en masse.

The air was foul, the water was foul, and the earth was foul. In the foulness of death, with its attendant terror and fear, every known type of inhumanity, sacrilege and perversion reared its head. Friend shunned friend, brother abandoned brother, husbands and wives deserted each other, and even mothers fled in terror from their own sick children. Infants were abandoned and left suckling on the poisoned breasts of their dead mothers.

Over the centuries time has dimmed the horrors of the plague, but through the writings of contemporaries the terrifying tale of this disastrous disease is recorded forever. The Black Death of 1348 can never be forgotten, for its chroniclers include such famous writers as Petrarch, and Boccaccio. In one of his famous letters, the great Italian poet Petrarch exclaims "Oh happy posterity, who will not experience such abysmal woe and will look upon our testimony as fable." It was an embittered Petrarch who survived the Black Death, for in the early morning of April 6, 1348, the body of Petrarch's Laura lay among the plague victims of Avignon.

Giovanni Boccacio, the famed Italian novelist who achieved his place among literary immortals as the "father of the short story," gives an excellent description of the plague. His Decameron remains one of the most widely read books in the world, although not because of its epidemiological data. This book is not merely a random collection of disconnected stories, but is an organic unit built upon a logical framework. There are ten leading characters in the book, seven ladies and three gentlemen, who have taken refuge from the horrors of the plague in a carnival of immagination. They knew no sense of public responsibility, and when the plague broke out in Florence in 1348 they did not feel obliged to remain in the city and help the victims. They found it safer and pleasanter to move behind the walls of a villa in the country. Here they spent their days in eating, drinking, flirting and telling spicy tales to one another. Each of the ten refugees narrates one story on each of ten days. Thus there are ten stories for every day, or a hundred stories in all.

Boccaccio starts his story of the plague as follows:

> In the year of our Lord 1348, there happened at Florence, the finest city in all Italy, a most terrible plague—which whether owing to the influence of the planets, or that it was sent from God as a just punishment for our sins, had broken out some years before in the Levant, and after passing from place to place and making incredible havoc all the way, had now reached the West.

In writing of the onset, symptoms, and treatment of the plague Boccaccio said:

> It began to show itself in a sad and wonderful manner, and different from what it had been in the East, where bleeding from the nose is the fatal prognostic, here, there appeared certain tumors in the groins or under the armpits, some big as a small apple, others as an egg, and afterwards purple spots in most parts of the body—the usual messengers of death. To the cure of this malady, neither medical knowledge nor the power of drugs was of any effect. They generally died the third day from the first appearance of the symptoms.

The high degree of contagiousness of the plague was noted and Boccaccio relates:

> The disease being communicated from the sick to the well, seemed daily to get ahead and to rage the more as fire will do, by laying on fresh combustibles,—and one instance of this kind I took particular notice of: namely, that the rags of a poor man just dead, being thrown into the street and two hogs coming by at the same time and rooting amongst them and shaking them about in their mouths, in less than an hour, turned round and died on the spot.

He further relates how some people did everything to avoid the sick, and isolated themselves or fled to the country. Some lived, temperately avoiding all excesses, while others went to the opposite extreme and "would baulk no passion or appetite." A third group tried to live in their usual normal fashion and for prevention depended upon "odors and nosegays to smell—for they supposed the whole atmosphere to be tainted." That none of these methods were effective in preventing the plague is shown by his statement that, "Divided as they were neither did all die nor all escape, but falling sick indifferently."

Commenting on the disintegration of society under stress of the plague, Boccaccio wrote, "And such at that time was the public distress, that the laws, human or divine were not regarded, for the officers, to put them in force, being either dead, sick, or in want of persons to assist them; everyone did just as he pleased." He recorded the terrific morbidity and mortality of the plague as follows:

> . . . fell sick daily by thousands, and, having nobody to attend them, generally died: some breathed their last in the streets, and others shut up in their own houses, when the stench that came from them made the first discovery of their deaths to the neighborhood. And indeed every place was filled with the dead . . . . they were forced to dig trenches, and to put them in by hundreds, piling them up in rows, as goods are stored in a ship . . . . such was the cruelty of Heaven, and perhaps of men, that between March and July following, it is supposed and made pretty certain, that upwards of a hundred thousand souls perished in the city only; whereas before that calamity, it was not supposed to have contained so many inhabitants.

There are only a few good contemporary medical accounts of the great plague of 1348 and probably the best of these is that of the famous French surgeon, Guy de Chauliac. Such was the lack of knowledge and the thinking of the times that he ascribed the origin of the plague as due to "the grand conjunction of the three superior

planets, Saturn, Jupiter, and Mars in the sign of Aquarius." It was
to be many centuries later before physicians were to know that the
Black Death was caused by the more ominous conjunction of rats,
fleas, the bacillus pestis, and man.

Guy de Chauliac described the outbreak of plague at Avignon in
1348 as follows:

> The said mortality commenced with us in the month of January and
> lasted the space of seven months.
>
> It was of two kinds: the first lasted two months, with continued fever
> and expectoration of blood. And they died of it in three days.
>
> The second was, all the rest of the time, also with continued fever and
> apostems and carbuncles on the external parts, principally in the armpits
> and groin: and they died of it in five days. And was of such great
> contagiousness (especially that which had expectoration of blood) that
> not only in visiting but also in looking at it, one person took it from
> another: so that the people died without servants and were interred
> without Priests.
>
> The father did not visit his son, nor the son his father.
>
> Charity was dead and hope destroyed.
>
> I call it great because it spread out through all the world or very
> little was spared.
>
> For it commenced in the Orient and so throwing its arrows against
> the world passed through our country towards the Occident.
>
> And it was so great that it scarcely left behind one quarter of the
> population.
>
> So it was useless and shameful for the physicians, since they did not
> dare visit the sick for fear of being infected: and when they visited
> them, they did not make them well, and gained nothing: for all the
> sick died, except a few at the end, who escaped it with mature buboes.
>
> The carbuncles were cupped, scarified and cauterized. And I, to
> avoid infamy, not daring to absent myself, with continual fear, I treated
> myself as much as I could, using the said remedies.
>
> Nevertheless, toward the end of the mortality, I fell into a continued
> fever, with an apostem on the groin, and sick nearly six weeks, and was
> in such great danger that all my companions believed that I would die,
> but the apostem becoming mature, and treated as I have said, I escaped
> by the will of God.

As can be seen from this the medieval physicians were a sorry lot,
and proved to be totally inadequate in trying to grapple with the
drastic onslaught of the Black Death. Many physicians fled before
the plague, to what they regarded as safer locations, and justified

their cowardice with the excuse that medical care was futile. It makes one wonder who was more frightened, the physicians or their patients.

Those physicians who remained and tried to help the plague victims adopted a special outfit designed to protect them as much as possible from contact with their patients. They clothed themselves in flowing dark gowns which covered them from head to foot, and wore long gloves to protect their hands and arms. They wore a hood or mask having a long beak protruding from it containing spices and perfumes. By breathing through this they believed that they were protected from the deadly tainted atmosphere. Because the customary medical procedures of cupping, purging and bleeding were of no avail, there was little they could do for their patients, except to comfort them and to spray the room and house with supposedly protective perfumes and odors.

Many terrible tales are told of the plague, such as the boy who returned to his native village and met an old man who said, "I am the only survivor"; of ghost ships that drifted through the seas with lifeless crews; of wolves living in houses in which all of the people had died; of beggars in possession of untold wealth and living in palaces left empty through death. Stories are told of the blind, terror-stricken flight of people in their futile attempts to flee the plague; of priests, princes and physicians fleeing in panic along with the others. Strange stories are told of hysterical merriment and unbridled debauchery occurring in the midst of universal destruction: sex and all of its perversions being indulged in until the last moments of life; women running naked through the streets; violation of dying women and of their bodies even after death; how some, in their hysteria, indulged in singing and dancing on the corpses of relatives and friends.

At the height of the terror and because of ignorance as to the cause of the plague, the common people sought a scapegoat. The rabble at first blamed the nobility for causing the plague. However, the nobility in self-defense, and because they were heavily indebted to the Jewish money-lenders, incited the mob against the Jews. They claimed the Jews had polluted the wells, poisoned the food and even tainted the air. Thus terror and avarice joined hands with disease and very nearly destroyed the Jews of medieval Europe.

In Basle all Jews were locked into a wooden building which was set afire and burned to the ground. At Strasbourg 2,000 Jews were burned alive on their own burial ground, and at Mayence 12,000 Jews perished in a gigantic bonfire.

Where there were no Jews, the gravediggers were accused of causing the plague, because they profited from the dead. Elsewhere the rabble turned upon the cripples and beggars, believing they caused the disease through envy and malice. They called them the "accursed of God" and slaughtered all who did not flee.

It has been said that nothing before or since has so nearly accomplished the extermination of the human race as did this great pandemic of bubonic plague. Some said it killed one-half of the world's population, others said not so many and set the figure at one-fourth. When Pope Clement VI asked for an accounting of the number of dead, he was finally given a figure totalling 42,836,486 corpses. However, it is believed that the total mortality of the Black Death was over 60 million. Over 13 million are said to have died from it in China, while India was said to have been practically depopulated, and Tartary, Mesopotamia, Syria and Armenia were literally covered with dead bodies.

In Europe alone 25 million are said to have perished. Florence and Venice are each said to have lost 100,000. At the height of the epidemic Strasbourg is said to have lost 9,000 daily, while in Vienna the daily death toll was 1,200. France was so hard hit that in some places not more than two out of twenty people were left alive. In Avignon nine-tenths of the population was exterminated, and the Pope found it necessary to consecrate the River Rhone so bodies could be thrown into it for Christian burial, as the churchyards could no longer hold the bodies. Crossing the channel, the plague is said to have killed one-fourth to one-half of the population of medieval England.

Despite the erroneous beliefs of the authorities that the plague was due to divine or cosmic origins, it was definitely recognized that the disease was "catching," or contagious. It was also gradually recognized that epidemics traveled and spread over the routes of trade and especially by sea. This knowledge led to groping attempts to control and prevent the spread of the plague. Quarantine procedures were born out of this knowledge, and were implemented by the ravages and fears that the Black Death produced. During the years of 1377 to 1403, Venice, Ragusa, Marseilles and Genoa, which were the chief maritime cities of the Mediterranean, adopted and enforced a forty-day detention period for all vessels entering their ports.

The word quarantine literally means forty days, and is derived from the Italian word "quaranta," meaning forty. While this period of time does not seem logical to us now, a number of factors may have influenced their selection of a forty-day detention period. The fortieth day of a disease was one of the critical days named by Hippocrates. Other possible factors may have been the familiar Biblical period of forty days, the forty days of Lent, the custom of having a truce last forty days, or the legal period of forty days allowed a widow to dwell in her deceased husband's house.

The banning of infected ships and travellers from entering cities and the detention of those coming from plague-infected areas, or those suspected of having plague, for a period of forty days was a historical landmark in public health and represented the beginning of communicable disease control procedures.

In addition to maritime quarantine, communities passed laws requiring the reporting of cases of plague. To enforce these laws "searchers" were employed to find and report new cases. Carrying white wands, they searched the community, street by street and marked infected houses with a sign. They barred the doors and sealed the windows, thus completely isolating the victim and his family. These unfortunates were completely cut off from the world, and had to depend upon the municipal authorities or the uncertain kindness of friends and relatives to bring them food and drink. The dead were passed out through the windows and removed for burial outside of the city by carts. When a victim of the plague died, the house was fumigated and his clothing and personal effects were burned. Later most cities forcibly isolated suspected cases or victims of the plague in a "pest house," located on the outskirts of the town.

Thus, the impact of the Black Death created a system of quarantine, sanitary control and disinfection, which was to serve as a pattern for combating epidemics and contagious diseases for many centuries to come.

This terrifying pandemic of plague which occurred in the mid-fourteenth century was not the last of the Black Death. Plague continued to ebb and flow like a deadly tidal wave, periodically washing over the world for almost 400 years before it began to decline at the end of the seventeenth century. London in 1603 lost one-sixth of its population and was hit as hard again in 1625. Ireland had a disastrous epidemic in 1650, as did Denmark in 1654. The plague returned to Italy again in 1657. London was again visited by the Black Death in the years of 1664 and 1665, losing 70,000 people out of a population of 500,000. Spain had epidemics in 1677 and 1681 and Germany in 1679 and 1681. In 1759 about 70,000 died on the island of Cypress, and during 1790 Marseilles and Toulon each lost about 91,000.

Probably the most widely known and best recorded of these various epidemics is the one that occurred in London during 1664 and 1665. Daniel Defoe, the famed author of *Robinson Crusoe,* ably described this outbreak in his work, *A Journal of the Plague Year.* Another account of this epidemic is contained in Pepy's Diary.

Various explanations have been offered to explain the retrogression of plague from the world at the end of the seventeenth century. Progress of civilization in general, with improved sanitation, better housing and cleanliness is considered an important factor. The instituting of strict quarantine measures and the isolation of plague victims in pest houses undobutedly helped control the disease. Some historians say that the disappearance of the plague was connected with a change in the rat population. Others say the Agrarian revolution which led to better housing and the exclusion of rats from human dwellings produced the decline of the plague. None of these explanations is entirely satisfactory and it may be that the plague subsided because it merely followed the natural law of the rise and decline of all epidemic diseases.

Chapter 10

OTHER MEDIEVAL EPIDEMICS AND DISEASES

Hardly had the first great epidemic wave of the Black Death subsided when its fantastic companion the "Dancing Mania" over-ran Europe. This peculiar malady was a form of mass hysteria and undoubtedly was the queerest emotional disorder ever to affect large groups of people. Assuming epidemic proportions, this mental contagion caused men and women to dance hand in hand in circles for hours, until they fell exhausted, some fainting, some having hysterical visions, while others had epileptiform seizures.

Originating out of the terror and horror of the "Great Plague," this strange phenomenon was the direct result of the mental and emotional trauma produced by that great disaster. Although the bodies of the millions of plague victims had been burned or buried, the minds of the survivors were still haunted by terrifying memories of death and disease. In addition, the periodic reappearance of the plague had a widespread emotional effect upon people, producing in them tremendous feelings of insecurity, fear and panic. There is a limit to what men's minds can endure and still remain rational, and during medieval times this limit was exceeded.

The people, mentally shocked and physically worn out by the repeated disasters of war, famine, plague and pestilence, believed that they had incurred the anger of God and were being punished for their sins. Believing that they were poisoned by demons and ascribing their misfortune to the "work of the Devil," they had deep feelings of guilt and contrition. The churches were filled with repentant sinners and the towns and villages resounded with cries and lamentations. As religious mania and mass hysteria spread, fanatics were commonly to be seen publicly inflicting chastisements upon themselves and calling on others to repent.

One expression of the religious mania of the times was manifested by a company of flagellants known as the Brotherhood of the Cross. Arising in Hungary they sent forth missions of brothers robed in somber garments with large red crosses on their chests. Carrying triple thonged scourges tipped with lead, they marched into towns with down-cast eyes and covered heads. Summoning the townsfolks by the ringing of bells they would scourge themselves in an act of public penance. Repeating this performance twice daily for several days they would make as many converts as possible and then march on to a new town.

However, the major manifestations of the mass hysteria that afflicted the emotionally troubled people of medieval Europe was the widespread explosive eruption of the Dancing Mania.

Apparently this strange emotional storm first broke out in the town of Aix-la-Chapelle in 1374. It supposedly began one morning when a strange band of people, coming from some unknown place in Germany, somberly and silently marched through the streets of the town until they came to the public square. Here, they formed a circle, joined hands and began to dance. Slowly at first, then faster and faster, they increased the tempo of their dance, until it climaxed in a frantic frenzy of convulsive contortions. The assembled spectators responding to mass suggestion and falling under the hysterical spell cast by this wild and weird dance, let loose their pent-up emotions and joined in the mad melee.

This was a dance such as no one in the city had ever seen before. Like the public acts of penance of the Brotherhood of the Cross, the performance was regularly repeated and was always started in the public square by a comparatively small number of people. News of this strange phenomenon spread like wildfire throughout the town and countryside. Spectators flocked to the public square by the hundreds to witness this wild and weird dance. The mere sight of the dance seemed to spread the mania and the spectators would soon be seized with a strange compulsion to join the mad dance.

Having once started to dance the dancers seemed to lose all self-control. As though possessed, they continued to dance for hours, their bodily movements increasing until they were flinging themselves about in a hysterical frenzy. Screeching and screaming they would finally fall to the ground, one by one, in sheer exhauston. With fixed

eyes and foam flecked lips, they would lie there wriggling and writh-
ing, while the emotionally aroused spectators frequently trampled them
in a wild rush to join the delirious dance.

Leaving Aix-la-Chapelle the dancers and their converts visited other
towns and cities repeating their mad performance. Soon processions
of dancers were to be found marching along all of the country roads
of Europe, going from town to town and city to city. As the madness
spread, the dance became more licentious and sexual in character.
Shops were closed, farms deserted and families neglected as the crowds
followed or joined the dancers. Frequently children were lured from
their parents, or parents deserted their children.

The Dancing Mania engulfed the cities of Cologne, Metz and
Erfurt, to mention just a few. In 1418 this mental turmoil reached
a climax in the city of Strasbourg. Here the church took a hand
and the priests tried to comfort and soothe the victims. Special masses
and services were organized for the expulsion of the devil and to
cure the mania.

The sufferers took St. Vitus as their patron saint and prayed to
him to save them from their wild outbreaks of uncontrolled dancing.

Although the Dancing Mania was first manifested on a large epidemic scale after the visitation of the Black Death, it was not exactly
a new phenomenon. Outbreaks of this type of mental and emotional
disturbance had occurred previously in earlier periods of history.
There are records of its occurrence during the tenth century and even
earlier. Undoubtedly some of the spasmodic hysterical convulsive
disorders recorded in Greco-Roman medical history were outbreaks
of this type.

The Dancing Mania was frequently called Chorea Sainti Viti or
Saint Vitus Dance. Saint Vitus was a Sicilian youth who suffered
martyrdom in 303 A.D. during the reign of the Roman Emperor
Diocletian. On the eve of his martyrdom he prayed to God to protect all those afflicted with Chorea. Just before his execution he
proclaimed that Heaven had answered his supplications and that all
who commemorated his death would be protected from convulsive
dancing disorders. Hence he came to be considered the patron saint
of the sufferers of this disorder and cures were sought at Shrines
erected to his memory.

Confusion existed about the use of the term Saint Vitus Dance and it was loosely applied to various types of twitching convulsive disorders. In 1686 Sydenham applied the Greek word for dance (chorea) to the nervous infectious disease we now know by that name. This further confused the use of the term Saint Vitus Dance and to clarify this the Dancing Mania became known as chorea magna. The infectious nervous disease which we now know to be a manifestation of rheumatic fever is also called Saint Vitus Dance, but is more properly termed chorea minor.

The Dancing Mania was also sometimes called the Dance of Saint John or Saint John's Disease because this Saint's day was traditionally celebrated with Bachanalian festivals of drinking and dancing. These became so excessive that eventually Saint Augustine had to take action against them.

As Italy was smitten by the Dancing Mania, the people, not knowing why they danced, sought an explanation. They went back to the ancient belief, half knowledge and half superstitution, that the bite of a venomous insect caused madness. They believed that spiders bit them and that the poison of the bite caused them to twist and squirm. Thus the medieval myth of the "Dance of the Tarantula" or "tarantism" was born. Tarantulas are large hairy spiders named after Taranto, a city in southern Italy where they were first closely studied. The superstitious belief that the bite of a tarantula caused a peculiar dancing disease called tarantism became firmly entrenched in Italy. It was found that music soothed and healed the victims. Hence the village musicians were called upon to treat the Dancing Mania supposedly caused by the spider bites. With flutes, oboe and Turkish drum they played lively whirling musical tunes which became known as Tarantellas. This superstition lasted for over 300 years and to this day there is an Italian dance still called the Tarantella which is performed to this lively type of music.

Outbreaks or epidemics of the "Dancing Mania" continued for several centuries. In the sixteenth century Paracelsus became particularly interested in this phenomenon and he loudly protested against any disease being attributed to the devil or being named after a Saint. Following the rational reasoning of Hippocrates he insisted that all diseases could be ascribed to natural causes. Disbelieving the power of Saint Vitus to cure this affliction, Paracelsus evolved his own harsh but effective treatment. He treated the victims of the Dancing Mania with such heroic measures as immersion in cold water, fasting, and solitary confinement. As his treatment gained acceptance the hysterical outbreaks of the Dancing Mania began to subside. Whether the cure or the fear of it brought about the cessation of these peculiar dances is a question still unanswered. By the seventeenth century these outbreaks had almost completely subsided.

Another strange disease that occurred in a series of severe, sporadic epidemics during the Middle Ages was Saint Anthony's Fire. First recorded in 857 in the Chronicles of the Convent of Zanten, medical historians have listed thirty-seven major outbreaks as having occurred between then and 1486.

Also known as "Ignis Sacer" or the sacred fire, the name of this disease was due to the intense burning sensation felt in the limbs of the victims. Cruelly burning as though the "Fires of Hell" raged within them, the fingers, toes, and even the whole extremities of the victims would turn black and become gangrenous. Then as the affected parts grew cold and lifeless they would spontaneously amputate. The unfortunate victims, if they lived, were left horribly and hopelessly crippled.

This cruel and crippling malady commonly affected the very poor. However, sporadically, at intervals of about twenty years it would occur in widespread epidemic form. During 1128 and 1129 widespread outbreaks occurred in France, England, Germany and the Netherlands. A particularly great outbreak occurred in 1373 and was most severe in France, especially in Lorraine and the Loire districts.

Strange and mysterious, the disease would occur during a season when the rains were heavy and the summer was damp and foggy. Then at harvest time, the rye from which the bread was made would be scanty and the grain would be spotted, swollen and blighted with a fungus smut. Later in the fall as the diseased grain was ground into flour, baked into bread and eaten, the disease would strike.

Gradually, victim after victim would appear, crying out in pain and fear as his fingers or toes, arms or legs burned with the pain of "Ignis Sacer." As the fearful news spread, the towns and villages were terror-stricken and people, believing the disease to be contagious, fled in terror from the victims. Only the good monks of Saint Anthony would come to the aid of the afflicted, carrying them to their monastaries where they prayed and cared for them. Because these monks devoted their lives to aiding and caring for the victims of this cruel disease and prayed to their patron saint for help, this disease became known as Saint Anthony's Fire.

As the epidemic moved through the land, scarcely a home would escape. Men, women and children were stricken indiscriminately, some dying, while others recovered. Those that recovered would be crippled, having lost either some fingers or toes or even an arm or a leg. Some unfortunate victims of this vicious disease would lose all of their extremities and their maimed bodies would be left with only a head and a trunk.

An epidemic would last only for a year at a time. Then the next year when a new harvest of rye was available it would cease, unless that year, too, had been wet and foggy. The cause of Saint Anthony's Fire lay before everyone's eyes, the simple fact being that rye blighted with fungus from a wet season was poisonous. The disease was ergotism and was caused by a fungus which grew on the rye. This fungus produced a black purplish granule resembling a cock's spur and hence was called "ergot" from the old French word argot, meaning a cock's spur. Ergot is poisonous and taken in large enough quanties it constricts the blood vessels, especially in the extremities, so that little or no blood flows through them. This lack of blood causes tissue death with gangrene, followed by subsequent loss of the affected part.

All that men needed to know to prevent Saint Anthony's Fire was to follow the simple rule, "Do not eat blighted rye." Yet it was not until 1597 that men guessed at the cause and it was not until 1630 that Thullier correctly traced Saint Anthony's Fire or ergotism to the ingestion of grain smut. Thus while a great victory had been won for preventive medicine, it took almost two more centuries for this knowledge to be put fully into effect.

During the Middle Ages the terms Saint Anthony's Fire and Ignis Sacer were employed for a variety of diseases which were diagnostically undifferentiated. Confusion existed between ergotism, erysipelas and diabetic gangrene. Finally Thullier in the seventeenth century correctly traced ergotism to the ingestion of grain smut and in the eighteenth century Cullen, a Scotch physician, fully described and identified erysipelas.

Another malady which appeared in epidemic from during Medieval times was the mysterious "Sweating Sickness." Commonly called the English Sweat, the Sudor Anglicus, or the Sudor Britanica, this was an obscure, noneruptive, febrile disease, with an unusually high fatality rate. It derived its name from the fact that it first occurred in England and had as its chief characteristic symptom a "severe stinking sweat."

Attacking mostly strong and robust men in the prime of life, the disease struck with terrifying suddenness and was often fatal in twenty-four hours. It began with fever, nausea, and headache, followed by cramps in the extremities and pains in various parts of the body. Profound anxiety, difficult breathing, and irregularity of the pulse occurred. Severe cases had an extremely high fever accompanied by delirium, hallucinations and stupor. Cases generally came to a crisis in twenty-four hours and at the end of that time, either the patient or the disease came to an end. The crisis was accompanied by a profuse malodorous sweat which drenched the victims.

Apparently this was a new disease and was either unknown or unrecorded prior to the fifteenth century. Because many of the disease entities described in the early literature are difficult to identify records of this disease are scarce and confusing. Perhaps the first record of what may have been an outbreak of the Sweating Sickness is the account given of a peculiar epidemic that occurred in Touraine, France in 1482. Here large numbers of people were stricken with a high fever and a curious delirium which frequently ended in death or caused the victims to commit suicide.

The disease first appeared in England in 1485, and Grafton in his *Chronicles of England* gave the following account:

> A new kynde of sickness came sodainly through the whole region . . . which was so sore so paynefull and sharpe that the like was never hearde of, to any man's remembrance before that tyme. For sodainly a deadly and burning sweate invaded their bodies and vexed their blood, and with a most ardent heat infested the stomache and the head grieviously by the tormenting and vexacion of which sickness men were sore handled, and so painfully plagued that if they were laid in their bed being not able

to suffer the importunate heate they cast away the sheets and all the clothes lying on the bed.

History relates that early in August of 1485, the army of Henry Tudor, then the Earl of Richmond, landed from France at Milford Haven. Later that month he overthrew Richard III at Boseworth Field. Scarcely had the victor entered London to ascend the throne of England as Henry VII when the disease broke out among the soldiers of the victorious army; it decimated their ranks and spread rapidly to the surrounding civilian population. A pall of fear and terror fell upon the capitol as the epidemic mounted and it was necessary to postpone the king's coronation. The epidemic was so severe that thousands perished and it killed two successive Lord mayors and six aldermen in one week. From London the epidemic spread rapidly to other parts of England. However, strange as it may seem, it did not invade Scotland, Ireland or the Continent at this time.

When the force of the epidemic wave of 1485 was spent this mysterious disease vanished for some twenty years. It then reappeared in England for three successive years. However, these epidemics which occurred in 1506, 1507, and 1508 were relatively benign. Then once again the English Sweat vanished only to reoccur approximately ten years later in a short severe epidemic extending from July through December in 1517.

Continuing to follow this peculiar epidemiological pattern the Sweating Sickness disappeared for another ten-year period. Then in 1528 it erupted in its most severe and violent outbreak. This epidemic not only spread rapidly throughout England, but also invaded the continent. It ravaged Germany, Austria, the Low Countries, Denmark, Sweden, Poland, and Russia. There were hundreds of deaths in Strasbourg, and Hamburg reported over a thousand deaths in a few short terror stricken days.

Then after a quiescent period of twenty-three years, the last recorded epidemic of the English Sweat occurred in 1551. As swiftly and mysteriously as it had come and for reasons unknown, the Sweating Sickness then vanished completely and has never returned to plague the world again.

Strangely very little about this mysterious disease and the impact of its devastating epidemics is to be found in the contemporary English medical literature of the fifteenth and sixteenth centuries. This lack of reference to the disease can perhaps be explained by the fact that the English physicians could find no description of this disease in the revered works of Hippocrates and Galen. They therefore disbelieved their own observations and were generally too ignorant to give an original account of the disease. Hence, they simply ignored it and left it out of their medical writings.

There is, however, a classical contemporary account of this disease given by John Caius. A most remarkable physician, Caius also spelled his name Cayus, Kees, and Keese, but pronounced it Keyes. He studied medicine at Padua and was a fellow lodger with Vesalius, who was then writing his *De Corporis Humani Fabrica,* the publication of which revolutionized the study of anatomy.

Arriving back in England Caius practiced medicine in London. He was successful and became president of the College of Physicians and also served as physician to King Edward VI, Queen Mary, and Queen Elizabeth. He introduced the study of anatomy into England and carried out public dissections.

His book describing the English Sweat was published in 1552 and was entitled, "A boke or conseile against the disease commonly called the sweate or sweatying sickness made by Jhon Caius doctour in phisicke." Caius reviewed the various epidemics of this disease, beginning with the one in 1485. He speculated upon its previous existence, but apparently could find no other disease with which to compare it. He carefully described the symptoms and course of the disease and wondered about its possible cause.

His graphic description of the suddenness and severity of this disease reads as follows: "As it founde them so it took them, some in sleape some in wake, some in mirthe some in care, some fasting and some ful, some busy and some idle, and in one house sometyme three sometyme five, sometyme seven sometyme eight, sometyme more sometyme all, of the whyche, if the halfe in everye Towne escaped it was thoughte great favour."

Medical historians have not agreed as to whether the English Sweat was a new disease entity which first appeared in the fifteenth century and then vanished or changed its form or whether it was a variation of a previously known disease. It is thought by some to have been a severe form of influenza, while others have tried to identify it with military fever, or even encephalitis. Because none of these contentions can be proven, the appearance, occurrence and disappearance of the English Sweat remains an interesting medical mystery.

Chapter 11

THE RENAISSANCE AND THE REBIRTH
OF MEDICINE

The Renaissance is generally considered to be the "Bridge of Time" between the Middle Ages and Modern Times. It is a period of approximately three hundred years which historians have variously placed as beginning anytime from 1300 to 1500. It eventually merges into the "Modern Era" of history somewhere between 1600 and 1700. It is that period of time during which mankind slowly emerged from the darkness and disorder of the Middle Ages into a new era of social, economic, cultural and scientific advancement.

The terrific mortality of the plague and other medieval epidemics upset the entire socioeconomic system of the times. Labor became scarce, the feudal lords died, and land changed hands with bewildering rapidity. All of this broke down the feudal system, freeing men from the land and giving rise to the growth of cities. While these disastrous diseases also struck damaging blows to the urban way of life, they did not stop the steady advancement of civilization. The revival of trade in the fourteenth century increased the importance of the cities, while the power of the feudal manors and the monasteries declined. Cities continued to rise and grow and there was a steady expansion of commerce and industry which ultimately broke through all feudal restraints. Thus the plague paved the way for the Renaissance.

In plague-ravaged Italy the people recovered with remarkable resilience and experienced a revival of interest in the forgotten teachings of ancient Greece and Rome. Beginning in the fourteenth century this interest continued to grow, and it stimulated the people to search for beauty, truth and wisdom. This interest in the classic past and the avid search for the wisdom of the ancients received great stimulus and aid from an unexpected quarter.

When Constantinople fell before the Turks in 1453, the Greek scholars fled to Italy, bringing with them their knowledge and culture. Here they performed the valuable task of editing and translating their original Greek manuscripts. They thus supplied their new hosts with an accurate and readily available source of Grecian wisdom. This definitely launched the "Revival of Learning" and established Italy as the "Cradle of the Renaissance."

The revival of classical learning was an event of great importance. The intellectual life of the world which had run in one narrow channel for many centuries now found inspiration in the rediscovery of the classic past. This produced an awakening from the intellectual lethargy of the Middle Ages and people began to think for themselves. A spirit of doubt and inquiry arose and men were no longer content to accept the answers of tradition or the blind rulings of the Church.

Religious dogma was questioned and the medieval concept that man's earthly trials were only a preparation for heavenly redemption was challenged. Of vital importance was the acceptance of the idea of the "Dignity of Man" and the realization that man is a reasoning, willing, and knowing being. Thus a whole new concept of life was born and the stage was set for a great awakening.

Representing the dawn of a new era, the Renaissance has been called the "Age of discovery of the world and man." It was a period of transformation, change and human progress. Art, literature, philosophy and science burgeoned forth with tremendous vitality.

It was an age of daring exploration and great discovery. Columbus discovered America and the Old World made contact with the New. Vasco da Gama rounded the Cape of Good Hope and discovered the sea route to India. Thus vast new lands and colonies were brought under European domination. The half-forgotten trade routes to China and the East Indies were reopened and a great expansion of trade occurred between Europe and Asia.

As exploration and discovery continued at a rapid pace, new world markets were created. Commerce and industry grew and expanded to meet the demands of these new markets, radically changing the economic and social order of the times.

With the expansion of commerce and industry the population of

Europe continued its shift into the urban areas. As cities grew into large commercial and industrial centers, they became more powerful. Their increased economic activity and power produced an evolution in the national state with a resultant growth and consolidation of central government.

A new social class, known as the bourgeoisie or middle class, arose. Composed mainly of merchants and skilled craftsmen, it soon began to acquire wealth, political power and social standing. A new concept of wealth known as mercantile wealth was created. Wealth no longer consisted solely of land, but of money or commodities of trade that were measurable in money.

The practical needs of the times could not be ignored and there was a growing urgency to know more about science. This produced an intellectual climate favorable for scientific discovery and advancement. The development of mines, salt works, foundries, glass factories and other industrial enterprises called for a better understanding of chemistry and physics. Navigation required a more exact astronomy and a better understanding of the natural laws of the universe. In the sixteenth century the Polish astronomer Copernicus was the first to realize that the earth was not the center of the universe. In the seventeenth century the great Galileo invented the telescope.

In the fifteenth century the invention of printing emancipated knowledge from the inaccuracies of oral transmission and the limited use of laborious handwritten manuscripts. Printing gave wings to knowledge and sped the dissemination of learning, both old and new, to the thinking people of every land. It was now possible to enrich the minds of hundreds of thousands of people by the exchange of knowledge and new ideas, as speedily as books could be run off the press.

Although brilliant and colorful, the Renaissance was not entirely a period of historical glamour. Progress is never painless and the changing social and economic order created grave problems. Along with their rise and growth the cities produced both wealth and squalor.

The patricians and wealthy merchants ruled the cities. The skilled craftsmen freed from feudal taxes and churchly restraint advanced both socially and economically. They banded together in powerful guilds, each trade having its own guild. There was even a physician's guild, as well as a beggar's guild. The guilds played an important part in town life, supervising their own members and helping to administer the city government.

However, the abandoned serfs found a new and terrible kind of poverty and filth. Many of the older serfs continued to stay on the land in hopeless despair and lived in rural poverty. The younger serfs desperately seeking work or bread went to the cities. Here with no trade or craft and no fields to till they lived in abject poverty, frequently joining the ranks of beggary.

Confronted with congested living they camped in dark and airless rooms, tossing their slops and offal through the windows with little regard to passersby. Bringing their pigs and chickens with them, they let them roam at will, further adding to the all-prevading stench and filth. Because of the lack of washing facilities, personal cleanliness was almost nonexistent and they all became vermin infested.

The old Roman custom of having public baths which had been kept alive in some areas, was now revived. Cruder, smaller, and on a much less grand scale than the Roman baths, the public baths of the late Middle Ages and the Renaissance nevertheless flourished. Men and women flocked to them in order to scrub and scour the dirt and vermin off of their itching, filthy bodies. Modesty was no problem and mixed bathing between the sexes was readily accepted by a society where the custom was for whole families to sleep together in one bed without the benefit of night clothes.

Although built with the good intentions of fostering cleanliness and health, the public baths soon became centers for the spread of contagion. They were highly unsanitary, with many people bathing in the same tubs, hence diseases were readily disseminated. In addition the evils of drink, debauchery and prostitution flourished at the public baths. Finally at the end of the fifteenth century, when syphilis became a new public health problem, this type of communal bathing fell into great disrepute. The public bath house was then recognized as a focus of infection and it gradually vanished from the urban scene.

During the Renaissance few real advances were made toward improving and protecting the public health of the people. The patterns of public health protection which had been set during the Middle Ages as a result of the fear and terror of the plague were followed. Strict quarantine measures were invoked when epidemics occurred, and pest houses were used to forcibly isolate the sick.

City councils carried on the routine administration of a city and dealt with health and welfare problems. Most of them tried to secure an adequate clean water supply and to protect it from contamination. There was a slowly growing emphasis on community cleanliness and city councils began to enact and enforce sanitary rules and regulations. They undertook to empty and clean ponds, ditches and cesspools and to secure the proper collection and disposal of garbage, offal and rubbish. Communities became interested in food sanitation and began to require the supervision and inspection of food markets. In general public health administration was carried out by laymen and not by physicians.

Despite the great advancements of this age the physicians of the Renaissance barely held their own. While they acquired some dignity and self assurance, their practical medical knowledge showed little or no improvement. For diagnosis they still relied on the pulse and the urine flask. They continued to explain all diseases on the basis of the Four Humors, and blood letting, cupping and purging were the only treatments used by them.

However in addition to the nobility they now had a new class of patients to treat, composed of the wealthy merchants and the skilled craftsmen. The great mass of the poor as always, were left without adequate medical care. A few cities however provided and paid for municipal physicians who were charged with the care of the sick poor.

Preventive medicine and public health received little from the Renaissance. However, during this age bursting with art, commerce and scientific advancement, the basic knowledge was being acquired upon which the foundations of modern preventive medicine were eventually to be erected.

It was the artistic genius of the Renaissance that gave birth to modern anatomy. Once again, as in the classic past, artists took delight in the beauty of the human form. No longer content to imitate the hackneyed illustrations of medieval times they turned directly to nature for inspiration. In order to represent the human body more faithfully on canvas or in marble they found it necessary to have a greater understanding of its anatomical structures and functions. With a passion for observation and research they not only studied external anatomy, but also began to dissect the human body, so as to be able to study the deeper structures.

It was the versatile genius of Leonardo da Vinci (1451-1519) that spearheaded the correlation between art and anatomy. A great artist with decided medical leanings, he dissected over thirty bodies in the Santo Spirito mortuary in Rome. In secrecy and by candle light he produced a magnificent series of notes and drawings on the structure and function of the human body. He did not confine his attention to the more superficial structures and musculature, but also studied the heart, lungs, blood vessels, brain and uterus. By astutely using his powers of observation and with a corpse as his only text, Leonardo da Vinci found that many of the anatomical descriptions given by Galen were gravely in error.

Fear, superstition and the theologic concept of the sanctity and resurrection of the human body had hampered the study of anatomy, and perpetuated the errors of Galen. But now as artistic and scientific interest centered on man and his body, the prohibitions and fears of dissecting the human body were ignored.

About this time Andreas Vesalius (1514-1564) began his brilliant and phenomenal anatomical career. Born in Brussels, Vesalius studied medicine at Louvain and Paris. Disgusted with hearing his professors read long passages from Galen, he decided to go to Padua, the leading medical school of Europe. A certain amount of actual dissection of the human body was being performed there.

Vesalius proved to be such a brilliant student that he was elected professor of anatomy at the age of twenty-four. His lectures became so popular that students flocked to him from all over Europe. In 1543 at the age of twenty-nine he published the first complete text book on human anatomy, *De Humani Corporis Fabrica.* Using the human body as his text he made anatomy a living working science and corrected over two hundred of Galen's errors.

Abandoning his anatomical career because of jealousy and opposition, Vesalius left Padua to become court physician to Phillip II of

Spain. While there he supposedly conducted a postmortem examination upon a Spanish nobleman who was not quite dead. To atone for this error he went on a pilgrimage to the Holy Land. On the return journey he was shipwrecked on the Island of Zante, where he died of exposure and hunger at the age of fifty.

Remembered as the "father of modern anatomy," he was the most commanding figure in medicine after Galen and before Harvey. His magnificent work overthrew the Galenical tradition and blazed the way for the many skilled anatomists who were to follow.

Michael Servetus (1509-1553), a friend and fellow student of Vesalius, made the observation that the blood moved from the heart through the lungs. He stated that here it is "made red" and then after a long detour is returned to the left ventricle.

In 1553 he published the *Christianismi Restitutio,* a book in which he discussed the nature of the Holy Spirit as well as giving his account of pulmonary circulation. This book offended the religious authorities of the day and he was forced to flee from Catholic France. Fleeing to "reformed" Switzerland he was nevertheless delivered to the Inquisition by Calvin. Sentenced to death for "heresay" he was burned at the stake in Geneva, along with all traceable copies of his book. He thus became a martyr to medical progress.

Gabrielle Fallopius (1523-1563), a loyal pupil of Vesalius, carried on the work of his teacher. In 1551 he succeeded to the Chair of Anatomy at Padua. An accurate dissector, he is remembered for his precise descriptions of the ovaries, round ligaments and the oviducts. The latter are called the Fallopian tubes in his honor. His only book, *Observationes Anatomicae,* was published in 1561.

Another great figure of Renaissance anatomy was Bartolommeo Eustachius (1524-1574). He served as professor of anatomy at Rome and was a careful observer and investigator. He discovered the auditory or Eustachian tube, the thoracic duct, the abducens nerve, the cochlea, and the pulmonary veins, as well as numerous other anatomical structures.

The "Renaissance of Surgery" was brought about by Ambroise Paré, the greatest surgeon of the sixteenth century. Taking up the knife from where Guy de Chaulaic had dropped it some two hundred years before, he salvaged surgery from the quacks and the academicians. He was destined to have as great an influence on surgery as Vesalius had upon anatomy.

Born in 1510, Paré started his career as a humble apprentice to his brother Jean, who was a master barber-surgeon at Vitre. In 1532 or 1533 he became apprenticed to a barber-surgeon in Paris. After completing his apprenticeship he became *compagnon Chirugien* (similar to a resident surgeon) at the Hotel Dieu in Paris. Attempting to enter the University of Paris he was disqualified because he knew neither Latin or Greek. So instead of studying Latin he studied nature and learned surgery by use of the "eye and the hand."

Paré lived in troubled times and during the greater part of his lifetime France was at war against either Italy, Germany or England. Because these wars produced a great need for barber-surgeons to accompany the troops and care for the wounded, Paré soon joined their ranks. War has ever been a great teacher of surgery and thus Paré finally found his university on the battle fields of France. Spending thirty-odd years as a field surgeon he served four French kings and became the ablest surgeon of his age.

In 1536 while serving as surgeon to Mareschal de Montejan, colonel-general of the French infantry, Paré made his first great discovery. At that time the treatment of the wounded was crude and cruel. The belief existed that all gunshot wounds were "envenomed" and must be promptly cleansed by sousing them with boiling oil so as to counteract the poison. Paré wrote of this campaign and his observations, as follows:

> Now all the soldiers at the Chateau, seeing our men coming with a great fury . . . killed and wounded a great number of our soldiers with pikes, arquebuses, and stones . . . I wish to know first, how the other surgeons did for the first dressing, which was to apply the said oil (of elder, mixed with a little theriac) as hot as possible, into the wound . . . At last my oil lacked and I was constrained to apply in its place a digestive made of the yolks of eggs, oil of roses, and turpentine. That night I could not sleep . . . beyond my hope, I found those upon whom I had put the digestive medicament feeling little pain, and their wounds without inflammation or swelling, having rested fairly well throughout the night; the others to whom I had applied the said boiling oil, I found feverish, with great pain and swelling about their wounds. Then I resolved with myself never more to burn thus cruelly poor men wounded with gunshot.

Paré was admitted to the Community of Barber-Surgeons in 1541 and wrote a volume on the treatment of wounds made by arquebus fire in 1545. In 1549 between wars, he wrote a handbook of anatomy in simple French for surgeons who were ignorant of Latin and Greek.

The Arabian surgeons had taught the Western World that hemorrhage could only be arrested by cauterization. It therefore was the custom to treat amputations and bleeding wounds by the brutal use of a red hot cautery iron. Paré made his most important contribution to surgery in 1552. During the seige of Danvilliers he amputated an officer's leg and used a "new method" to control hemorrhage. Having learned to tie off arteries at the points where they were torn or cut, he had rediscovered the ligature. Although known to Hippocrates, the ligature had been long forgotten and abandoned.

Paré also fought against the practices of dressing wounds with unpleasant plasters composed of vile ingredients such as ground-up frogs, vipers and dung. Instead he advocated clean dressings, hot fomentations and the free incision of wounds to drain infection. Like Hippocrates he continuously protested the use of harmful remedies that interfered with nature's healing process.

Once a severely wounded soldier, foredoomed to die by his companions, was treated out of pity, by Paré. Under his competent and kindly care, the soldier made a miraculous recovery. His grateful comrades were so impressed, that they collected and publicly presented Paré with a purse. Paré humbly responded to this presentation with his immortal reply, "I dressed him and God healed him."

Paré not only reformed the treatment of gunshot wounds and introduced the ligature as a substitute for cauterization, but also invented a number of new surgical instruments, including the artery forceps. He was interested in rehabilitation and designed ingenius artificial limbs and used trusses to treat hernias. His interest in medicine extended beyond the army and he perfected a method of version of the child in utero and also correctly observed that syphilis was a cause of aneurism.

Remembered as the "father of modern surgery," Paré revitalized this art by linking the new anatomical teachings of Vesalius to the mainstream of practical surgery.

The critical, rebellious spirit of the Renaissance found expression medically in the person of Phillipus Aureolus Theophrastus Bombastus von Hohenheim. A small slight man with unruly hair framing a large bald skull set with blazing eyes, he fiercely attacked the errors and follies of medieval medicine. Boastfully calling himself Paracelsus, a name meaning greater or better than Celsus, he tried to reform medicine by exposing the errors of Galen and Avicenna.

Born in Einsiedeln, Switzerland in 1493, Paracelsus was the only child of a physician and was distantly related to the nobel "House of the Bombasts." He attended medical school at Vienna but soon became a traveling scholar. As a student or teacher he visited all of the more important centers of learning in Europe. Disappointed with the ancient bookish teachings of Galen and Avicenna offered by the universities, Paracelsus clashed with the authorities wherever he went. He refused to blindly follow the teachings of traditional medicine but followed Hippocrates in the belief, that "experience is the best teacher," and thus acquired his medical knowledge at the bedside.

Becoming a traveling doctor, Paracelsus practiced medicine throughout southern Europe. Introducing and using metals, metallic salts and mineral compounds as drugs, he founded iatrochemistry and thus dimly foreshadowed modern chemotherapy. A tremendous showman and part quack, Paracelsus mixed his new medical knowledge with alchemy and magic. He claimed to have distilled a quintessence of metals that possessed universal health giving properties. He fostered the belief that this "universal arcanum," which was capable of curing all diseases, was hidden in the handle of a large sword that he always carried with him.

As he traveled about practicing his art, he won fame and acclaim everywhere—in humble homes, wayside hostels, and palatial palaces. His cures were called miraculous by his patients, but he always clashed with his medical colleagues, publicly calling all who differed with him imbeciles and idiots. Thus while he won ardent friends, he also made bitter enemies. His tremendous ego, irritable temper and quarrelsome nature led him to use his tongue and pen to violently attack the established authorities. As a result he always succeeded in antagonizing so many influential people that he was forced to move on, again and again. As Paracelsus himself said "I pleased no one, except the sick, whom I healed."

After ten years of ceaseless wandering Paracelsus settled down to practice in Salzburg. However, he become involved in the intrigue of the "Peasants War" and had to flee the city. He then went to Basle, Switzerland, where fortune smiled upon him.

Johann Froben or Frobenius, the famed Renaissance humanist, printer and publisher, was ill with a persistent leg infection and the leading surgeons of Basle advocated amputation. Froben sent for Paracelsus who cured him of the infection and saved his leg. In gratitude Froben influenced the city council to appoint Paracelsus to the office of municipal physician and professor at the University of Basle.

The outraged faculty of the university was in no mood to accept this rebellious semi-quack and Paracelsus promptly antagonized them further. He insisted on lecturing in the Swiss vernacular instead of the traditional Latin, and stated that he left Latin to the old grey-beards, who clothed their ancient thoughts in an ancient tongue. He also publicly burned copies of Avicenna's *Canon* and Galen's texts in a student's St. John's Day holiday bonfire. He vehemently attacked the old theoreticians whose views were gradually being discredited by the rational investigations of the Renaissance.

By act after act and pamphlet after pamphlet Paracelsus continued to attack everyone. He finally created such furor and animosity that he had to flee in the night in order to save his life. In 1540 the Prince Bishop of Salzburg offered asylum to Paracelsus and here he spent his remaining days in relative quiet, dying September 24, 1541 at the age of forty-eight.

A controversial figure in medical history, Paracelsus has been revered and vilified, alternately praised as the leader of the medical reforms of the Renaissance, or damned as one of its greatest quacks. However, the facts remain that he was the first to abandon Latin and to lecture on medicine in a modern language. He attacked witchcraft and superstition, broke with the traditions of Galen and Avicenna, and attempted to return medicine to nature and the bedside.

The advocacy of the use of chemical agents for the treatment of specific diseases was one of Paracelsus' greatest contributions. He recommended mercury for the treatment of syphilis; introduced powdered tin as an anthelmintic; brought antimony into vogue; and employed zinc, lead, arsenic, copper, and iron compounds. Wherever he went, Paracelsus left "chemical kitchens" behind him and thus inaugurated an era of iatrochemistry that served as a forerunner of modern chemotherapy.

Clinically he suggested the hereditary transmission of syphilis, observed the close relationship between endemic goiter and cretinism, and recognized mental illness as a disease.

In 1524 he wrote one of the first works on occupational medicine describing the pulmonary and other diseases of miners, smelter workers, and metalurgists. He also recognized and described the toxic effects of mercury and its compounds. He not only discussed the etiology, pathogenisis, diagnosis and therapy of these diseases, but also discussed their prevention. These books had a definite influence on the development of occupational and preventive medicine.

In England, Renaissance medicine moved forward under the influence of Thomas Linacre (1460-1524). Known as the "restorer of learning," Linacre was a humanist-doctor who gained fame through his flawless translations of Hippocrates and Galen. He thus gave English medicine its first accurate body of ancient medical knowledge, thereby correcting the errors of previously garbled versions.

Serving as physician to Henry VII and Henry VIII, he used his influence at court to fight mountebanks and quackery. In 1518 he obtained a patent from Henry VIII to form a body of physicians to supervise the practice of medicine in London. From this supervising group the Royal College of Physicians was born, bringing with it medical advancement and greater professional competence.

John Caius (1510-1573), who is remembered for his classic account of the English Sweat, succeeded Linacre as president of the Royal College of Physicians. While a student at Padua, Caius had roomed with Vesalius while he was writing his great *Fabrica*. Upon his return to England, Caius was appointed reader of anatomy at the Barber-Surgeons Hall, where he initiated the Renaissance of English Anatomy.

Chapter 12

SYPHILIS–SCOURGE OF THE RENAISSANCE AND A NEW CONCEPT OF CONTAGION

THE GREAT SCOURGE of the Renaissance was syphilis which exploded in epidemic form at the end of the fifteenth century. Carried by the invading armies of various nations, it swept rapidly throughout Europe. The great voyagers, explorers and traders soon took it with them to every corner of the world. Thus syphilis became the "calling card of civilized man" and he left it everywhere he went.

Despite centuries of patient research the mysterious origin of this dread disease is still in dispute. The question remains unanswered, as to whether syphilis existed in Europe prior to Columbus' discovery of America, or whether it was an unwelcome gift from the New World to the Old.

Most medical historians accept the so-called Columbian theory which believes that syphilis was brought to Europe in 1493 from the Island of Haiti by Columbus and his crew. The story is that in the course of rejoicing over their homecoming, during their feasting and carousing, Columbus' sailors sowed the seeds of an epidemic. Starting in Spain in 1493, syphilis was carried to Italy by the troops of Gonzalo de Cordoba, who had been sent to defend Naples. Cordoba's troops, some of whom had sailed with Columbus, promptly passed their disease on to the obliging ladies of Naples.

In 1494 Charles VIII of France set out to conquer Northern Italy with an army of 30,000 which was accompanied by 900 camp followers, a large percentage of whom were low class prostitutes. When the French troops conquered Naples, they conquered the Neopolitan women along with the city. These agreeable ladies promptly proceeded to present the victorious French troops with syphilis. Erupting explosively, syphilis soon spread like wildfire throughout Naples, the French calling it the "Italian Disease and the Italians calling it the French Disease."

One year later, as the French soldiers were driven off, they returned home, carrying syphilis along with them. In less than three years, epidemics of syphilis had broken out in France, Germany, Switzerland, Holland and all the rest of Europe. Exploration, war and trade soon completed the worldwide dissemination of this disease and thus made syphilis the scourge of the civilized world, which it has remained ever since.

According to another school of thought, syphilis is considered to be of great antiquity and was known to the ancients. They refer to the Columbian theory as the "Haitian Myth" and state that the disease is as old as mankind. Unfortunately documentary evidence for this view-point is not too clear-cut. However, its exponents state that syphilis was formerly confused with leprosy, skin cancer, scabies, gonorrhea and other skin and venereal diseases. They believe that some of the lepers mentioned in the Bible were actually syphilitics.

Because syphilis leaves evidence of its disease process in the bones, experts have checked leper cemeteries for its evidence. They contend that they have found bones showing signs of syphilitic infiltration. However, no one has been able to set a date on these and prove conclusively that they predated Columbus.

The exponents of the pre-Columbian theory cite a Latin translation of Avicenna which describes dysuria and a penile sore as a sign of a form of "lepra" which was contracted during intercourse. They also point out that Roger of Salerno in 1170 reported that lepra may be contracted during sexual intercourse.

Nicolo Leoniceno, professor at Ferrara and one of the most eminent physicians of his age, wrote a classic account of the "French Disease" in 1497. He was at the height of his reputation when the outbreak of syphilis occurred in Italy and he insisted that the disease was of great antiquity and was known to Hippocrates.

In 1863 a Captain Darby wrote a history of medicine in China and gave a startling account of syphilis which presumably was taken from the writings of Huang Ti in 2637 B.C. However Okamura later studied these ancient records and flatly stated that syphilis did not appear in China until after its introduction from Europe in the sixteenth century.

The proponents of the pre-Columbian theory further argue that the outbreak of syphilis in Naples, attributed to the troops of Gonzalo de Cordoba, actually began before Columbus returned from America. They further state that this outbreak occurred two years prior to the arrival of Charles VIII in Italy.

Regardless of whether syphilis had existed previously in Europe or had been newly introduced from America, the fact remains, that it had attracted no general attention until the end of the fifteenth century. There is also no question about the fact that the Spanish sailors as well as the sea-faring men and soldiers of many countries were instrumental in causing syphilis to break out into a great conflagration during the late fifteenth and early sixteenth centuries.

The facts of history seem ready-made to explain how Columbus and his sailors imported this disease from the New World and were so effective in sowing the seeds of syphilis that within a few years Europe reaped a whirlwind of disease.

Direct historical evidence favoring the Columbian theory is found in the writings of Gonzalo Fernandez de Oviedo y Valdes, (1478-1557) who was in Spain when Columbus returned and who later made several trips to the West Indies himself. In his two books on history, published in 1525 and 1535, he specifically stated that syphilis was brought to Spain by the ships of Columbus. He further stated that it was spread from Spain to Italy by the troops of Gonzalo de Cordoba.

The most direct early support is found in the writings of Rodrigo Ruiz Diaz de Isla (1462-1542). Reputed to have been the first to describe syphilis, which he observed among the returning sailors of Columbus' squadron, this Spanish surgeon reported that he had treated several of the diseased sailors himself.

If syphilis had existed prior to Columbus' voyage it must have lacked the great virulence that characterized its behavior in the decades following Columbus' return. In all probability, because the disease had been previously unknown to the populations of Europe, it struck with great severity. The victims ran high fevers and experienced intense headaches, bone and joint pains, severe skin symptoms, prostration and frequently early death.

Many of the physicians of the times at first tried to ignore syphilis and refused to examine and treat "a disease that began in the most degraded and ignoble place of the body." However the widespread extent and severity of the outbreak soon forced them to study, diagnose and treat the disease.

Since mercury ointment had been used by the Arabians for many centuries to treat any and every kind of skin disease, it was soon seized upon to treat syphilis. Proving efficacious, it came into widespread use and was highly praised by Paracelsus as the best of antisyphilitic drugs. Unfortunately physicians used it in such heroic doses that many of their patients came down with mercury poisoning. Francois Rabelais, the famous satirist, poet, and physician described these poor people, who had the mucous membranes of their mouths eaten away by mercurial stomatitis as follows: "their face sharp as a butcher knife, their teeth rattling like a keyboard of a broken down spinet."

The sexual transmission of syphilis was noted from the beginning, but because tolerance in sex matters was characteristic of the Renaissance, no stigma was attached to the disease. No one thought of concealing a syphilitic infection. In fact, it was considered a "gentlemen's disease," and became a popular topic for discussions and articles. As a result innumerable articles on syphilis were written in the late fifteenth and early sixteenth centuries.

In 1496, Theodore Ulsenius, the city physician of Nuremberg, wrote a treatise in Latin about the venereal plague which was then raging. He ascribed it to an astrological forecast of 1484 which predicted the conjunction of Jupiter and Saturn. The famous Renaissance artist Albrecht Dürer illustrated the pamphlet with what was undoubtedly the first illustration of syphilis. Appropriately enough this depicted the figure of a soldier showing the skin manifestations of secondary syphilis.

A Spanish physician, Juan Almenar, also was one of the first to write on syphilis. His treatise, *De Morbo Gallico,* which was published in 1502, advocated mercury for treatment and recognized the sexual transmission of the disease. However as a loyal son of the church, he felt that the clergy did not get it sexually, but contracted syphilis from the corruption of the air.

Perhaps the most remarkable book ever to be written on syphilis was Ulrich von Hutten's, *De Morbo Gallico,* which was published in 1519. One of the most picturesque and pathetic figures ever to make a contribution to medical literature, von Hutten was an impoverished poet, humanist and reformer.

Coming from a poor but knightly family and being of a slight and sickly physique, his father sent him to a Benedictine cloister near Fulda. He apparently had scholastic aptitude and literary ability, but finding the restrictions and dullness of monastic life unbearable he soon fled the confines of the cloister.

Wandering through Germany and Italy for approximately nine years, he served for a time as a soldier in the army of the Emperor Maximilian. During his adventuresome wanderings he acquired syphilis while still in his early twenties. In the years that followed he kept a diary of his disease, carefully recording his case history.

He eventually found a patron for his literary ambitions and poetic gifts in the person of Albert, the Archbishop of Brandenburg and Elector of Mayence. However this pleasant mode of life came to an end when von Hutten espoused the Lutheran Reformation and unwisely used his pen to attack the Papal cause in Germany. This caused the Archbishop Albert to dismiss him, while Pope Leo X issued orders for his arrest.

Von Hutten fled to Basle, Switzerland and sought aid and refuge from Erasmus. However this famous scholar feared von Hutten's loathsome disease and denied him aid. Going on to Zurich, von Hutten received aid from the reformer Zwingli and together they found refuge on the Island of Ufnau in Lake Zurich. Here in 1523, Ulrich von Hutten died at the age of thirty-five. Poor and penniless, he left nothing behind him except the remarkable account of his disease.

Because syphilis was considered a "gentlemen's disease" and no stigma was attached to it, von Hutten dedicated his book to his patron, the Archibishop Albert. In his book, *De Morbo Gallico,* von Hutten completely and painstakenly described syphilis, not only as he knew of it himself as a victim and sufferer, but also as he observed it in others.

He commented on the origin of the outbreak as follows:

> It hath pleased God, that in our time sickness should arise, unknown to our Forefathers, as we have come to surmise.
>
> In the year of Christ 1493, or thereabout this Evil began amongst the People, not only of France, but originally at Naples in the French

Camp . . . the French disdaining that it should be called of their country (the French Pox), gave it the name of Neapolitane or the Evil of Naples . . . the Divines imputed this disease to the Wrath of God, sent from Heaven as a scourge for our Wickedness.

On its mode of transmission he wrote:

This disease in our Days ariseth not, unless by infection from carnal contact, as in copulating with a diseased Person, since it appears now that young children, old men and others not given to Fornication or bodily lust, are very rarely diseased. Also the more a Man is addicted to these pleasures, the sooner he catcheth it, and as they manage themselves after, either temperately or otherwise, so it the sooner leaves them, holds them a long time, or uterly consumes them.

Von Hutten described the lesions and symptoms as follows: "They had Boils that stood out like Acorns, from whence issued such filthy stinking Matter, that whosoever came within the Scent believed himself infected." He further stated: "In Women the Disease resteth in their secret Places, wherein as little pretty Sores, full of venomous Poison, being very dangerous for such as unknowingly meddle with them." He further described the progression of the disease as follows:

Sometimes the Disease transforms itself into the Gout, at others, into a Palsy and Apoplexy, and infected many also with a Leprosy . . . After this there will appear small Holes and Sores, turning cankerous and fistulous which the more putrid they grow, the more they will eat into the Bones, and when they have been long corrupted the Sick grows lean, his flesh wasting away, so that there remaineth only the Skin as a cover for them: and by this many fall into Consumption, having their inward Parts Corrupted.

From some of his writings it is known that von Hutten had suffered from syphilis for about ten years before his book appeared. He graphically described the mercurial ointment therapy that was used: "They anointed the joints of the arms and legs, some also the spine and neck, some even the temples, likewise also the navel and others again the whole body, some once a day, some twice, some again three or four times. The patient was shut up in a hot room which was steadily and most vigorously heated, some keeping him there for twenty days, some for thirty."

He cried out against this type of treatment by saying: "Cure was indeed so terrible, that many chose rather to die than to be eased thus of their sickness." He told how he had struggled with his disease for nine years and had undergone this vigorous treatment, "eleven times, with great Peril and Jeopardy of Life." In the autumn of 1518 he took the guaiac treatment at Augsburg. After forty days of treatment on guaiac juice he falsely, but confidently considered himself cured. Loudly singing the praises of guaiac, he helped glorify it as the medical triumph of the age.

Guaiacum, the "holy wood" was the miracle drug of the Renaissance and soon came to be considered a "sure cure for syphilis." Because guaiac wood came from America, as did syphilis, people readily accepted the old belief that, "the Almighty always provides a cure for an ailment in the place where it originated." Unfortunately guaiacum, the "holy wood," contained few if any curative properties.

Ulrich von Hutten's *De Morbo Gallico* became extremely popular and was widely read. Soon after its appearance it was translated into German, English and French. It was copied from by many physicians of the times who wrote on syphilis. The book definitely influenced the therapy of syphilis by promoting the use of guaiacum and pointing out the abuses of overtreatment with mercurial ointments.

The variety of names which the sixteenth century writers applied to this venereal outbreak offers the advocates of the Columbian theory another argument in favor of their theories. They claim that syphilis must have been a new disease because no specific name for it existed prior to Columbus' time. Each of the nations of Europe tried to pin the blame for syphilis on the other. It was variously called the French Disease, the Italian Disease, the Neopolitan Evil, or the Spanish Complaint. They also pointed out that the disease we now call smallpox was simply called the pox. When this new venereal disease appeared with its larger sores or "pocks," it was called the Great Pox and the other disease was renamed the smallpox.

Jacques de Béthencourt, a physician of Rouen, being a loyal Frenchman resented the name of the "French Disease." Therefore in his book a *New Litany of Penitence* published in 1527, he suggested that since the disease arises from illicit love, it should be called "the Malady of Venus" or venereal disease. He observed that the disease can be transmitted to the offspring, but fell into the serious error of confusing syphilis with gonorrhea.

The disease did not receive the name of syphilis until about 1530, when Girolamo Fracastoro composed the most famous medical poem of all times and gave the disease its present name. This poem was entitled "Syphilis Sive Morbus Gallicus," and presented the origin, symptoms, course and treatment of the disease in polished Latin Verse. The poem became so famous that the word "syphilis" gradually became the universal term for the disease and displaced all other designations.

The hero of Fracastorius' famous poem was a mythical shepherd boy named Syphilis. According to legend he was the first to suffer from this disease. However, he did not contract it in the orthodox manner, but was plagued with the disease by the god Apollo as a punishment for having blasphemed against the Sun.

The word "syphilis" is of curious origin and comes from the Greek words, "suis or sys" meaning swine, and "philos" or loving. Therefore some historians feel that perhaps Syphilis, the hero of the poem, was actually a swine-herder rather than a shepherd. However, others believe that the name stems from the theory that the disease was brought to Italy by the Spanish Moors and Jews who were expelled from Spain for refusing to adopt Christianity. These unfortunate refugees were inelegantly called "Marrenes" or hogs. Fracastorius may have chosen the name Syphilis or swine-lover for his shepherd hero in support of this theory.

Born in Verona in 1483 of a noble family, Girolamo Fracastoro supposedly had such a small mouth at birth that it was necessary to enlarge it surgically so that he could nurse. One day while his mother carried him in her arms, she was struck by a thunderbolt and killed. Surviving these misfortunes of infancy, Fracastoro grew up to attend the renowned University of Padua. Here he studied philosophy, mathematics, belles lettres and medicine.

After his graduation he practiced medicine at Verona and although medicine was his chief interest he found time to engage in many other activities. Extremely versatile and talented, he was not only a physician but a mathematician, astronomer, physicist, geologist and a gifted poet. His famous poem, while probably written in his lighter moments, summarized all of the then known knowledge of syphilis.

It set forth its history, fact or fable, its symptoms and diagnosis. In regards to treatment he touched upon both the mercury and guaiac cures. First published in 1530, Fracastoro dedicated his poem to his old friend and former classmate, the illustrious Cardinal Bembo.

Fracastorius' poem was undoubtedly the most famous publication to come out of the welter of the "syphilis" literature that appeared in the early sixteenth century. It must be remembered that most of this literature was written before a precise delineation of the characteristics of syphilis had been attained. Undoubtedly many of these writer-physicians were overwhelmed by the venereal epidemic of their times. With their limited knowledge they probably failed to differentiate mixed venereal infections and also frequently confused leprosy, skin cancer and even smallpox with syphilis.

There can be no doubt about the fact that Columbus' sailors brought back a venereal infection from the West Indies. However this could have been lympho-granuloma inguinale, chancroid or yaws, as well as syphilis. It is even quite possible that they had acquired some mixed venereal infections.

Another interesting possibility as to the origin of this disease exists in the fact that it is now known that the spirochete of syphilis is practically indistinguishable from that of the related disease, yaws. The West Indies have probably always had yaws and even now in some of these islands 70 percent to 90 percent of the population is infected. Although yaws is generally considered to be a non-venereal disease, a number of physicians believe that yaws is merely an uncivilized form of syphilis.

Despite all this confusion syphilis emerged as a separate disease entity in the sixteenth century. It was also recognized to be a different venereal disease from the previously well known and ancient disease of gonorrhea. However this distinction was soon lost and even the astute Paracelsus confused the two diseases and called syphilis the "French Gonorrhea." Many other physicians of the sixteenth century also fell into this error and believed that gonorrhea was only the initial stage of syphilis.

From the time that syphilis first appeared great efforts were made to combat and control it. These efforts followed the traditional patterns of protection that had been laid down to combat leprosy and plague. In 1496 the barbers of Rome were forbidden to serve syphilitics. In many cities and towns the victims of syphilis were forcibly expelled and banished. In others they were isolated in the old pest houses that formerly had been used for lepers. In Germany and Italy special hospitals were established for syphilitics.

Due to the loose and tolerant sexual standards of the Renaissance, brothels were an accepted institution and prostitution was widely practiced. Because the sexual transmission of syphilis was recognized early, prompt but harsh and cruel actions were taken against infected prostitutes. Prostitutes who were unfortunate enough to become infected were banished, whipped and even branded. In 1507 a statute of Faenza ordered that all women wishing to serve as prostitutes had to be examined first and those with the French disease could not serve. Similar regulations were passed in numerous other communities of Europe. However, it was to remain for later periods of history to bring forth humane, rational and effective measures for the control of syphilis.

Girolamo Fracastoro's studies on syphilis led to more than the writing of his famous poem. His interest in this disease stimulated him to make a thorough, brilliant and practical study of all contagious and infectious diseases. These studies culminated in 1546 with the publication of his classic work, *De Contagione*.

This book came very close to expressing the modern conception of infection and offered some amazing inklings of bacteriology, long before the discovery of bacteria. He grasped the fact that infection was a cause and epidemic a consequence. He advanced the idea that contagion was caused by infective seeds or "seminaria" which were so minute that they were not perceived by the senses (*insensibilibus particalis*). He further stated that these seeds are specific for individual diseases and that like seeds produced like diseases. He believed that these seeds were transmissable and self propagating and that disease occurred when they acted upon the humors and vital spirits of the body.

Fracastoro recognized three modes of contagion: (1) by direct contact, person to person; (2) by intermediate agents such as fomites, a word he used for the first time; and (3) by infection at a distance, for example through the air.

Through careful observation, Fracastoro recognized the contagiousness of smallpox, measles, tuberculosis, rabies, and syphilis. He was one of the first to recognize typhus and gave accurate descriptions of the great Italian epidemics of this disease that occurred in 1505 and 1528. He also noted the immunity which ensues after attacks of measles and smallpox.

Fracastoro's great work on contagion consisted of three books; the first presented his theory of contagion, the second discussed various contagious diseases, and the third dealt with their treatment. This book is one of the great landmarks leading to the development of a scientific concept on contagion.

Girolamo Fracastoro died in 1553 of apoplexy. He was of such great repute and was held in such esteem that in 1559 a statue was erected to his memory at Verona. The inscription on this statue eulogizes him as the author of "that divine Poem Syphilis." However his greatest claim to fame probably rests upon the fact that he was the "world's first epidemiologist."

The doctrine of animate contagion was not exactly new, and had been advanced by others, notably, Varro, Columella and Paracelsus. Fracastoro, however, presented the first consistent theory of contagion, and while he did not discover bacteria nor predict their existence, he did logically observe the facts surrounding the transmission of infectious and contagious diseases. Unfortunately his keen insight did not keep him from believing in astrology. Thus the influence of the stars as a cause of epidemics was as real to him as bacteria are to a modern scientist.

During his lifetime, and for many years after, his concepts on contagion were widely accepted. Unfortunately as time went on all that he had achieved was gradually lost. His concept of contagion was supplanted by the erroneous "miasmatic" theory of disease spread, and it was not until the nineteenth century that his observations and concepts were rediscovered.

On the whole, the cultural and scientific advances of the Renaissance had cut only a narrow path through a worldwide wilderness of ignorance and superstition. At the end of the sixteenth century alchemy, astrology, witchcraft and sorcery were still universally believed in. Philosophers and sages continued to wander down the roads of fantasy leading nowhere. Alchemists still sought the secret formula which they firmly believed would change baser metals into precious gold; while explorers financed by aging men of wealth seriously searched the world for the "Fountain of Eternal Youth."

The sixteenth century had witnessed a great religious revolt and upheaval. Martin Luther had ushered in the Reformation and Protestantism had advanced across Europe breaking the universality of Papal power. Although the Catholic Counter-Reformation and the rise of Jesuit power later checked the advance of Protestantism, the religious universalism of the middle ages was replaced by the religious diversity of modern times. However most people still believed that the devil had a personal existence and led a very active life under many different forms. Torture continued to be the universal technique for eliciting information. Free thought was heresy to the theologians and the Inquisition continued to imprison and mutilate disbelievers, while supposedly heretical books were banned or burned.

Politically the universal power of the medieval empire had given way to a differentiation into Nation-States. The City-States which emerged and grew wealthy and populous, found their sphere of action too small and failed to perpetuate themselves. Hence, the Nation-States continued to grow in power, strengthened by their geographical environment and a common language. National integration was further strengthened, as the nobility and the clergy, the traditional medieval rivals of royal authority, had their power curtailed and were brought under more complete control of the monarchy. Progress had been made in the establishment of national armies and navies, systems of central taxation and courts of law.

Economic life had undergone rapid expansion and development along with the increase in travel and trade. City dwellers discovered the power of capital in their affairs and used it. Merchants and bankers lent their powerful support to help the monarchies in their plans for centralization of power. The rural masses were raising themselves from serfdom to freedom and European society had largely escaped the confines of medieval times.

The Renaissance had ushered in an intellectual revolution and there had been a tremendous awakening in learning, art and science. The knowledge of the ancients had been rediscovered and scholars had taken a fresh outlook at men and nature. The great authorities of the middle ages had been questioned, and their faulty reasoning and numerous errors exposed. The printing press continued to disseminate knowledge ever more quickly and widely, while improved transportation facilitated the movement of scholars from country to country. However even at the end of the sixteenth century the medieval mentality still prevailed and scholars continued to have too much respect for the Ancient Greeks. They had not yet discovered that Aristotle and the other ancients were sometimes ignorant and in error.

During the sixteenth century medicine had made great gains when the anatomists led by Vesalius shook off the authority of Galen. The medical students of Europe at last were ready to recognize the facts of nature and to rely for their knowledge on what their own eyes could see. Yet progress was slow, because the authorities still frowned upon and frequently forbade dissection of the human body.

The extensive travel and exploration which had characterized the Renaissance resulted in the introduction of a profusion of new herbs and plants from all parts of the world. Botanical gardens were established and these new medicinals brought about the use of a wider range of effective drugs. However the old humoral theory of disease continued to be blindly accepted and treatment consisted of purging, blood-letting and cunning psychology. Anyone could become a doc- if he knew the "Four Aphorisms of Hippocrates" and a dozen passages from Galen along with the names of various diseases. There was not yet a valid basis for science and medicine existed in a dim half-world of magic and superstition.

The disease pattern of the Western World had changed significantly and hitherto prevalent diseases such as leprosy had declined and diminished. This along with increased clinical observation had made way for the recognition of new and previously unrecognized diseases such as syphilis and typhus. The newer concepts of contagion developed by Fracastoro during the sixteenth century had brought about a better understanding of epidemiology. However it was still believed that the stars controlled the destinies of men and that unfavorable astrologic conditions caused the devastating and deadly epidemics that still swept the world.

Thus while a dark mantle of ignorance still hovered over the world at the end of the sixteenth century, the cultural, socioeconomic and scientific advances of the Renaissance had been great enough to set the stage for the rise of modern civilization.

Chapter 13

THE SCIENTIFIC AND MEDICAL ADVANCES
OF THE SEVENTEENTH CENTURY

THE SEVENTEENTH CENTURY heralded the emergence of Modern Europe and the rise of Western Civilization. Although it was a period of unprecedented progress, it was also a century of conflict. It was a world of political and religious turmoil, marked by civil, international and religious wars.

In England these were the years of the fall of the monarchy and the rise of the Commonwealth under Oliver Cromwell, followed by the Restoration.

For France the seventeenth century fell almost entirely within the reigns of Louis XIII and XIV. France was ruled for seventy-two years by Louis "The Grand" from the most splendid court the world had ever seen, and war, art, literature and science flourished.

Spain's decline of power which had started with the defeat of the Spanish Armada in 1588 continued during the seventeenth century.

During the Thirty-Years' War, Germany became the battleground of the nations. Beginning in 1618 as a Civil War between the Protestants and Roman Catholics this series of wars eventually became a general struggle for territory and power. Most of the nations of Europe were involved before this war ended in 1648. It left Germany exhausted and virtually destroyed.

During the seventeenth century Holland became a great sea power and the Dutch merchants became the wealthiest in the world. A policy of toleration made their land an asylum for English Catholics, Puritans, Spanish Jews and French Huguenots. Many of these people were skilled artisans and thus Holland became the center for many highly skilled crafts such as lens-grinding and clock and instrument making. Refugee scholars helped make the University of Leyden the foremost institution of learning in Europe. In the fine arts this was the age of Rubens and Van Dyke, followed by Rembrandt, Van Ruisdael and Van Steen.

The economic pressures and religious persecutions of the seventeenth century started the great migration to the New World. The building of overseas empires and the colonization of America became important factors in European politics and economics. Trade with the New World, population growth, increased travel and the need of materials for exploration and war all produced an expanding commerce. This increased need for goods brought about the first stage of the industrial system.

The population of seventeenth century Europe was still relatively small. Russia, which had not yet emerged as a European state, had approximately 13 million people as did Germany. France had approximately 18 million and the Italian Peninsula about 13 million. Spain was estimated to have 8 million people while England had about 4½ million and Holland approximately 3 million.

Even though cities had grown constantly in number and size, seventeenth century Europe had fewer than one hundred cities of 10,000 or over. Paris was the largest with a population of about one-half million, while London was a close second. City dwellers lived in small rickety wooden houses, built along narrow winding streets or dark alleys. The houses were vermin infested and rat ridden while the streets were muddy and refuse strewn. Basements and cellars were used as stores, food shops, and work places. Sanitary arrangements were lacking or primitive and people lived in an accumulation of filth. The cities of the seventeenth century had all of the horrors of civilization and none of its niceties.

European society still had its traditional three-fold division into clergy, nobility and commerce. One of the most important developments of the century was the growth of the middle class, which was composed of merchants and skilled craftsmen. This increase was greatest in Holland and England. However, in all of Europe the middle class was not much larger than the combined clergy and nobility. The vast majority of the seventeenth century population was still composed of the peasants who lived on the land. While serfdom had vanished, the large landowners with their harsh policies of sharecropping kept the peasants' lot a hard one. Agricultural tools and methods had not yet advanced and the peasants had to labor from dawn to dusk. Living in poorly built one-room cottages, they rarely travelled more than a few miles from the place of their birth.

Despite the political and religious turmoil of this unsettled time, the seventeenth century was an age filled with a flood of intellectual treasures. Art, literature, philosophy, and science flowered and flourished. It was a disputatious age that witnessed an intellectual revolution whereby new theories replaced the old. There was an unheaval of thought and a disregard for traditional opinion. Mysticism, astrology, witchcraft, and the appeal of ancient writings were under critical scrutiny. Aristotle, Galen and the other ancients were finally placed upon the marble pedestal of antiquity.

The seventeenth century was a "Golden Age" for European science. During its course, scientific inquiry replaced superstition and fantasy. Scholars turned from the blind acceptance of traditional authority to the methodical study of nature. The world of practical affairs with its dual pressures of war and expanding commerce placed a premium upon scientific discovery. New worlds were thus opened up for the advancement of philosophy, science and medicine.

It was a century of genius that produced a whole galaxy of philosophic and scientific stars. All the leading nationalities of Western Europe contributed to the achievements of this new age. The catalog of names includes Bacon, Harvey, Boyle and Newton from England; Descartes and Pascal from France; Galileo and Malpighi from Italy; the Dutch-Jewish philosopher Spinoza and Huygens and Van Leeuwenhoek from Holland; and Kepler and Leibnitz from Germany. Thus the seventeenth century gave birth to modern thought and science and from this century on the advance of knowledge continued in an almost unbroken chain.

The century opened in 1600 with the publication of Gilbert's classic treatise *De Magnete* which laid the foundations for the study of modern electricity. Dr. William Gilbert (1540-1603) was president of the College of Physicians and practiced on the London aristocracy. His work on magnetism exploded the myth of the "loadstone" which had been considered of medical value because of its supposed ability to "pull or draw" diseases out of the body. Although most of Gilbert's work was on physics, his methods of scientific investigation were of value to medicine.

The English philosopher, statesman and jurist, Sir Francis Bacon (1561-1626), contributed more to real scientific progress than any other man since the days of the Greek philosophers. His chief renown rests upon his development of the inductive method of reasoning. Undertaking the tremendous task of trying to rearrange the whole system of human knowledge he did much to destroy the medieval mentality of his generation. Insisting that most existing knowledge was based on false premises he urged scholars to forsake the "Four Idols" they had worshipped in previous centuries, namely authority, popular opinion, legal bias, and personal prejudice. Emphasizing the necessity of "dwelling purely and constantly among the facts of nature," he underlined the need of noting these facts carefully and drawing conclusions from experiment and experience and not from speculative theory.

As an exponent of the "experimental method," Bacon acted as a scientific scout, setting forth the methods which others were to use. He pointed the way leaving scientific verification to others.

In 1609 the great Galileo began to sweep the starry heavens with an instrument of his own making. Although not the actual inventor of the telescope, he was the first to put it to extended practical use. Acting upon the ideas and suggestions of various Dutch opticians, Galileo constructed a telescope capable of magnifying objects a thousand times. He thus became one of the first scientific astronomers, discovering that the moon was not a sphere shining by its own light and that the milky way consisted of myriads of individual stars.

He stated his belief in the theory of Copernicus, and despite the animosity and persecution of the church, continued his study of the laws of the universe. One of the first to see clearly the unchangeable relations between cause and effect, he stated that "Nature is written in mathematical symbols."

Galileo was born at Pisa in 1564 and at the age of eighteen made his great discovery of the principle of the simple pendulum by watching the lamp hanging from the roof of the Cathedral of Pisa swinging "too and fro." Beginning the study of medicine, he soon abandoned this branch of science for mathematics. His mathematical achievements soon won him renown and he was appointed professor of mathematics at the University of Pisa. Here he conducted his famous studies from the Leaning Tower of Pisa that led him to the discovery of the law of falling bodies.

Later Galileo went to Padua where he lectured on mathematics. Among his students was Sanctorius, who borrowed his instruments and made comparative studies of the human temperature and pulse. Toricelli, another of his students, discovered that the height of mercury in a tube is a measure of atmospheric pressure and thus provided the principle for the modern barometer. A young English medical student named William Harvey who was later to become world famous for his discovery of the circulation of the blood was also among his students.

Galileo exerted a tremendous indirect influence on medicine and is important to the history of medicine for two reasons. First, he urged the men of medicine to apply to their research the scientific tools of experiment and exact measurement. Secondly, while engaged in constructing his telescope, he produced as a by-product an elementary type of microscope. This instrument later was to become of tremendous importance to medical progress. Galileo was one of the world's great original thinkers and his investigations and discoveries made him one of the founders of experimental science.

With the sciences making such great progress, it was only natural that medicine would follow along in the same rational manner. Once and for all, the men of medicine turned their backs on the old dogmas and moved forward following the progressive pathways of investigation and experimentation.

The foundation for the accurate knowledge of the structure of the human body had been created by the observations of Andreas Vesalius in the previous century. Although the anatomists had cast off the fetters of Galenic authority, the great puzzle of how the blood flowed through the body still remained unsolved.

For 1,500 years, Galen's erroneous concepts regarding the function of the heart and the movement of the blood had prevailed. It was believed that new blood welled up in an incessant ebb and flow from the liver and was transported by the veins to the right side of the heart and then seeped into the left chamber via invisible pores in the septum. Although Michael Servetus had described the pulmonary circulation in 1533 and Realdo Colombo had demonstrated that the pulmonary vein contained blood, they all believed that the septum of the heart was porous.

Vesalius had challenged this concept in his monumental book on anatomy when he wrote, "I do not see how even the smallest amount of blood could pass from the right ventricle to the left through the septum." Unfortunately, he did not advance a theory of his own in explanation and it remained for a small bearded English physician named William Harvey to solve this age-old puzzle.

A turning point in medical history was reached in 1616 when William Harvey, in a Lumleian lecture before the Royal College of Physicians in London, quietly outlined his theory on the circulation of the blood. His epoch-making discovery revolutionized medical thought and gave birth to the modern era of medicine.

Born April 1, 1578 at Folkestone, England, William Harvey was the eldest of seven sons of a well-to-do merchant and town official. Given every educational advantage, he was entered at the age of ten to the Kings' Grammar School at Canterbury. At fifteen, he went to Caius College of Cambridge University, graduating four years later with a Bachelor of Arts degree.

In 1598, Harvey left England to enroll in the famed medical school of the University of Padua. Here, where Vesalius had done his most brilliant work, Harvey studied the human body under the tutelage of another famous anatomist, Fabricius of Aquapendente. He also was inspired by the lectures of the great Galileo, who urged his students to apply to medical research the scientific tools of experiment and exact measurement. Winning his diploma as "Doctor of Physic" from Padua, Harvey returned to England and received the degree of "Doctor of Medicine" from Cambridge in 1604. After marrying a daughter of the physician to King James I, he began his medical practice in London.

Harvey was an active practitioner of medicine all of his life. He served as physician to the poor, the great and to two kings. In 1615, he was appointed "physician to the poor" at St. Bartholomew's Hospital. As his fame grew, he treated many of the most eminent persons in England including the Lord Chancellor, Sir Francis Bacon.

Scientific research was actually an avocation with Harvey, which made his discoveries all the more remarkable. Appointed Lumleian lecturer, he became a teacher and demonstrator of anatomy. It was as a part of this series of anatomical lectures that Harvey in 1616, at the age of forty-two, first outlined his theory on the circulation of the blood. A hard-working, incessant and methodical researcher, Harvey spent twelve years setting down his experiments and conclusions. Using observation and logic, he undertook his experiments, as he wrote, "for the purpose of discovering the motions and functions of the heart by actual inspection and not by other peoples' books."

In 1628 he published his famous book, *De Motu Cordis et Sanguinis.* A slender volume consisting of seventy-two poorly printed pages, this was one of the most important books ever published in the history of medicine. Clearly and concisely, he set forth how the blood circulates throughout the body and how the heart functions as a pump. This basic concept of physiology founded modern medicine and made it possible to understand, treat and prevent disease from within the body as well as from without.

Fortunately, Harvey lived to see his work accepted by the great majority of medical men throughout the scientific world. However, as usual, a minority refused to abandon their obsolete concepts and attempted to discredit him with falacious arguments and bitter personal attacks.

Despite the controversy his work created, Harvey attained great eminence. In 1618, he was appointed "Physician Extraordinary" to King James I and thereafter moved largely in court circles. He attended the coronation of Charles I in Scotland in 1633 and became his personal physician and close friend. He was a frequent companion of the King on hunting trips and had the privilege of dissecting the kill for scientific study. Harvey continued to loyally serve the crown until the King's tragic death in 1649.

Following the beheading of King Charles and the rise of Cromwell, Harvey led a quiet life of semiretirement. He saw few patients, but devoted much time to the welfare of the College of Physicians and continued to record many experiments in natural science and embryology. In 1651 he published a work on embryology entitled "Concerning the Generation of Animals."

Remaining true in his devotion to the advancement of medicine, one of Harvey's last acts was to endow a library and museum for his beloved College of Physicians. Death finally closed William Harvey's remarkable career in his eightieth year on June 3, 1657.

The seventeenth century was a time of great medical advancement and witnessed the return of medicine to the patient's bedside. It was a period during which the foundations of modern clinical medicine were laid by direct observation and the application of the powers of reason to the patient and his disease. This gave impetus to the study, recognition and description of individual diseases.

Out of the morass of medical misconception surrounding disease, and the welter of confusion on contagion, the figure of Thomas Sydenham arose. Towering head and shoulders above his contemporaries, he became the greatest clinician of the century.

The fifth son among the ten children of a well-to-do Puritan landowner, Sydenham was born in Dorsetshire in 1624. At eighteen he entered Magdalen Hall at Oxford, but left his studies when Civil War broke out to enlist in the Army of Parliament. An enthusiastic soldier of Cromwell's Army, he rose to the rank of Captain and was demobilized at the age of twenty-two, following the defeat of the Cavaliers.

Returning to Oxford in 1647, he transferred to Wadham College to study medicine. Six months later he received his degree as a Bachelor of Medicine by order of the University's Chancellor, the Earl of Pembroke. This was a highly irregular procedure in view of the fact that he lacked a degree in arts and had studied medicine for only a few months.

Appointed a Fellow at All Souls College, Sydenham served in this capacity until 1655. However, when Prince Charles landed in Scotland he interrupted his fellowship and again entered the Parliamentary Army. During this period, he was reputed to have both led and doctored his troops with distinction. Following the Royalists defeat, Sydenham received a grant of 699 pounds for his services. With this, he was able to both get married and start a practice in London. Being a competent physician he soon developed a successful practice, despite the fact that his detractors called him a "trooper turned physician."

Interrupting his practice in 1659 in order to further his knowledge of medicine, Sydenham attended Montpelier and studied under the famous French teacher and consultant, Barbeyrac. Resuming his London practice in 1661, he became a licentiate of the Royal College of Physicians, but never attained the higher mark of Fellow. Later after having attained success and fame, he obtained an M.D. degree from Cambridge in 1676, while his son was a medical student there.

Sydenham was an active, successful and respected practitioner with all the patients he could possibly care for. Garbed in his plain Puritan costume in contrast to the rich raiment of many of his colleagues, he immediately commanded respect. With his honest practical approach and common-sense methods of treatments he easily inspired his patients with confidence. Suspicious of academic science and theoretical medicine, Sydenham modeled himself after Hippocrates and became the greatest exponent of clinical medicine in England.

Primarily a practical physician, he tried to protect his patients from the poly-pharmacy of his day and at times refused to use drugs, writing, "I have consulted my patients safety and my own reputation most effectively by doing nothing at all." However, he was not sparing of drugs where indicated and was one of the first clinicians in England to use chincona in the treatment of fevers. He was not above using such quaint practical procedures as placing a puppy dog or kitten on a patient's abdomen to serve as a form of hot water bottle, or to place a young person in bed with an elderly patient for the purpose of providing warmth.

Sydenham made no new medical discoveries, but like Hippocrates, he charted the natural course of disease. A keen observer, he made a systematic study of symptoms, assigning them to specific illnesses, and thus differentiated many diseases. Objectively observing disease at the patient's bedside, he developed the concept that the various diseases were separate entities that could be described, recognized and classified. From this he advanced the idea that treatment must be rationalized in terms of specific illness.

Like Hippocrates, Sydenham believed that "patients were a physician's best books." The following anecdote serves as an interesting illustration of this belief. After Sydenham became famous, Sir Hans Sloan, who later founded the British Museum, came to London as a young physician to see the great clinician. Sloan's letter of introduction described himself as "a ripe scholar, a good botanist, a skillful anatomist." After reading the letter, Sydenham turned to his would-be disciple and exclaimed, "This is all very fine, but it won't do—anatomy, botany! Nonsense! Sir, I know an old woman in Covent Garden who understands botany better, and, as for anatomy, my butcher can dissect a joint full as well; no, young man, all this is stuff: You must go to the bedside, it is there alone you can learn disease."

Sydenham made a number of important contributions to the differentiation and understanding of contagious disease and thus helped lay the foundations of preventive medicine. He studied the various fevers and epidemics of London from season to season and year to year.

In 1666 he published his first medical treatise, a book on fevers, a term which included a multitude of diseases. This was written in 1665 during the time that Sydenham and his family had fled London in order to escape the plague. Strangely enough, a physician's flight from the plague was not considered unethical at this time. Although not present during the height of occurrence, Sydenham gained a wide experience and cause for much thought from the Great Plague of 1665.

His book was well received at home and was reprinted in many countries. A second enlarged edition was published in 1668 and in 1676 his largest and best known book, *Medical Observations,* appeared. In a short chapter in this book entitled "Febris Scarlatina" he gave a classic description of this disease as well as naming it. He also differentiated and gave accurate accounts of measles, smallpox, influenza, dysentery and plague. His clinical descriptions of chorea and gout are medical classics. Chorea minor is still called Sydenham's Chorea, while his masterly work on gout reflects his own personal and painful experience with this affliction.

Sydenham's writings on epidemic disease were masterpieces and he is frequently given credit for initiating the science of epidemiology. He denied that the stars either produced diseases or influenced their course. He believed that the acute febrile diseases fell into two groups: the epidemic distempers produced by atmospheric and climatic changes, and the intercurrent diseases which were due to the susceptibility of the body.

Sydenham believed that the atmospheric changes that caused epidemics were due to miasmas that arose from the earth. He thus gave birth to the atmospheric miasmatic theory of contagious disease spread, a concept which was to influence public health thought well into the nineteenth century. Although this concept was erroneous, it was to serve the public health well. It gave rise to the idea that "dirt and disease go hand in hand" and that decaying organic materials gave off noxious odors and effluvia which in turn created the disease producing miasmas. Thus for approximately two hundred years, this erroneous concept served to initiate many much needed sanitary reforms that helped promote environmental cleanliness.

Less esteemed at home than abroad, Sydenham's own colleagues while respecting him, bestowed no honors upon him. In later years, he suffered from severe attacks of gout to which were added the tortures of urinary calculus. He died December 29, 1689 and was buried in St. James Church, Westminster.

His fame spread rapidly after his death and he became known as the "Father of English Medicine" and the "English Hippocrates." It is said that the great Dutch clinician Boerhaave so admired Sydenham that he respectfully removed his hat whenever he mentioned his name.

Another physician who left us some classic descriptions of infectious and contagious diseases was Guillaume de Baillou (1538-1616). A skillful physician, brilliant teacher and masterful writer, he was dean of the Medical Faculty in Paris. He gave excellent descriptions of whooping cough, diphtheria, plague and rheumatic fever.

Numerous other anatomical and medical advances were made during the seventeenth century. Thomas Wharton (1614-1673) was an eminent English physician and one of the few who remained at work during the Great Plague of London in 1665. He is famed for having described the duct of the submaxillary gland which is still called Wharton's duct.

A great friend of Wharton's was Dr. Francis Glisson who is remembered for his description of the fibrous (Glisson's) capsule of the liver in 1654. Glisson, who was Regius Professor of Physic at Cambridge, also remained at work during the Great Plague. He wrote the original classic account of infantile rickets and was the founder of England's Royal Society.

Thomas Willis (1621-1675) was a successful and wealthy physician who also managed to find time for study and writing. In 1664, he wrote his famous *Cerebri Anatome* which accurately described the network of arteries at the base of the brain, which has ever since been called the "Circle of Willis." He also described the eleventh cranial nerve and wrote on both typhus and typhoid fevers. He wrote a treatise entitled *Diabetes or the Pissing Evil,* and was the first in England to draw attention to the sweet taste of diabetic urine.

During this century three generations of the Danish family of Bartholin taught anatomy at the University of Copenhagen from 1613 to 1738. Thomas Bartholin discovered the thoracic duct and gave the first full description of the whole lymphatic system. His son, Casper Secundus, described the vestibulo-vaginal glands as well as the sublingual duct, and both structures are named for him.

Also from Copenhagen came Niels Stensen (1638-1686) who discovered and described the duct (Stensen's duct) of the parotid gland. An amazing anatomist, Stensen examined other glands and proved that all secretory glands have ducts. He also described the lachrymal apparatus and the mechanism of lacrimation. Before his time it was believed that the tears were formed in the brain and were led through the nerves to the eyes. Stensen studied and dissected the head of a shark sent to him from Leghorn, Italy and demonstrated that shark's teeth were a component of certain fossils. His treatise resulting from this study is acclaimed as having laid the foundations for the science of paleontology. At the age of thirty-six, he took holy orders after being converted from Lutheranism to Catholicism. He soon rose to the rank of Bishop, but unfortunately died at the early age of forty-eight.

This century also witnessed Holland's rise to medical fame. Nicolaas Tulp (1593-1674) achieved immortality as the teacher and central figure in Rembrandt's famous painting, "The Anatomy Lesson." However, Tulp was famous in his own right and was a distinguished clinician, teacher, and anatomist. He wrote on diphtheria, gave one of the earliest accounts of beriberi and described the ileocecal valve.

Franciscus Sylvius (1614-1672) was professor of medicine at Leyden where he popularized Harvey's ideas on the heart and circulation. He was one of the first great workers on tuberculosis and wrote a classic description of this disease. He described the cerebral aqueduct, which is frequently called the Aqueduct of Sylvius and also described the lateral cerebral or Sylvian fissure.

Regnier de Graaf (1641-1673) was one of Sylvius' students at Leyden who achieved fame as an anatomist. He is remembered for his classical studies on the anatomy of the genital organs. In 1668, he published an excellent treatise on the testes. His great work on the female generative organs was published in 1672. He demonstrated the process of ovulation and discovered the vessicle of the ovary which was later named the Graafian follicle. De Graaf was a friend and fellow townsman of Van Leeuwenhoek's and called the attention of the Royal Society of London to his friends' great work. Unfortunately De Graaf's brilliant career was cut short when he died from the plague at the early age of thirty-two.

During the seventeenth century, mathematicians were sometimes physicians and physicians sometimes mathematicians. This gave rise to the Iatromathematical School as exemplified by Descartes, Borelli, Sanctorius and others who regarded man as an earthly machine. They believed that although man's actions were directed by a rational soul, they could be interpreted mathematically and that the mathematical-physical laws which governed the universe also governed the human body.

Chief among the proponents of this concept was Rene Descartes. A true genius, his brilliant mind embraced many disciplines, chief among which were mathematics, philosophy, theology, astronomy, psychology and medicine.

Although famed chiefly for his contributions to mathematics and philosophy, he contributed to medicine by authoring one of the first textbooks on physiology. He embraced and popularized Harvey's concepts on the heart and circulation. Attempting to reduce all physiology to physics, he treated locomotion, respiration and digestion as mechanical processes. Along with the other proponents of the Iatromechanical School, he compared the various organs of the body to a machine. Skeletal and muscular actions were explained on the theory of levers, the teeth were likened to a pair of shears, the chest to a bellows and the stomach to a flask.

The scientific advances of the seventeenth century included notable progress in both chemistry and pharmacy. Chemistry which had long been hampered by its association with the magic of alchemy finally emerged as a scientific discipline.

One of the founders of modern chemistry was the English physicist and chemist, Robert Boyle (1627-1671). In his book, *The Sceptical Chemist*, he differed with the alchemists by maintaining that the baser metals could not be transmuted to gold.

He attacked the concept of "phlogiston," and the accepted concept of matter, including Aristotle's "four elements" by stating that an element is a pure substance and cannot be broken down. He studied air and the gases and in 1622 formulated Boyle's Law regarding the pressure of gases. In 1669 he made an important contribution to our knowledge of respiration by demonstrating that air is necessary for life.

Quinine, one of the world's most important curative and prophylactic drugs, was introduced during the seventeenth century. According to legend, the Countess of Chinchon, wife of the Spanish Viceroy of Peru was stricken with malaria while in Lima in 1630. An Indian supposedly arrived in the nick of time with some powder made from the fever-bark or quina-quina tree and miraculously cured the Countess. She subsequently was said to have introduced the drug into Europe.

Chinchona or quinine was also called Jesuit's bark or Cardinal's bark after the Jesuit Cardinal Lugo, who in the 1640's promoted use of the bark in Europe after he had successfully treated Louis XIV with it. Many physicians refused to prescribe the drug because it was not mentioned in the texts of the ancients. However, Sydenham was one of the earliest clinicians to adopt it and he helped popularize its use.

In England during the first part of this century, the guild of grocers and apothecaries was officially separated and a pharmacopoeia appeared in London which introduced a set of recognized standards by which medicines could be compounded. It contained about two thousand remedies, some of which were rather bizarre, such as oil of ants, oil of wolves, dried fox's lungs and lozenges of dried vipers.

The first manufacturing pharmaceutical chemist was Johann Rudolf Glauber. In 1656, he artificially made and sold sodium sulphate or Glauber's salt, the curative properties of which he had discovered in a natural spring at Neustadt. He was able to manufacture hydrochloric acid on a large scale and distilled ammonia from animal bones. Glauber became quite famous, manufacturing many other compounds and authoring over thirty books. He was so revered by the pharmacists of Europe, that for about one hundred years, his gilded bust placed over the doorway served as a sign of their calling.

Chapter 14

VAN LEEUWENHOEK'S TINY LITTLE BEASTIES
AND
THE INVISIBLE WORLD OF
THE MICROSCOPISTS

T HE SEVENTEENTH CENTURY witnessed the beginning of the "microscopists," a group of "many-talented" men, who became fascinated with the invisible world of tiny things. Mankind had long searched for instruments to aid the eye and extend the sense of sight. The ancients were known to have used lenses for the magnification of small objects and Roger Bacon was familiar with and used magnifying glasses in the thirteenth century. However, the first notable advances in optometry were made during the Renaissance by the lens grinders and spectacle makers of Holland.

The telescope which had been developed by the Dutch opticians had been perfected and put to practical use by Galileo. The microscope was also the work of the Dutch opticians, but just exactly who invented this instrument is not clear. However, it is generally conceded that Hans and Zacharius Janssen of Middleburgh, Holland in about 1590 were probably the first to construct a compound microscope. This information reached Galileo in about 1610 and he experimented with a type of microscope. Many other scientists including Francesca Fontana, Cornelius Van Drebbel and Rene Descartes contributed to its development. The word microscope is said to have been coined by Johannes Faber of Bemberg in 1628 and is a simple descriptive term composed of the Greek words, "mikros" (small) plus "skopein" (to view).

Just as the telescope opened the heavens to reveal the secrets of the distant stars, so the microscope opened a new universe to reveal a hitherto invisible world of tiny things. Once perfected, this instrument became "a miracle leading to countless other miracles." Almost simultaneously, men in three different countries—Holland, Italy and Germany—began to use this fascinating new instrument to study all manner of small things. The development of the microscope gave birth to several important new branches of medicine, namely, histology, pathology, bacteriology and eventually preventive medicine.

The first man to peer curiously and carefully into this hitherto invisible world was an amateur scientist with a hobby of grinding lenses and a passion for making things look bigger. Antony Van Leeuwenhoek, a Dutch linen-draper and janitor, discovered how to use a small biconvex lens to magnify things. He was thus able to view structures and organisms never before seen by men. Becoming the world's first microscopist, he was also the first to observe and record microscopic organisms which he called "tiny little beasties."

Van Leeuwenhoek was born in Delft, Holland, October 24, 1637. He came from a family of respectable burghers most of whom were brewers and basketmakers. His father who was a basketmaker died when Antony was five. Hence Van Leeuwenhoek's formal education was scant and he left school at sixteen to be apprenticed to a linen-draper in Amsterdam. At twenty-two, he returned to Delft, bought a house, married and set up a shop of his own. He was to remain in Delft for the rest of his life, continuing in business as a linen-draper and haberdasher.

Van Leeuwenhoek entered civic affairs and enjoyed a minor degree of success. He held an office comparable to that of an alderman, served as official wine-gauger and was a licensed surveyor. For over forty years, he held the post of janitor or custodian of the City Hall and served as the "Bedellus" or chamberlain to the sheriffs of Delft.

Antony Van Leeuwenhoek was not the inventor of the microscope. Hand lenses had been used before his day and a compound microscope had been built before he was born. However, he was a masterly meticulous grinder of precision lenses. Just how or when he became interested in grinding lenses and using them to study the secrets of nature is not known. Nor is there any record of how or where he acquired his technical knowledge and mechanical skill. Working entirely by himself, he kept his methods a closely-guarded secret throughout his entire life.

Avidly pursuing his avocation, he turned out hundreds of tiny lenses within the confines of his "closet" or workroom. He laboriously ground his lenses by hand and mounted them between thin sheets of silver or brass (and occasionally gold) so that he masked all but the central area. Thus, at a fixed focal distance the object under scrutiny could be brought into view, and at a distance of eight inches, a maximum magnification of two hundred diameters was possible. He mounted solid specimens before the lenses on needle points, using adjustable thumb-screws to regulate height and distance. Other microscopes he designed held small glass vials or capillary tubes so that liquids could be studied.

Possessing a boundless curiosity, Van Leeuwenhoek placed all manner of things under the probing eyes of his microscopes. Selecting his specimens from his surroundings, he studied rain water, the scum from stagnant ponds, the tartar from his teeth, scrapings, secretions and excretions of all sorts, various human and animal tissues, and a wide variety of mineral and vegetable matter. In order to preserve an interesting specimen which he found to his liking, Van Leeuwenhoek would leave it attached to the microscope and fashion another instrument. Thus, over the years, he accumulated many of these, keeping them in pairs in small lacquered chests.

Undoubtedly the father of microscopy, Van Leeuwenhoek was also the first man to observe and record protozoa and bacteria. Scraping a bit of tartar from his ill-kept teeth and placing it under his microscope he discovered a whole world of tiny little living creatures, smaller than what the human eye could see. Calling them tiny little beasties or "animalcules," he used a grain of sand as his standard of measurement. Describing their various sizes, he estimated that it would take a thousand to a million of his tiny little beasties to equal the bulk of a grain of sand. He wrote, "there are more animalcules living in the scum of the teeth in a man's mouth than there are men in a whole kingdom."

Van Leeuwenhoek made observations and drawings of various protozoa, bacilli, cocci, and spirochetes. He described the fantastically rapid multiplication of his tiny little beasties, after observing this phenomenon in specimens left standing for several days. He also noted the purity of rain and snow water in comparison to the teeming life found in stagnant waters. He discovered spermatazoa as a regular constituent of semen, studied the structure of the crystalline lens and noted the striped character of voluntary muscle. Later, after becoming famous, he frequently demonstrated capillary circulation by focusing his microscope on the transparent tail of a small eel or fish. He was visited by many celebrities, including Peter the Great of Russia, who purposely came to Delft to see the tiny little beasties.

Van Leeuwenhoek's first report of his scientific studies was made in 1673 at the age of forty-one. His friend and fellow townsman, the famous Dutch physician Regnier De Graaf, had written to the Royal Society of London describing Van Leeuwenhoek's great findings and enclosed a letter from him. Over the years and until the end of his life, Van Leeuwenhoek continued his observations, recording his findings by correspondence to the Royal Society. He sent approximately 250 such letters to them and in 1680 was honored by being elected to Fellowship. Although handicapped by failing eyesight, Van Leeuwenhoek faithfully continued to send his famous letters and it is reliably recorded that he dictated his last letter to the Royal Society just thirty-six hours before he died at the ripe old age of ninety-one.

Antony Van Leeuwenhoek was not a physician, or a scientist or even an educated man in the commonly accepted sense of the term, yet he contributed greatly to the advancement of medicine and was one of the great benefactors of the human race. Although recognized by his contemporaries as the epoch-making discoverer of a hitherto invisible world, the full implication of his observations were not recognized for approximately 150 years.

Van Leeuwenhoek had no concept of bacteria as disease producers, nor did he make any attempt to correlate them with contagious or epidemic diseases. He was not aware of the fact that some of his tiny little beasties were fearsome, ferocious creatures capable of annihilating whole races of men. He did not realize that they were the silent assassins that murdered babes in their cradles and indiscriminately killed poverty-stricken peasants in their hovels or wealthy kings in their palatial palaces. However, his observations and discoveries laid the foundations for the development of bacteriology and the practical applications growing out of this science eventually led to effective preventive medicine and the ultimate control of contagion.

The first physician to fully use the microscope in scientific medical research was the great anatomist, Marcello Malpighi (1628-1694). Four years after Harvey's death, Malpighi solved the mystery of the union of the blood vessels. He placed the simple transparent tissue of a frog's lung under his microscope and observed how the blood passed from the arteries to the veins. Thus, in 1660, he discovered the capillary circulation and provided the final link which confirmed Harvey's thesis on the circulation of blood.

Marcello Malpighi was born near Bologna and studied at the University there. He became qualified in medicine at the age of twenty-five and three years afterwards was appointed professor of medicine at his alma mater. His reputation soon spread and Ferdinand II, the Grand Duke of Tuscany, following the tradition of the Medicis as patrons of learning, appointed Malpighi to the chair of theoretical medicine at the University of Pisa. However, after three years at Pisa, Malpighi returned to Bologna, where with the exception of a period of four years that he spent at the University of Messina, he remained for the rest of his professional career.

He did outstanding studies on the anatomy and physiology of the kidney and is best known for his discovery of the Malpighian corpuscle or body. He described the red corpuscles of the blood, discovered the rete mucosum of the skin and proved that the papillae of the tongue are organs of taste. In fact, there is hardly an organ or structure of the body which he did not examine under his microscope. By the use of his microscope, Malpighi became the founder of microscopic anatomy and the father of the sciences of histology and embryology.

Malpighi terminated his brilliant career as a microscopist and teacher in 1691, when he accepted the summons of Pope Innocent XII to become physician in chief and chamberlain to the Papal Court. He died in 1694 at the Quirnale Palace and in true keeping with his scientific spirit, he made an antemortem request that an autopsy be performed upon his body.

Probably the first man to employ the microscope to investigate the causes of disease was Athanasius Kircher (1602-1680). A versatile Jesuit priest from Fulda in central Germany, Kircher was professor of philosophy at Wurzburg. He acquired an outstanding reputation in physics, optics, mathematics and music as well as medicine.

Due to the troubles of the Thirty Years' War, Kircher was driven from Wurzburg to Avignon and subsequently taught mathematics at the Collegeo Romano in Rome. While in Rome, he observed and described how maggots and other "small animals" developed in putrescent material. He microscopically examined the pus and blood of plague victims and found it filled with countless "little worms," which he believed to be the cause of plague. In his treatise, *Scrutinium Pestis,* published in 1658, he set forth his observations and probably was the first to propose a doctrine of "Contagion Animatum." It is doubtful that his microscope was powerful enough to detect the "Pasteurella Pestis." In all probability, his observations were incorrect and most likely the little worms and animals that he detected were red blood corpuscles, pus cells and rouleaux of erythrocytes. However, Kircher's work was important to the advancement of preventive medicine because he pioneered in pointing the way toward the establishment of the bacterial origin of disease.

In 1665, Robert Hooke, a London botanist who was probably the first botanical histologist, observed cellular structure and introduced the term, "cell." After microscopically studying cork, he described its structure as bearing a fancied resemblance to the cubicles or cells used to house monks in the monasteries.

Thus the pioneer microscopists of the seventeenth century lighted a torch of knowledge that has burned brightly ever since. After thousands of years of invisibility, their inquisitive minds and searching microscopes discovered a whole new world of tiny things never before revealed to human eyes.

Chapter 15

THE BOOKKEEPING OF LIFE
AND THE
BIRTH OF VITAL STATISTICS

PREGNANT AND PERTINENT to the development of modern preventive medicine and public health was the birth of the science of vital statistics. Prior to the seventeenth century, there had been no organized statistical and analytical methods of studying the health status of a population. While other sciences had advanced through the methodical steps of collecting and analyzing facts and data, there had been no significant attempt to apply these numerical methods to the study of the epidemic and contagious diseases that had so long plagued mankind.

In 1662 a small book entitled, *Natural and Political Observations Mentioned in a Following Index and Made upon the Bills of Mortality*, was published by Captain John Graunt, citizen of London. Vital statistics in the modern sense of the term may be said to take its origin from the publication of this remarkable work.

Weekly "bills of mortality" consisting of lists of burials, marriages and baptisms had been compiled by parish clerks for more than a century before Graunt's time. They had their origin and stemmed from an order issued by the London City Council in 1532, requiring that a record be kept of deaths occurring from the plague. The earliest such known "plague bill" was issued for the week of November 16-23, 1532. It is still extant and is preserved among the Egerton Manuscripts in the British Museum.

Graunt is historically considered to be the founder of vital statistics because he was the first to conceive of the idea of carefully observing and analytically studying the bills of mortality for the purpose of trying to determine the basic laws of human mortality, natality and population movement.

From the confused and long neglected contents of the bills of mortality for the city of London and adjoining parishes, Graunt discovered four basic demographic principles. First, he clearly showed the regular occurrence of certain vital phenomena which appears to be the mere play of chance when occurring individually. Second, he pointed out that male births exceed female births, but that females constitute approximately one-half of the population. Third, he demonstrated that mortality rates are highest in the early and the late years of life. Finally, he discovered that the urban death rate normally exceeds the rural death rate.

Graunt, the son of a haberdasher and linen-draper, was born in Hampshire, England, April 24, 1620. Receiving a sound English education, he was bound as an apprentice to a haberdasher of small wares, a trade he mostly followed, though "free of the Drapers' Company." Building a reputation for integrity, he soon became a prosperous tradesman and acquired considerable wealth.

Early in his career, he entered politics and after successfully passing through the various ward offices of the city, he was elected a member of the Common Council of London, where he served for a period of two years. He acquired his title of Captain by serving as a leader of the "Trained Band" for a number of years.

Graunt's energy, success and ability soon won him recognition and he achieved considerable social standing. He was admitted to the Royal Society upon the personal recommendation of King Charles II and was one of the first members recruited from the merchant class. It was a real mark of distinction for a shopkeeper to become a Fellow of the Royal Society.

Graunt had studied the bills of mortality for several years before he conceived of the idea of publishing his findings. His *Natural and Political Observations* is said to have first appeared in 1661; however, the earliest edition in the British Museum is dated 1662.

Graunt constructed the first London life table, classified deaths and death rates by causes, noted the seasonal and annual variations in the death rate and suggested that "populousness" may influence the death rate. He noted that fertility is influenced by the sex and age composition and the health of the population, as well as other social and physiological factors. He also observed that the rural natural increase of population contributes to the urban growth.

His book created considerable interest and was reprinted four or five times during his lifetime. In 1676, two years after his death, another edition appeared which was enlarged and edited by his good friend, Sir William Petty. This probably led to the erroneous statement that has frequently been made that Petty was the real author and that Graunt deserves little or no credit. This claim has been critically examined and the overwhelming weight of expert opinion is that Graunt was the main, if not the sole author of his remarkable book.

Graunt had been raised as a Puritan and for a number of years took down the sermons he heard by means of a clever and dextrous method of "short-writing" which he had developed. Later he changed his religion and became converted to Catholicism. He eventually resigned all of his public appointments in consequence of his change of religion.

Having acquired considerable wealth, Graunt retired from business fairly early in life. After his retirement, he was admitted to the management of the New River Company, a firm which supplied water to the City of London. Because of this and also because of the antagonism he had aroused by his conversion to Catholicism, Graunt was accused of having had a hand in the Great London Fire. He was charged with contriving to stop the supply of water to the city on the night before the outbreak of the fire, Sunday, September 2, 1666. There was no truth to this story because the records show that Graunt was not associated with the New River Company until twenty-three days after the Great Fire.

Graunt died of jaundice on April 18, 1674, just a few days short of the age of fifty-four. An ingenious, successful and studious person, this "shopkeeper turned statistician" found a place in history as the founding father of the science of vital statistics.

Besides the intrinsic value of its results, Graunt's remarkable book served as the stimulator for further work and progress in the same general field. Graunt was a close personal friend of Dr. (later Sir) William Petty and undoubtedly influenced and stimulated Petty in his statistical studies.

In 1669, seven years after the publication of Graunt's book, Christian Huygens, the famous Dutch mathematician and astronomer, took up the problem of determining mathematically the probable expectation of human life at any given age.

In 1693, Edmund Halley, the great English astronomer, published a "life table" that was directly applicable to the calculation of life annuities. When the first life insurance companies were established in the eighteenth century, they made use of Halley's life tables.

Many of those who initially began to use numerical and statistical methods concerned themselves with what is commonly called the "bookkeeping of state." Their efforts were directed toward ascertaining the basic quantitative data of national life in the belief that this knowledge could be used to increase the prestige, power and prosperity of the state. This new field of endeavor was founded by William Petty, who christened it "political arithmetic."

William Petty (1623-1687) was born in Hampshire, the son of a clothier. After receiving his preliminary education in England, he studied at Caen. Upon his return to England, he served in the Royal Navy for several years. Going abroad again in 1643, he remained in the Netherlands and France for a period of three years and was enrolled as a medical student at the University of Leyden.

In 1647, Petty obtained a patent for his invention of double writing, a method using a type of copying machine. The following year, he was appointed deputy professor of anatomy at Oxford and in 1649, obtained his degree of Doctor of Physic.

A versatile individual, Petty engaged in commerce and industry, setting up iron works, opening lead mines and marble quarries as well as engaging in a trade in timber.

Petty also entered politics and public life, serving as Commissioner of Distribution of Lands and secretary to the Lord Lieutenant Henry Cromwell. In 1652, he was appointed Physician General of the English Army in Ireland. He was elected to Cromwell's Parliament in January of 1658. After the Restoration, Petty was favorably received and later knighted by King Charles II.

Petty by virtue of his training and experience as a physician, politician and economist was keenly aware of the importance of collecting and analyzing numerical data on population, diseases, education and revenues as well as on agriculture, commerce and industry. He repeatedly urged the collection of such data in the firm belief that its analysis was of vital importance in the formulation of national policies that would contribute to the nation's progress and growth. He aptly named this new field of endeavor, "political arithmetic" and employed mathematical calculations whenever possible in the analysis of his collected data.

In his "Essay on Political Arithmetic" population data was of central interest because of its basic political and economic importance. Death and disease rates and problems of health were considered chiefly in the light of how they affected the population. Petty demonstrated what individual industrialists had already suspected, that industry as a whole was the loser by the high sickness and death rates of its workers. He suggested that government should be concerned with the health of its most productive members, such as farmers, manufacturers, merchants and seamen. He concluded that epidemic diseases were not only a question of life and death for the individual, but that they were also socially and economically disabling, affecting the entire life of the community and the nation. In 1676 Petty stressed that it was the duty of the state to foster medical progress. In 1687 he proposed the formation of a health council to deal with the health problems of the city of London.

Petty was one of the first members of the select Royal Society and was a close friend and associate of Graunt. They probably influenced and collaborated with each other in some of their statistical studies.

Petty presented his "Essay on Political Arithmetic" in manuscript form to Charles II, but because it contained matter likely to be offensive to France, it was kept unpublished until 1691 when it was edited by Petty's son, Charles.

From the promising beginnings made by Graunt and Petty, the "art of reasoning by figures" continued to develop during the following centuries. The application of the numerical method to the analysis of health problems was destined to be extraordinarily fruitful for the future development of public health and preventive medicine.

Chapter 16

PLAGUE–FIRE–PEOPLE AND PROGRESS

THE BEGINNING of the seventeenth century found bubonic plague still smouldering throughout Europe. As the century advanced, plague continued to spread from country to country increasing in frequency and deadliness.

The continent was severely ravaged and almost one-half of the population of Lyon, France was swept away in the terrible epidemic of 1628-1629. The plague then swept northward invading Dijon in 1636, where it almost depopulated the entire region. According to Corradi, approximately one million deaths from plague occurred in Northern Italy between 1630 and 1631. After the Thirty Years' War, Germany and the Netherlands were severely stricken.

Under the Tudors and Stuarts, the plague visited England at frequent intervals, reaching a frightful climax in the Great Plague of London. In 1664 and 1665, London was stricken with one of the most frightful and violent epidemics that the world had witnessed since the original onslaught of the Black Death in the mid-fourteenth century.

Daniel Defoe of *Robinson Crusoe* fame, gave a classical account of this outbreak in his *Journal of the Plague Year*. His description of the Great Plague of 1665 is written in such tragic and masterly detail that it obviously seems to be an eyewitness account of a person living in London during that dreadful year. Although Defoe did live through the plague, and possibly in London, history shows that he was only five years old at the time.

The seventeenth century's newly discovered science of medicine proved to be entirely helpless before this frightful onslaught of plague. Most of the city's physicians fled, seeking personal safety along with their wealthy patients. A small heroic remainder, garbed in fantastically designed protective clothing, treated the stricken with a wide variety of ineffectual methods and medicines. As Defoe put it, "The plague defied all medicines. The very physicians were seized with it, with the preservatives in their hands." It was common practice to open the buboes by cautery or knife so that the "peccant humors" could escape. Apparently because many victims died while asleep or in coma, sleep was considered fatal and it was customary to awaken the victims every four hours.

Defoe says, "that of the doctors who stayed behind, few cared to stir abroad to sick houses; one fortified himself throughout with drink and in consequence became a sot." Dr. Nathaniel Hodges, one of the physicians who stayed behind throughout the visitation, attended throngs of plague victims both in his office or at their homes. His personal precautions included the sucking of lozenges and the burning of disinfectants on hot coals. Hodges also frequently fortified his body and rejuvenated his spirits by consuming "heavy draughts of sack." He survived to write *Loimologia,* the best medical account of the Great Plague.

So many physicians fled London, that the Royal College of Physicians closed its doors. However, before the college closed, the Lord Mayor requested that they recommend an antiplague remedy so as to protect the public from quacks, charlatans and astrologers. They promptly obliged and speedily concocted "The Royal College of Physicians' Plague Water." This useless nostrum contained twenty-one ingredients and consisted of two varieties, one for the rich containing onyx and unicorn's horn, and another for the poor composed of less costly substances.

When the Royal College of Physicians were asked by the aldermen of London for recommendations as how to best combat the plague, they were given nothing better than a weak rehash of fourteenth century procedures. To meet the medical emergency, four city physicians were employed to care for the plague-stricken poor and an apothecary was assigned to distribute anti-plague water.

The authorities invoked harsh and frequently senseless quarantine measures, trying desperately to isolate nests of infections. When one member of a family caught the disease, the entire household was quarantined for weeks on end, a procedure which made their infection a virtual certainty. A cross was painted on the doors and the house was securely locked and closely guarded. The windows were fastened shut and the key holes plugged so as to keep the "miasmatic air" inside. It was ignorantly believed that the escaping air endangered passersby and was so deadly that it could even strike down the birds in flight. Fires were burned in the streets to clear the air. Official dog catchers were employed to destroy stray dogs and cats while the real culprits, the flea-bearing rats, were left unharmed.

The bills of mortality were frequently falsified because families feared the long lock-up and harsh quarantine. Therefore, official searchers were employed to ferret out plague-infested households. Death carts made daily morning rounds through the city streets calling out the terrifying cry, "Bring out your dead." The dead were stacked like cordwood on the carts and hauled off to be buried or burned en masse. All measures proved futile and the city became one vast mortuary, a reeking prison house of the living, the dying, and the dead. By the year's end, 68,596 Londoners out of an approximate 500,000 were dead. This was according to an official but not very accurate tabulation.

The next year saw a rapid decline of the plague due in most part to the Great London Fire of 1666. Destroying most of the city and along with it vast numbers of the plague-bearing rat population, the Great Fire of London did more than any doctor or government to halt the plague. It eradicated the septic conditions that bred infection by destroying much of the overcrowded rat-ridden housing of the congested city.

The Great Fire thus presented the authorities of London with an excellent opportunity for planning and rebuilding the city, not only with an eye toward architectural beauty, but also with due regard to the health and welfare of its citizens. Sir Christopher Wren, a many-talented physician of London, had visions of such a well-planned city. A most remarkable and extraordinary individual, Wren was not only a skilled physician, but was also an excellent mathematician and philosopher, as well as being highly accomplished in the theory and practice of architecture. Soon after the Great Fire, he was appointed to the office of Surveyor General and had much to do with the planning and rebuilding of London. He gained great fame for the architectural beauty with which he designed many of London's public buildings, chief among which was St. Paul's Cathedral.

After the plague and fire, the general sanitary environment of London was greatly improved. Housing was better, the streets were kept cleaner, waste and refuse disposal was improved and the offensive trades came under closer scrutiny. Throughout all of Europe, sanitary conditions slowly and steadily improved toward the end of the seventeenth century.

Although there was an increased recognition of the need for improved sanitation, the ever-growing cities and ports of Europe were overcrowded and had extremely poor and congested housing conditions. Dirt and squalor were everywhere and the streets were still narrow, winding and unpaved. There were no sewers or drains, hence, they were muddy, filthy and refuse littered. Sanitary arrangements were primitive and people lived and worked together in filth and congestion. Water supplies were generally contaminated and were correctly regarded with suspicion. In fact, most people were so suspicious of the disease-producing properties of water that the last thing they thought of was to drink it. Hence, wine and beer were the commonly accepted beverages. In England, beer was the people's drink and records show that in 1688, 12 million barrels of beer were brewed for a population of less than 5 million.

While plague declined markedly throughout Europe during the latter part of the seventeenth century, the other epidemic and contagious diseases continued to take a heavy toll. Malaria was prevalent in Italy, typhus was epidemic in many countries and smallpox occurred in disastrous outbreaks not only in Europe, but also on the American continent. Scarlet fever, diphtheria and other contagious and infectious diseases had been recognized and identified, but little was known as to how they could be treated or controlled.

In England, public health had advanced to the point of recording the cause of death, but in the same country and in the same century Parliament placed a tax on windows and so deprived a major portion of the population of sunshine and light.

Thus, despite the tremendous scientific advances of the seventeenth century, it was apparent that the public, the politicians and the physicians had not yet discovered or grasped the fundamental concepts of preventive medicine and public health.

The lot of children in medieval times and throughout the seventeenth century was a harsh and unpleasant one. Few provisions were made for the care and treatment of orphans and foundlings. The hordes of children left orphaned by the ravages of war, plague and other epidemic diseases were left by a cruel and indifferent society to shift for themselves. It was common practice for unscrupulous people to horribly exploit these children by deliberately crippling them and sending them forth to beg. This pernicious practice was so open and flagrant, especially in Paris, that St. Vincent de Paul in about 1629 was able to enlist the aid of wealthy and influential people to establish an asylum for children. His movement brought about the founding of the Sisters of Charity or Mercy who were devoted to caring for sick and orphaned children.

This movement spread and gained support, not only in France, but throughout Europe. It led to better provisions for the care of foundlings and orphans and brought about the passage of laws providing for the punishment of crimes against children.

Although scientific medicine had been born during the seventeenth century, general medical practice as usual remained old-fashioned. The brilliant discoveries and activities of the scientific world failed to penetrate the complacency and ignorance of most medical practitioners. Popular medicine was still based on the medieval concepts of the humoral theory of disease. The physicians covered their ignorance by self-confidently swaggering about in their robes of office with their square caps set firmly on their powdered wigs. There was no clear-cut distinction between physicians and charlatans because both groups believed in occult powers and the superstitions of the times and routinely dispensed panaceas and secret remedies. It has been said that the physician rode into the seventeenth century on horseback sitting sidesaddle like a woman, and out of it in a carriage. However, he apparently acquired little real scientific medical knowledge on his passage through this century.

Great as were the advances of civilization during the seventeenth century, it was not a civilization of or for the masses. The increased prosperity, enlightenment, culture and scientific benefits did not extend below the upper middle classes. Manners had grown more elegant and people in good society no longer helped themselves at the table by dipping their hands into a common dish. The fork, an Italian invention, had come into use during this century. However, even among the upper classes, life was still crude and in spite of luxurious clothing, furniture and carriages, personal hygiene was generally unpracticed. Even among the lords and great ladies, with perhaps the exception of the rich bourgeois of Holland, bathing was no longer customary and there was a general lack of sanitary conveniences.

New worlds had been opened up by the advances of science and medicine during the seventeenth century, and great things had taken place. Yet all this meant little in the day-to-day lives of the great masses of people who lived, ate, sickened and died as always.

Chapter 17

THE EIGHTEENTH CENTURY

INTELLECTUALLY AND PHILOSOPHICALLY the eighteenth century was known as the Age of Enlightenment. The Enlightenment was an international philosophical movement that gave a tremendous impetus to learning and thereby stimulated social change and progress. It was characterized by rationalism and fostered a spirit of skepticism and empiricism in social and political thought. Basic to the Enlightenment was the acceptance of the belief that human intelligence was of supreme social value; the movement placed great confidence in the capacity of human reason to produce social progress. Its heritage stemmed from the works of Locke and Newton and it grew out of the social and economic ferment of late seventeenth century England.

As the Enlightenment grew and gained momentum, its intellectual leadership became French. It flourished and reached its height at or about midcentury, and the brilliant writings of the French philosophers Diderot, D'Alembert, Voltaire and Rosseau were typical of the movement. The Enlightenment provided the seed-bed which germinated a whole new set of ideas on social progress and human welfare. It did much to bring about and speed up the humanitarian and democratic movements which started their march during this century.

Historically the eighteenth century was characterized by a series of great political upheavals and crucial changes that exerted a profound effect upon the development of Western Civilization.

It was a time of great colonial expansion for England—she expanded into the British Empire. India was acquired in 1757 when Clive founded the British Indian Empire. In the Seven Years' War which lasted from 1756 to 1763, England and Prussia defeated Austria, France, Russia, Sweden and Saxony. The French and Indian Wars in America, which were a part of the Seven Years' War, caused

[132]

France to lose her American possessions and thus all of Canada became British.

Prussia's victorious emergence from the Seven Years' War established her as a power and enabled Frederick the Great to make her one of Europe's leading nations.

The eighteenth century also raised Russia to a first class power. Peter the Great's victory at the Battle of Poltava introduced Western Civilization into Russia. Catherine the Great, who ruled Russia from 1762 to 1796, was a capable ruler despite her personal capriciousness. She extended the borders of her country both in Asia and Europe, fostered progress and made Russia into one of the great nations of the world.

The latter half of the eighteenth century witnessed the occurrence of the great political revolutions in America and France. These two great revolutionary upheavals broke the age-old shackels of "royal tyranny" and spread the principles of democracy and the rights of the common man throughout the world.

The dawn of the eighteenth century witnessed the birth of occupational medicine. Progress, population growth and colonial expansion had led to an expansion of commerce and trade which in turn had stimulated industrial development. However, scant attention was given to the health of the workers; working conditions in the factories, mines and shops were abominable. Little or no recognition existed regarding occupational hazards and industrial diseases.

While at the University of Padua Bernardini Ramazzini in 1700 wrote the first comprehensive text book on occupational diseases and thereby qualified himself historically as the "father of industrial medicine."

Originally practicing in Modena, Ramazzini established a scholarly reputation through his controversies and correspondence with other physicians on exceptional cases that came to his attention. He was fortunate in being able to pursue his medical practice in a scholarly fashion by virtue of receiving patronage from the noble House of Este. Ramazzini conducted the first scientific survey of industrial diseases. He collected information concerning the hazards of various occupations by carefully questioning his patients regarding their occupations and personally visiting their places of work. From these studies and visits as well as from correspondents he collected information concerning a wide variety of occupations ranging from athletes to zinc miners. Out of this collection of observations came his famous book *De Morbis Artificum* or *The Diseases of Workers*.

Ramazzini dedicated his book to the moderators of Padua who had proferred him the chair of practical medicine at the University. He also gave credit to numerous observers who had furnished him with reports on various occupational diseases and disorders. In this comprehensive work he studied a total of fifty-three different occupations. He not only reported on the diseases that these occupations were liable to produce, but also gave recommendations as to their cure and methods of avoiding them. He recognized that prevention was of the utmost importance and noted that it was often impossible to persuade workers to take even the simplest of precautions.

That Ramazzini's insight and professional attitudes were far in advance of his times can be seen by the following quotation from his book.

> . . . in our own times also laws have been passed in well-ordered cities to secure good conditions for the workers; so it is only right that the art and science of medicine should contribute its portion for the benefit and relief of those for whom the law has shown such foresight; indeed we ought to show peculiar zeal, though so far we have neglected to do so, in taking precautions for their safety, so that as far as possible they may work at their chosen calling without loss of health. I for one have done all that lay in my power, and have not thought it beneath me to step into workshops of the meaner sort now and again and study the obscure operations of the mechanical arts . . .

Ramazzini summarized his work with recommendations for a general improvement of diet and less arduous work. His recommendations also included such prophylactic measures as bathing, frequent change of clothing, correct posture and covering the mouth in dusty trades. He concluded: "Pecuniary gain is worthless if it entails the loss of what is best worth having, health." He also stated: " 'Tis a sordid profit that's accompanied with the destruction of health."

His book was so well received that it was followed by a second edition in 1713. Originally written in Italian, it was translated into other languages and an English edition appeared in about 1750.

Because this work was so far in advance of its time, it remained as a standard reference for a long period.

Ramazzini also wrote *De Principum Valetudine,* a work expressing his views on the health of princes. This treatise on the medical care of the privileged classes was enthusiastically received all over Europe and Lancisi, the physician to Pope Clement XI, called it a work of gold.

Ramazzini lived to a ripe old age and suffered a fatal stroke shortly after his eighty-first birthday. During this terminal illness he was attended by his young friend, Morgagni. During his lifetime Ramazzini had deplored the barbaric customs of burial within churches and had written of this as follows: . . .

". . . the corpse-bearers have to go down into those terribly fetid caverns full of decomposing corpses and lay in them the bodies that have been brought there: hence they are exposed to very dangerous diseases, especially to malignant fevers and to sudden death . . ."

However, despite his feelings on this matter, he was buried in the Church of the Nuns of St. Helena in Padua.

At the close of the Seven Years' War, much remained in Europe to remind one of the Middle Ages. Feudalism and serfdom, although modified, still lingered and actually little industrial progress had been made. Tools and implements were little better than in ancient times and all manufacturing was done by hand. However during the second half of the eighteenth century there was a tremendous "Industrial Awakening."

The Industrial Awakening was ushered in by a number of great inventions which were destined to give Great Britain more wealth than her possession of Canada, Australia and the Indian Empire. One of the epoch-making inventions of history was the steam engine which is attributed to the Scotch inventor James Watt in about 1770. The spinning jenny was invented by Hargreaves in about 1765 and the power loom by Cartwright in 1785. Watt's engine was soon applied to these machines and steam power took the place of the tedious methods of hand spinning and weaving that had been in use since the dawn of history. Thus one person could now do what required more than a hundred before the time of the great inventions.

These great inventions and the many others that followed made Great Britain for the time being the workshop of the world. This leadership in manufacturing was brought about partly by the fast growing commerce that followed British colonial expansion.

The problem of motive power was solved when the steam engine by the use of shafts and cranks was made to turn the wheels of all sorts of machinery. Improvements in the production of iron soon followed. The use of coke made from coal took the place of charcoal in the smelting of iron and this with the improvements in mining reduced the cost of steam engines and increased their use.

The tremendous change in the industrial world brought about by the invention of machinery was not an unmixed good. It increased the wealth of the nations by leaps and bounds, but it brought distress rather than happiness to the common workers. The domestic system was replaced by the factory system. The rural homes of the spinners and the weavers, who had lived on their little farms, owned their own looms and wheels and sold their own products, were broken up. The workmen could not afford to purchase the expensive machinery nor could they, with the old methods, compete with the products of the new. In some places the people rose in riot against the new order, declaring that the new inventions took the bread out of their mouths. They attacked factories and destroyed machinery. Hargreaves, inventor of the spinning jenny, was mobbed by his fellow workmen and driven from his home.

The new machinery was costly. Only the rich could afford to purchase it. Factories were built in the cities and equipped with the necessary machinery. Thereby two new classes were added to society —the rich manufacturer or capitalist, and the common laborer who worked in his factory.

The spinners and weavers, unable to compete with the factory, had to give up their cottage homes and move to the city and become factory workers.

Working conditions in the factories were not organized or planned to protect the workers' health. On the contrary, machines were set up in any available shed or cellar and the workers were herded into them to toil long and hard for low wages.

The prosperity of eighteenth century England was founded upon its vast supplies of coal. The fires to drive British industry were lit in this century and were kept burning by the worldwide clamor for English goods. Soon forests of chimneys rose in the grey skies of English cities. Long monotonous rows of tenement homes were built to house the workers. Smoke from the belching chimneys blackened everything. Evylyn, a London diarist, wrote that Londoners were never free from coughs and that almost one-half of them died of "phthisical and pulmonic distempers."

Although industrial diseases were nothing new, the eighteenth century workers' burden of suffering was unequaled in history. Thousands of lead workers suffered from paralysis, while mercury and its vapors poisoned many more in a variety of trades. Glass makers, felt workers, and metal refiners died or were disabled from inhaling the noxious fumes of their trades. Textile workers and workers of all kinds succumbed to a variety of complaints as a result of toiling long hours in dark, dirty and dusty workrooms. In order to supply the power for all these industries the coal miners toiled incessantly in hastily sunk pits that were unprotected against the constant threat of accidental death.

The factories employed great numbers of women and children as well as men. Childhood frequently came to an end at the age of five or six when many children were sent to work in the grim factories or mines so as to earn the pittance which was needed to help their families live. Many of these children failed to survive their hard apprenticeship, and illness and death frequently terminated their careers by or before the age of fourteen.

During the eighteenth century motherhood was hazardous and infant life was cheap. Infant mortality averaged four out of ten babies born alive and seven out of every ten died before their fifth birthday. This mass murder of children was not accomplished by the contagious diseases alone, but was aided and abetted by the deplorable social conditions of the times. This wastage of child life was not considered to be alarming and parents believed that the deaths of one-half to three-quarters of their children before the age of two was normal and according to nature's plan.

Children in general were considered to be a troublesome burden, but especially so to the poor, and to the large numbers of unmarried mothers. The grinding poverty of the poor frequently compelled them to abandon their infants, leaving them to die of exposure, because they lacked the means of rearing them. It was also a common custom for mothers to drop off their unwanted offspring on the doorstep of some rich woman in the hope that she would provide a home for the foundling. Another way of getting rid of unwanted children was for a mother to claim that "overlaying" had accidentally killed her child. Because it was the belief that maternal warmth was good for babies, it was the custom for a mother to sleep in the same bed with her baby. Hence it was easy for an unmarried mother to toss about in her bed and to "accidentally" suffocate or crush her unwanted child with little or no fear of being punished.

Strange as it may seem the man who cried out against this "massacre of the innocents" in England was neither a father nor a doctor. Thomas Coram (1668-1751), a maritime trader and bachelor, took practical action to protect abandoned, neglected, and suffering children by establishing the first children's hospital in London. Coram was a successful maritime trader who had spent a number of profitable years in America and then returned to his native England. Moved to pity by the heartrending sight of the many babies that were abandoned along the highways leading to London, he spent his old age fighting to save such infants.

In 1739, Coram was instrumental in establishing London's Foundling Hospital. He was successful in gaining popular and powerful support for his movement. Dr. Richard Mead, the leading physician of London, supported him and acted as one of the governors of the hospital, while Hogarth, the famous artist, volunteered his services as official artist. Although it was really a children's shelter and not a hospital in the modern sense, it received generous aid and support from the medical profession. Thirty years later Coram's work led the Government to pass an act which enabled dependent children to be cared for.

There was little or no understanding of proper infant care and ignorance and superstition ran rife. Wet nursing was popular, especially among the rich. Unfortunately, most of these wet nurses were ignorant, lazy and untrained, hence babies were frequently neglected or brutally treated. The nurses commonly gave them liquor, not only to soothe and quiet them, but to "harden their systems." Cow's milk was looked at askance because it was superstitiously believed to give a child cow-like characteristics. Bread and water was considered to be the proper diet after nursing and thus rickets was common and bandy-legs were inevitable. Probably the greatest hazard facing an infant was the common practice of tight swaddling. Babies were tightly wrapped in heavy airtight bandages so that they looked like little "mummies." The purpose of this swaddling was to keep the bad air out and the natural nourishing juices in. It was considered dangerous to change diapers too often.

By and large, the medical profession was not concerned or alarmed by the poor care and neglect accorded to children. Doctors in general believed children to be outside of their sphere of care and left the "little nuisances" to the care of their mothers and nurses. Children were viewed as "miniature grown-ups" and when doctors did treat them, they were bled and drugged just like adults.

However medical interest was finally aroused during the 1740's when some pioneer pediatricians made themselves heard. Among these was Dr. William Cadogan of London, who wrote his famous "Essay Upon Nursing" in 1748. Until this time England had more and better books on the cure and care of horses than upon the care of infants.

In his book Cadogan told mothers it was dangerous and harmful to use swaddling clothes. He advocated breast feeding and cried out against the "unwholesome messes" that were fed to infants. Cadogan's work increased pediatric interest and sparked the development of this vital branch of medicine.

In France the philosopher Jean Jacques Rousseau advocated that children should be allowed to grow up "free and straight as a tree," unimpaired by the hampering conventions of civilization. This idea found a medical counterpart when the science of orthopedics was founded by the French physician Nicolas André (1658-1742). André was the first to ever publish a book especially on orthopedics and was responsible for coining the term.

In 1741 he published a book called *Orthopaedia, or the Art of Correcting and Preventing Deformities in Children*. In this book, André gives the following explanation of the origin of this word: "I have formed it of two Greek words, viz. 'orthos', which signifies straight, free from deformity and 'paidos', a child. Out of these two words, I have compounded that of Orthopaedia, to express in one term the design I propose, which is to teach the different methods of preventing and correcting the deformities of children".

André not only was the founding father of orthopedics, but also tremendously influenced the current concepts of child care. He not only advocated child welfare, but also emphasized its preventive aspects by recognizing that society can be saved much suffering and expense if abnormalities are detected and corrected at an early age.

As industrialization and urbanization took place, numerous unhealthy social and environmental conditions developed which affected both the rich and the poor. Even as measured by eighteenth century standards, these conditions were deplorable. Poverty, thievery, contagion, child neglect, gin drinking and filth were widespread and rampant. As these deplorable conditions continued and grew worse they cried out for correction and reform. Sporadically they began to receive the thought and attention of some of the more enlightened citizens of the times.

Society as a whole gradually began to recognize its obligations toward the welfare of all of its members. The idea grew that all men were equal and imbued with reason and hence society should be concerned with the care of the poor, the crippled, and even its criminals. Medicine joined, and sometimes led, the fight for the more humane treatment of these unfortunates. Even the rich joined the movement, not only for charitable reasons, but because they recognized that sick and impoverished people created economic waste and loss. They realized that this economic loss reduced the ability to purchase and produce goods and thus undermined the nation's wealth.

In England, gin drinking became the chief escape from the problems and drabness of life. Drunkenness became so commonplace that it affected the national economy by upsetting the capacity and productivity of the workers. In an attempt to remedy these conditions, Parliament passed several Gin Acts during the eighteenth century. These acts limited the number of "pot-houses," which had numbered one to every six dwelling places, and relegated them to every street corner. Despite these regulations, drunkenness, squalor and poverty continued to be prevalent everywhere.

One of the outstanding sociomedical reformers of the times was the Quaker physician, John Coakley Lettsom (1744-1815). The son of a Quaker planter, Lettsom was born in the British Virgin Islands, but at an early age was sent to London for his education. He studied medicine under the famous Quaker physician John Fothergill at St. Thomas' Hospital. Upon completion of his studies, Lettsom returned to the Virgin Islands and began the practice of medicine. When his father died, leaving him a few slaves and a small tract of land, Lettsom freed the slaves, parcelled out the land, and gave the slaves the tools they needed to cultivate the crops.

Lettsom then returned to England to study with Cullen at Edinburg, but shortly after went on to Leyden where he received his M.D. degree in 1769. After some further travels on the Continent, Lettsom returned to London, married a woman of wealth and established his medical practice. Soon the combination of a wealthy wife and a profitable practice gave him financial security and enabled him to participate in various philanthropic and reform movements.

In 1787 Lettsom prepared an original account on alcoholism which was published in the *Memoirs of the Medical Society of London*. This excellent clinical treatise was one of the first accounts on this condition. In it he accurately described the symptomatology and physiological effects of chronic alcoholism and stressed its compulsive and addictive aspects. He concluded his account as follows:

> I would not, however, infer, that every spirit-drinker acquires the symtoms of disease above related, or that other diseases do not more frequently succeed this dangerous habit: hepatic affections, of various kinds, it is well known, usually result from intemperance, and dropsies often succeed: . . . There is something in spirituous liquors, so injurious to the human frame, that too much attention cannot be paid in discouraging the use of them . . . and it is from the most decided conviction of the injury, that I would guard every person from beginning with even a little drop of this fascinating poison, which once admitted, is seldom, if ever, afterwards overcome.

Lettsom was instrumental in founding the General Dispensary in

London. Ambulatory care had scarcely existed prior to this time
and hence the establishment of an outpatient clinic inaugurated a
new era in the care and treatment of the poor. Ambulatory cases
were treated by senior physicians in the clinic while those too sick
to attend were treated at home. The success of the General Dispensary
soon led to the setting up of other dispensaries. These outpatient
clinics afforded an excellent opportunity for the training of young
physicians and they soon were in competition with the teaching hospitals for student fees.

In 1773 Lettsom helped found the Medical Society of London
and the Royal Humane Society in the following year. He was active
in prison reform and promoted a summer camp for poor children.
Having sponsored smallpox inoculation prior to Jenner's work on
cowpox, he soon accepted the merits of this discovery and provided
Benjamin Waterhouse of Boston and others with dried lymphs for
vaccination.

Lettsom dressed himself in simple Quaker garb and throughout
his life advocated brotherly love, philanthropy for the poor and social
reform for all. He gave generously of both his time and money to
various charitable causes, not only in England, but in the Colonies
as well. Harvard, Dartmouth, Dickinson, and Bowdoin colleges were
recipients of gifts, books, and specimens of natural history. Pennsylvania Hospital sought his advice in the selection of books for the
medical library and, in turn, received suggestions and volumes from
his own library. The College of Physicians of Philadelphia elected
him a Fellow, and Harvard College honored him with a Doctor
of Laws.

Lettsom died in 1815 of an infection acquired while conducting
a postmortem examination. That he truly loved medicine and
especially his work in the outpatient dispensary is shown by the following excerpt from one of his letters:

> . . . this is the highest and most devine profession, that can engage
> human intellect. I have attended eighty-two-thousand patients, and what
> can equal the dignity of having so many lives intrusted to your decision;
> What more devine, than to soothe the afflicted, and soften agony! What
> more sublime than to restore to life the victim of disease! I envy not
> the prince on the throne, nor the sultan in his harem, whilst I enjoy the
> confidence of the sick chamber, and the blessings of the restored. I love

my profession, perhaps too much. It loves me, and I have no objection
to die in the chamber of malady, provided I can mitigate it in a fellow
creature—and so every other physician would, I doubt not, reason.

Perhaps the most appalling of all social conditions existing in
eighteenth century England was that of its jails. The prisons were not
only disgracefully neglected and overcrowded, but were downright
dirty and filthy, with an almost complete lack of sanitary facilities.
Bad social conditions on the outside plus the pressures and struggles
of a highly competitive society forced more and more people down-
ward so that many of them either resorted to a life of crime or
landed in a debtor's cell. The debtor's cells housed many hundreds
of poor innocent men and women, many of whom succumbed from
various diseases and debilities induced by poor food, overcrowding and
bad hygienic conditions.

A newcomer to the prison population would find himself locked in
a small dirty room along with thirty to fifty other wretched people.
Men, women and children were often locked up together with neither
beds nor covers provided for their rest and comfort. Sanitary facilities often consisted of one malodorous and filthy privy. All of the
prisoners soon became louse infested because the clean and the
verminous were forced to lie down together. Hence outbreaks of
"jail-fever" were frequent, because it never took very long for
infected lice to convey typhus throughout these vermin-infested jails.

That "disease is no respecter of persons" and that "iron bars
do not a prison make" in so far as typhus is concerned, was demonstrated in 1750 during the Easter Session of the Old Bailey. The
Lord Mayor of London and numerous other important personages
sickened and died from the same contagion that was raging throughout Newgate Prison. Inquiry and investigation revealed that "the
whole prison of Newgate and all the passages leading thence were in
a very filthy condition and had long been so."

Thus the time was ripe and the ground was ready to receive the
seeds of prison reform that were to be sown by John Howard, sheriff
of Bedfordshire. This English philanthropist, social reformer and
hygienist, devoted a large part of his life to cleaning up jails and
introducing sanitary reforms.

Born at Hackney, England in 1726, John Howard was the son

of a wealthy upholsterer. After his father died and left him a fortune in 1742, he spent his time traveling extensively. Shortly after the death of his first wife, he sailed on a trip to Lisbon and in 1756 was captured by a French privateer and imprisoned at Brest. This captivity, although relatively short, left a lasting impression on him regarding the cruel and inhuman treatment accorded prisoners of war.

Following his release and return to England he married a second time and settled at Cardington, near Bedford. In 1773 he became the high sheriff for Bedfordshire and as a result of his duties became further interested in prison reform.

John Howard thus became well aware of the appalling conditions existing in the jails and recognized the fact that many prisoners were unjustly detained. Many were imprisoned without ever having had a trial, while others were held even after having been found innocent or having served their sentences, because they were unable to pay certain fees which were assessed against them. Jailers had no fixed salaries and earned their livelihood from fees assessed against their prisoners. Before release these fees had to be paid, either by the prisoner or his friends or relatives.

Howard made a series of tours throughout Great Britain and Ireland for the purpose of studying and investigating prisons and prisoners. He thoroughly studied the problem and reported to Parliament on the filthy conditions of the jails and the unjust and inhuman treatment accorded the prisoners. He advocated cleanliness and recommended that sanitary and bathing facilities should be available and that prisoner's clothes should be baked so as to destroy vermin and disease. He further recognized the need for isolation in order to keep the sick from spreading their diseases to the well.

Chiefly as a result of Howard's efforts, Parliament passed two acts in 1774, one providing for fixed salaries for jailers and the other to enforce cleanliness. Howard continued his visits and studies of British jails and in addition studied many prisons on the European Continent. In 1777 he wrote, *The State of Prisons in England and Wales, with an Account of Some Foreign Prisons.* In 1780 he wrote *An Account of the Principal Lazarettos in Europe.*

Howard also was interested in hospital reform. Eighteenth Century hospitals were an outgrowth of the old "pest houses" of the Middle

Ages and the charitable institutions founded by the Medieval Monks. Howard challenged public complacency by giving graphic descriptions of the deplorable conditions that existed in the hospitals that he visited. Many famous hospitals were exposed for being dirty, neglected and verminous. For example, St. Thomas' had no water closets, while at Middlesex Hospital the patients were crowded in wooden beds which were enclosed by suffocating hangings that excluded all fresh air. Hospital staffs were untrained, poorly paid and generally of low caliber, so that drunkenness and immorality were common.

Patients were neglected, badly treated and poorly fed. Many of the hospitals instead of curing patients, actually served as breeding places for the further spread of disease. Howard's exposé and indictment of the hospitals helped to bring about some badly needed improvements, reforms and rebuilding.

Ironically enough, John Howard died in 1790 at the age of sixty-four from "camp fever," contracted while attending an inmate at a prison he was visiting in Kherson, Russia.

John Wesley, the famous eighteenth century English preacher and founder of the Methodist Church, had a tremendous impact not only on the spiritual lives of his people, but upon the hygiene of his age. Born June 17, 1703, the son of the rector of Epworth, this remarkable man spent half a century carrying out his evangelistic mission. He travelled over 250,000 miles and preached over 40,000 sermons. During his itinerary crowds of from 10,000 to 30,000 people would wait patiently for hours to hear him. He gave his strength to the working classes and his converts were colliers, miners, weavers, foundrymen, and workers of every kind.

He produced a tremendous amount of literary work, including pamphlets, books, psalms and hymnals. His work and teachings dealt not only with the spiritual methods of living, but with the physical as well. Because he preached a methodical manner of living, his converts and followers were called "Methodists" from the strict regularity of their lives.

In about 1745 he wrote his famous book, entitled *Primitive Physick: or an Easy and Natural Method of Curing Most Diseases*. This book exerted a tremendous impact upon the health and hygiene of his age by giving a set of useful rules on personal hygiene. In this book Wesley gave to the world the famous aphorism "Cleanliness is, indeed, next to Godliness."

Science, which had taken tremendous strides during the seventeenth century, continued its unbroken progress throughout the eighteenth century. Medicine, however, had progressed more slowly and lagged behind the general advancement of science. The seventeenth century medical advances in physiology, chemistry and microscopy had given doctors a multiplicity of baffling facts which they were unable to apply in daily practice. The discoveries of Harvey, Boyle and Leeuwenhoek seemed to have no immediate bearing on medical practice and patients were unrelieved and continued to suffer from their same old diseases.

Thus, as the eighteenth century dawned, the time was ripe for medicine to take stock and assimilate this newly discovered scientific knowledge. The fundamentals of medicine needed analysis and correlation with the known basic scientific facts.

By the beginning of the eighteenth century the University of Leyden in Holland had become the leading medical center of Europe. Herman Boerhaave (1668-1738), a clinician of great intelligence and deep understanding, had acquired a reputation as the greatest doctor of his time. Hundreds of patients clamored to see him daily and students from all parts of Europe flocked to Leyden to attend his lectures. Like Hippocrates and Sydenham, Boerhaave brought medicine to the bedside and made the patient the center of medical attention by teaching in the hospital wards. A great orator who possessed personal warmth and great common sense, he was able to lecture with simplicity and clarity. Not since Galen had a clinician achieved such a wide reputation as a teacher. His fame was so great that a Chinese mandarin had supposedly sent a letter simply addressed to "Boerhaave of Europe" and it was promptly delivered to him. He systematized medical knowledge and classified medical theory through his excellent teaching and exemplary care of the sick.

A many-talented man, his interests included philosophy, chemistry, botany and physics, as well as clinical medicine. He held four professorships at once at Leyden, lecturing on medicine, chemistry, pharmacology and botany. In his lectures he set forth the new concepts of basic science and explained physiology and morbidity according to the laws of physics, mathematics and chemistry. He lectured not only at the bedside, but also in the postmortem room, and had the ability to make connections between different fragments of knowledge.

Boerhaave himself did not advance medicine by making any great discoveries or innovations. His fame rests upon his abilities as a medical leader and great teacher. His greatest success lay in the training and education of the "medically great." Many of his pupils were destined to advance medical science and to revitalize medical education.

A great pupil of Boerhaave's was the Hollander, Gerard van Swieten (1700-1772), who became physician to the Austrian Empress and was the initiator of the great medical school at Vienna. Among Boerhaave's disciples was Albrecht von Haller, a poetic Swiss physician who established physiology as a science while at Goettingen. Another Boerhaave pupil was Alexander Munro who founded the Munro dynasty at Edinburgh where for the next 126 years grandfather, father and grandson all occupied the chair of anatomy. Linneaeus, the great Swedish botanist, who was also professor of medicine at the University of Uppsala, studied under Boerhaave.

The influence of Boerhaave extended to America and his lectures and texts formed the essentials of every eighteenth century American physician's library. The practice of Benjamin Rush, as well as almost every physician in Philadelphia, was governed and influenced by Boerhaave's system of clinical medicine.

Not only was Boerhaave famous as a physician but he was extremely popular as a citizen of Leyden. On one occasion following his recovery from an illness the city held a public celebration in his honor. He gave freely of his skill to the poor and stated that they were his best patients "for God paid for them." He died at the age of seventy and legend states that he bequeathed to the world a large and elegant volume entitled *All of the Secrets of Physic.* However, upon opening the volume, every page was found to be blank, save one, upon which he summed up all of his medical knowledge with the statement; "Keep the head cool, the feet warm and the bowels open."

Although London ranked below Leyden as a medical center during the first half of the eighteenth century, it produced a number of physicians who contributed to the advance of clinical medicine. Dr. John Radcliffe was a wealthy and powerful physician who advanced medical education by bequeathing most of his fortune to Oxford University and endowing Radcliffe Observatory, Hospital and Library. He is credited with summing up the medical knowledge of his times by saying that as a young practitioner he knew ten remedies for every disease, but that in his old age he knew twenty diseases, but not one remedy.

Dr. Richard Mead succeeded to Radcliffe's practice and became the foremost physician of London. His practice was so successful that he reputedly earned 7,000 pounds annually, which would be the approximate equivalent of 100,000 pounds today. Although he lived lavishly in princely style, he never lost his humane touch. He was interested in sanitary reform and advocated that the government set up an agency similar in function to a national health council.

When a disastrous outbreak of plague struck Marseille in 1719, Mead was requested by the government to study the epidemic and to propose measures to keep it from striking England. In 1720 he wrote a treatise entitled *A Short Discourse Concerning Pestilential Contagion and the Methods to be Used to Prevent It.* This little book of 150 pages was concerned chiefly with plague and discussed its history, cause, control and prevention.

Although he attributed the cause of the plague to the contamination of the air, he discounted the idea that it was caused by Divine Providence. He recognized the importance of direct contagion and condemned the practice of quarantining and locking up the sick with their families. He recommended that plague victims be removed and isolated in "plague houses."

In general his book was full of common sense and proved so popular that it went through seven editions.

One of the great medical advances of the eighteenth century was the founding of pathologic anatomy by Giovanni Battista Morgagni, professor of anatomy at Padua. By establishing clinical pathology as a distinct part of medicine he gave physicians their present day concept of disease. He was the first to correlate anatomical appearances after death with the clinical features of disease during life. He carefully connected the symptomatology and clinical history of disease with the structural alterations and anatomic changes he found on postmortem dissection. He thus overthrew the ancient and erroneous concepts which ascribed illness and disease to a disturbance of the four humors or to an upset of atoms and pores.

Giovanni Battista Morgagni was born February 25, 1682 in Forli, Italy. At the early age of fifteen he began his medical studies at Bologna, where he was fortunate enough to be a pupil of the great anatomist Valsalva. He was granted his doctorate in medicine and philosophy in 1701. Morgagni continued on at Bologna as Valsalva's anatomical assistant and frequently filled his professorial chair when he was absent.

In 1706 at the age of twenty-five he published an anatomical text entitled *Adversaria Anatomica*. This book established his reputation as a great anatomist and attached his name to a number of anatomical structures which he was the first to describe accurately. Morgagni's reputation grew and in 1711 he went to the University of Padua where three years later he was elevated to the chair of anatomy. Thus at the early age of thirty-five he was following in the footsteps of such anatomical greats as Vesalius, Columbus and Fallopius and lectured from the most famous anatomical theater in the world.

Morgagni proved to be a great and enthusiastic teacher and his lectures and demonstrations became so popular that he attracted many students to Padua from all over Europe. He served as professor of anatomy for fifty-six years and became so famous that he was referred to as "His Anatomical Majesty."

Not until 1761 when he was nearly eighty did Morgagni publish his greatest work, *De Sedibus et Causes Morborum* or *On the Seats and Causes of Disease*. After nearly fifty years of teaching he assembled seventy of his epistles in which he described the findings of some seven hundred autopsies. This five-volume work embodied a lifetime of experience in dissection and observation and was one of the great scientific works of the eighteenth century. This work was carefully systematized and cross-indexed so as to correlate the clinical history with the postmortem findings. He gave the first descriptions of luetic lesions in the cerebrum and the cardiac valves as well as emphasizing the importance of visceral lues. In his reports of many autopsies, he proved that the cerebral lesions in cerebral vascular accidents were on the opposite side from the resulting paralysis. With his life and work, clinical pathology began to be established as a distinct part of medicine.

Pathology was thus removed from the realm of purely academic speculation. Whereas it had previously been pursued chiefly because of curiosity and the hope of findings bizarre monstrosities or gross abnormalities, it now acquainted physicians with the bodily ravages that the common diseases produced.

In 1761, the same year that Morgagni published his great work, an Austrian physician, Leopold Auenbrugger published a small significant book that inaugurated the art of physical diagnosis. In this ninety-five page book entitled *Inventum Novum* or *A New Invention,* Auenbrugger using only twelve hundred words described his discovery of percussion as a diagnostic measure.

Dr. Leopold Joseph von Auenbrugger was born in 1722, the music loving son of an Austrian innkeeper. He studied medicine at Vienna where he was a pupil of the great physiologist Gerard van Swieten. Like other eighteenth century physicians he had only two accepted methods for examining a patient. He could observe the patient's respiration and he could take his pulse. As an innkeeper's son, he had often seen his father and others tapping wine casks in order to find out whether they were full or empty. Auenbrugger therefore reasoned that the chest cavity has a different resonance when it is filled with air than when it is filled with liquid.

While serving as a physician at the Spanish Hospital in Vienna, Auenbrugger's knowledge of music and acoustics prompted him to explore percussion as a method for examining patients suffering from diseases of the chest. While his colleagues shook their heads in disbelief he methodically tapped his patients' chests and carefully noted the sounds produced. Seven years were required to develop his methods and to check on the autopsies and experiments he conducted at the Spanish Hospital. His discoveries on percussion included information concerning the size of the heart and the state, healthy or diseased, of the contents of the pleural cavity.

In the preface of his book, Auenbrugger stated: "I here present the Reader with a new sign which I have discovered for detecting diseases of the chest. This consists in the Percussion of the human thorax, whereby, according to the character of the particular sounds thence elicited, an opinion is formed of the internal state of that cavity."

Auenbrugger was aware that his book would make him unpopular with the conservative physicians of his time.

"In making public my discoveries," he stated in the introduction, "I have not been unconscious of the dangers I must encounter; since it has always been the fate of those who have illustrated or improved the arts and sciences by their discoveries to be beset by envy, malice, hatred, detraction and calumny."

He was not wrong. Soon after publication of his book, he was forced to resign his hospital post.

Dedicated to the welfare of his patients, grave, gentle and charitable, Auenbrugger seemed untroubled by the reception given his work. He continued with his large private practice in Vienna. He also pursued his interest in music which had probably contributed to his discovery of percussion and wrote the libretto to Salieri's opera, "The Chimney Sweep." Fortunately, Auenbrugger lived long enough to see his work win recognition. In 1808, a year before his death at eighty-seven and almost a half a century after the publication of his book, Corvisart, physician to Napoleon I and a leader of the French medical profession, published his own observations on percussion. Unlike many early physicians, Corvisart was generous with credit and praise for Auenbrugger's original contribution. This approval marked the beginning of medical acceptance for percussion as a diagnostic technique.

The eighteenth century witnessed the rise of surgery from the level of a handicraft to the respected height of a professional science. During the Middle Ages, medicine and surgery had been separated, much to the detriment of both of these branches of the healing art. Surgery had been left in the hands of uneducated craftsmen such as barbers, bone setters, bathhouse keepers and sow-gelders. The architect of the bridge between medicine and surgery and the founder of scientific surgery was John Hunter.

Hunter was born February 13, 1728 on a farm in Lanarkshire, Scotland, the youngest of ten children. His father died when he was thirteen and John grew up to be a rough, red headed country boy who successfully escaped almost all formal education. He was an unsatisfactory pupil at school and his ill temper made him personally unpopular. However, he apparently had an inquiring mind for in later years he said of himself, "When I was a boy, I pestered people with questions about what nobody knew or cared anything about."

John's older brother, William, his senior by ten years, had first studied for the ministry, but had later turned to medicine. Well educated and able, William had successfully established himself in London as an outstanding surgeon and obstetrician. He was also successfully operating a school of anatomy. In 1748, while still in his twenties, John became apprenticed to his brother. Here his talents flowered and he soon became a skilled dissector. Within two years he was supervising his brother's classes in practical anatomy. In the summers, when weather made dissecting impossible, John Hunter studied surgery under William Cheselden at Chelsea Hospital and later under Percival Pott, at St. Bartholomew's. Under these masters he walked the hospital wards, assisted at major surgical operations and learned the skill and art of sound, simple surgical technique. All the while he continued with his studies and dissections in his brother's anatomical laboratory. In 1753, along with the famous Dr. Percival Pott, he was honored by the Surgeons Corporation by receiving the degree of Master of Anatomy.

In 1789 a lung inflammation caused him to adopt another way of life. The war with Spain and France gave him the opportunity to become an army surgeon and then a naval surgeon. Thus, experience in the field supplied the foundation for the excellent work *A Treatise on the Blood, Inflammation, and Gunshot Wounds*. This milestone in the development of general pathology was published a year after his death.

In 1763 the Peace of Paris brought Hunter back to London where he embarked upon the practice of surgery in Golden Square. However, surgery was for him only a means to an end and he avidly pursued his studies in comparative anatomy and natural science. As soon as his surgical practice was sufficiently remunerative he moved from his Golden Square consulting rooms, first into his brother's house in Jerymn Street and then into a much larger establishment in Leicester

Square. He started his famous museum of comparative anatomy and his collection eventually contained over 13,600 specimens. He collected everything—plants, animals, monsters, mummies, skulls, diseased hearts, brains, spleens and kidneys, thousands upon thousands of specimens, preserved dry, in spirits or stuffed.

To further his study of living animals, he purchased two acres of land in 1764, "about two miles from London near Brompton, at a place called Earl's Court." Here he built a house and gathered an extensive menagerie of both domesticated and rare animals. If he could not obtain the rare beasts he required from circuses and zoos, he wrote begging letters to correspondents in Africa and Asia. To his good friend and former pupil, Edward Jenner, he sent requests for cuckoo eggs, salmon spawn and porpoise nipples.

Hunter's scientific curiosity knew no bounds and the records show that he dissected more than five hundred different species of creatures and "some thousands" of his fellow human beings. He pioneered a daring operation for popliteal aneurysm by tying off the main artery above the aneurysm and allowing the collateral circulation to supply blood to the lower leg. In the field of experimental surgery he caused a cock's spur to grow from its comb, and a cock's testicle to flourish in the belly of a hen. He wrote a book entitled *A Treatise on the Natural History of the Human Teeth* and after investigating the behavior of whales, wrote his *Observations on the Structure and Economy of the Whale*.

The great length to which Hunter would go to secure material for his collection is illustrated by the story of his acquisition of the skeleton of the Irish Giant. In 1783, he visited an exhibition of freaks and became interested in Charles Byrne or O'Brien, who was known as the Irish Giant. Byrne was nearly eight feet tall and was in poor health. In an interview, Hunter informed him that all giants had a short life expectancy and requested permission to dissect his body after death. The Irish Giant had a superstitious horror of being dissected and on his death bed left orders that his body was to be closely guarded and sealed in a lead casket. He requested that his burial was to be at sea and that the casket was to be dumped into the Irish Channel so that his body could never reach Hunter's dissecting table. However, Hunter bribed the undertaker's guards and had the body stolen from the casket. Thus John Hunter's persistence won out and the bones of the Irish Giant instead of lying on the bottom of the Irish Channel were articulated and still hang in the Museum of the Royal College of Surgeons in London.

Hunter studied the venereal diseases and accurately described the sore of primary syphilis which is still called the "Hunterian Chancre." It was in connection with his studies on these diseases that he made his greatest mistake. In order to find out whether gonorrhea and syphilis were separate diseases or merely differnt symptoms of the same disease, Hunter inoculated himself with the discharges from a venereal patient. Through bad luck he inadvertently selected a patient who was suffering from both diseases and thus unhappily contracted both syphilis and gonorrhea. This unfortunate error led him to proclaim that the two diseases were identical and his preeminence was so great that this error was generally accepted. This ill-fated experiment not only succeeded in holding back progress in the field of venereal diseases for almost a century, but also wrecked his health. He developed a syphilitic aortitis which later led to his dramatic death from an anginal attack.

Combining natural talent, insatiable curiosity and keen observation, John Hunter was one of the greatest comparative anatomists and naturalists of all times. However, his chief claim to fame rests upon the fact that he raised the status of surgery from a rough and ready craft carried on by men of doubtful reputations to an honorable and scientific branch of medicine.

Because of his angina, Hunter tolerated fools poorly, and his easily aroused anger frequently precipitated an attack. On October 16, 1793, during a heated board meeting at St. George's Hospital, Hunter's wrath was aroused to the point where he collapsed and died from an anginal attack. He was at first buried at St. Martins-in-the-Fields, but in 1859 his remains were reburied with great honors in Westminster Abbey. The brass plaque over his grave honors him with the simple inscription: "The Founder of Scientific Surgery."

The scientific interest and curiosity of the eighteenth century was so great that many classes and professions took an active interest in the world about them. Dukes, politicians and clergymen as well as physicians experimented in the fields of biology, chemistry and physics.

Many theologians were no longer content with philosophical speculations and, hence, actively conducted scientific experiments in an attempt to solve the mysteries of life. Therefore, it is not as strange as it may at first seem that several of the most important scientific discoveries of the eighteenth century were made by two English parsons whose avocation was physiology. The Reverend Doctor Stephen Hales discovered the measurement of the systemic blood pressure and the Reverend Joseph Priestly isolated oxygen and investigated respiration.

Although Stephen Hales was a conscientious English clergyman who never forsook his theological duties, he achieved everlasting fame as a physiologist. Born in 1677 at Bekesbourne, Kent, little is known of his early life until he entered Cambridge at nineteen. Here he studied physics and astronomy and participated in biological studies and experiments. He graduated with a Bachelor of Arts degree at the age of twenty-five and then went on to receive his Master's as well as a Bachelor of Divinity degree. In 1709 he was appointed curate of Teddington in Middlesex, a position which he held until his death and which earned him the title of "perpetual curate."

As an avocation, Hales continued to carry on his experiments in natural science. In 1727 he published a work entitled *Vegetable Staticks* which reported on the movement of sap in plants and trees. However, his great work dealing with the hemodynamics of the central and peripheral circulation, was described in *Haemastaticks,* published in 1733. These important investigations had been started some twenty years before their publication. His first circulatory experiments were performed on dogs and later on horses. Hales described his monumental experiment on the measurement of blood pressure as follows:

> Then laying bare the left Carotid Artery, I fixed to it towards the Heart and the Brass Pipe, and to that the Wind-Pipe of a Goose; to the other End of which a Glass Tube was fixed, which was twelve Feet nine Inches long. The Design of using the Wind-Pipe was by its Pliancy to prevent the Inconveniences that might happen when the Mare struggled; if the Tube had been immediately fixed to the Artery, wthout the Intervention of this pliant Pipe.
>
> There had been lost before the Tube was fixed to the Artery, about seventy cubick Inches of Blood. The Blood rose in the Tube in the same

manner as in the Case of the two former Horses, till it reached to nine
Feet six Inches Height. I then took away the Tube from the Artery, and
let out by Measure sixty cubick Inches of Blood, and then immediately
replaced the Tube to see how high the Blood would rise in it after each
Evacuation; this was repeated several times, till the Mare expired.

Thus, Hales introduced quantitative measurement into the study
of the circulation, progressing from the simple measurement of blood
pressure to the more complex circulatory interplay of pressure, flow
and resistance. These facts together with the scientific methods that
he used and his concept that a living organism is a self-regulatory
machine, assured Hales a place in history, second only to Harvey, as
a founder of physiology.

That Hales was a versatile man is shown by the fact that during
the sixth decade of his life, he became interested in various social and
hygienic reforms. This was typified by his invention of a bellows
type of ventilator, which could be operated manually or by a windmill, for improving the ventilation of jails, ships and hospitals. He
arranged to have a windmill type of ventilator installed on the roof
of Newgate Prison. The improvement in ventilation that it brought
about is said to have markedly reduced the death rate of the inmates
from "gaol fever." Hales also actively aided in the passage of the
Gin Act of 1736 and served as a trustee for the founding of the Colony
of Georgia.

A man of great genius and simplicity, the Reverend Doctor Stephen
Hales died in 1761 at the age of eighty-four, after leading a long and
busy life.

Like Stephen Hales, the Reverend Joseph Priestly's interests in
science were avocational. The vocation of each was theology with
the difference that while Hales remained as a "perpetual curate" in
one parish, Priestly moved about frequently in an attempt to better
his position. He gained most of his livelihood as a minister and teacher,
supplemented by royalties from his writings, and received some assist-
ance from friends for his scientific research.

Joseph Priestly was born in 1733 a few miles from Leeds in York-
shire and died in exile in Northumberland, Pennsylvania in 1804.
He was an avid reader and a prolific writer, with most of his writings
dealing with theology, natural philosophy and metaphysics. His scien-

tific presentations consisted of various experiments in chemistry, some original experiments on electricity, as well as a history on electricity and another on optics. Some of his experiments attracted worldwide attention and he received early recognition for his scientific accomplishments. Edinburgh awarded him an honorary LL.D. in 1764 and he was elected to Fellowship in the Royal Society in 1766.

From 1761 to 1767 he taught at Warrington Academy, one of the most influential dissenting schools in England. Here he introduced the teaching of modern history and political science. He subscribed to the doctrine of "philosophical necessity" which believed in a natural order of society in which the world of man was as ordered and regular as the Newtonian universe. He consequently believed that any effort to tamper with the social processes was contrary to nature and that attempt to provide relief from poverty and idleness by government "poor laws" was an obstacle to self help. He believed that the poor should be compelled to fend for themselves and stimulated to help themselves by being provident. Priestly expressed this belief by stating, "that individuals when left to themselves are, in general, sufficiently provident and will daily better their circumstances."

His next position was at the chapel at Leeds, which fortunately provided him with a salary adequate to support his family. Here he carried out some of his most notable experiments.

In 1774 Joseph Priestly heated mercuric oxide and recovered and isolated oxygen which he called "dephlogisticated air." Unfortunately, he attempted to fit his observations into the phlogiston theory and thereby failed to "discover" oxygen. Hence the first honors for the discovery of oxygen as a new gas went to Lavoisier by default. Priestly also studied a number of other gases, such as nitrous oxide, ammonia, chloric, sulphurous and fluor acid. He investigated the reaction of oxygen and metals, combustion, the respiration of lower and higher animals, putrefaction and the relationship of the vegetable and animal kingdom.

Priestly's home, meeting house, and laboratory were destroyed by rioters in 1791 because of his expressed sympathy for the French Revolution. His library and experimental laboratory were demolished and many of his unpublished manuscripts were burned. He fled to London under an assumed name and in 1794 left England to come to the newly organized United States. Here he passed up an offer to serve as professor of chemistry at the College of Philadelphia and retired to reside in Northumberland, Pennsylvania.

A great and kindly man who contributed much to science, Priestly found peace and refuge in the home state of his scientific colleague and good friend, Benjamin Franklin.

One of the most significant scientific contributions to medicine during the eighteenth century was the work of a young French chemist named Antoine Laurent Lavoisier. Although not a physician, Lavoisier unlocked one of the great medical mysteries of all times by demonstrating how we breathe. He proved what actually happens during respiration, how oxygen is utilized and carbon dioxide expelled. He thus opened the way to the scientific understanding of the physiology of human respiration and diseases involving the lungs.

The son of a middle class lawyer, Lavoisier was born in Paris on August 26, 1743. He studied law at Mazarin College, receiving his Bachelor of Laws degree in 1763. However, he was keenly interested in all of the natural sciences and soon revealed his special talents for chemical research. In 1765 he published his first paper on chemistry and in 1766 he won a medal from the King for an essay on metropolitan street lighting. Two years later, he was made a member of the Royal Academy of Science.

In 1768 at the age of twenty-five, Lavoisier bought a share in the Ferme Generale. This was a much-hated group of private financiers to whom the French government had given the profitable monopoly of collecting the national taxes. Later, during the French Revolution, this association was to cost him his life. Lavoisier married Marie Paulze, the daughter of a Ferme colleague, in 1771. A brilliant and talented woman, she aided her husband in his scientific work by taking notes, translating scientific papers and making sketches.

Undoubtedly, Lavoisier's greatest accomplishment was his discovery of oxygen which led him to an almost complete reconstruction of the science of chemistry. He proved that water is a compound rather than an element and completely overthrew the ancient theory of the four elements, air, earth, fire and water. He upset the phlogiston theory by proving that burning substances combine with oxygen and give off both heat and carbon dioxide. He summed up the newer concepts of chemistry in his work *Traite Elementaire de Chimie* published in 1789. His book included a new system of chemical nomenclature which with only minor revisions is still used today.

From chemistry, Lavoisier proceeded to physiology and respiration. He also applied his scientific knowledge toward helping solve many practical problems such as improvement of the Paris water supply, the ventilation and sanitation of prisons and hospitals, and other hygienic and public health problems. He was appointed to many scientific commissions and boards for the French government. He served as head of a committee to direct the Royal Powder Factory in an attempt to remedy a shortage of gun powder. He also served on the Commission on Weights and Measures which established the metric system.

As the French Revolution gained momentum, Lavoisier, his father-in-law Paulze and other members of the Ferme Generale were arrested and tried for "plotting against the people of France." They were condemned and executed on May 8, 1794. Lavoisier was beheaded at the age of fifty-one, long before his scientific researches were completed. He accepted his fate calmly and is supposed to have said "this probably saves me from the inconveniences of old age."

A most befitting epitaph was given by Joseph Lagrange when he said: "It took only a moment to sever that head, and perhaps a century will not be sufficient to produce another like it."

Pharmacology and hence medical treatment were advanced during the eighteenth century by the scientific contributions of Linnaeus and William Withering.

Carl von Linné (1707-1778) was a Swedish botanist and professor of medicine at the University of Uppsala who achieved world fame as the "father of scientific botany." His father, a pastor of modest means, was an amateur botanist and the rectory's fine garden gave Linnaeus an early introduction into this branch of science. Although his father had desired him to study theology, Linnaeus turned to medicine and natural science because of a belief that the Lord had chosen him to study and explore natural phenomena.

Despite the fact that medicine was his prime motive, a profound attraction for botany could not be suppressed and Linnaeus continued to work in this field while pursuing his medical studies. At Uppsala he studied under Professor Rudbeck, cataloging and classifying the University's large collection of botanical specimens. He interrupted his studies at the age of twenty-four to serve as a naturalist on a scientific expedition to Lapland.

Linnaeus went to Holland at the age of twenty-eight in order to secure his doctorate in medicine because this degree was not granted in Sweden at that time. While there, he studied under the great clinician Boerhaave, who soon recognized his talents and became his lifelong friend. Linnaeus lived and studied in Holland for two years, during which time he was in charge of an excellent botanical garden in Amsterdam. This was one of the most productive periods of his life and he published over a dozen treatises of great scientific importance. In 1735 he published his famous *Systema Naturae* which originated a scientific system for the classification of plants, animals and minerals.

Returning to Sweden he experienced an initial slow period of medical practice. However, he soon won scientific recognition and in 1741 was offered a professorship at Uppsala. His first appointment was to the chair of physic and anatomy, however, this was later exchanged for the chair of botany, a position which he held until his death in 1778. As a teacher he was immensely popular, with students flocking from all of Europe and America to attend his lectures.

A deep sense of orderliness led Linnaeus to his greatest scientific contribution which was the development of a system of binomial nomenclature for plants. Previously there had been little uniformity in assigning names to plants. He eliminated multiple terms and used a maximum of two, the first identifying the genus, the second, the species. The familiar "L" in botany stands for Linnaeus and refers to the binomial names of plants as set forth in his famous work, *Species Plantarum,* published in 1753.

Having contributed to the classification of plants, animals, shells and minerals, Linnaeus turned to the classification of disease. In his *Genera Morborum* published in 1759, he divided diseases into classes, orders and species similar to the classification of plants.

Although Linnaeus lived a century before Pasteur and Koch,

he believed that certain diseases—dysentery, whooping cough, small-pox, syphilis, leprosy, and consumption—were contagious and were associated with the entrance of small animals into the body. While these had not yet been discovered, Linnaeus wrote that there was

> . . . in the spread of infectious diseases a similarity to the mode of re-production and increase of many animals, especially insects. The smaller an animal, the more numerous and rapid its progeny; hence it is not difficult to conceive that some of these minute organisms by their exces-sively rapid multiplication may in a short time totally fill, as it were, the whole body.

Another physician, botanist, William Withering, scientifically intro-duced digitalis into clinical medicine during the eighteenth century.

Withering was a man of many talents; in addition to being a physician and botanist, he was an able mineralogist, chemist, musician, and meteorologist. He was born March 28, 1741 into a family of physicians. His maternal grandfather had delivered Samuel Johnson and his father was a successful physician.

Withering was graduated from Edinburgh at the age of twenty-five with the degree of Doctor of Physic. His early practice at Stafford afforded him ample time to study botany and his major scientific contribution was in that field.

While still engaged in his country practice, Withering heard of an old woman in Shropshire who possessed a miraculous medicine capable of curing the dropsy. He investigated and gleaned from her the ingredients of this remarkable remedy. His description and findings were as follows:

> In the year 1775 my opinion was asked concerning a family recipe for the cure of dropsy. I was told that it had long been kept a secret by an old woman in Shropshire who had sometimes made cures after the more regular practitioners had failed. I was informed also that the effects produced were violent vomiting and purging; for the diuretic effects seemed to have been overlooked. This medicine was composed of twenty or more different herbs; but it was not difficult for one conversant in these subjects to perceive that the active herb could be no other than foxglove.

The botanical foxglove or digitalis had been used empirically by herbalists for an unrecorded period of time in the treatment of epilepsy, the healing of wounds, and as an expectorant. This plant was called the fox glove or originally the folks or fairies glove because its blossoms bore a fancied resemblance to a lady's thimble. The Bavarian botanist Leonard Fuchs in 1541 had christened the plant digitalis, which is a Latin translation of its common German name "fingerhut" or thimble.

Withering continued to intensively study the properties of digitalis although he had relocated his practice in Birmingham, where he became famous as a practitioner and consultant. In 1776 he published a monograph on the flora of the British Isles. This was followed in 1785 by the publication of his monumental thesis entitled, *An Account of the Foxglove and some of its Medical Uses, with Practical Remarks on Dropsy and other Diseases.*

William Withering died of pulmonary tuberculosis on October 6, 1799 at the age of fifty-eight and was buried in a vault at Edgbarton Church. There is a tablet in this church adorned with the foxglove and the staff of Aesculapius to commemorate his discovery of "one of medicine's most useful drugs."

Several of Withering's biographers quote a pun that was supposedly composed at the time of his death and which reads as follows: "The flower of English medicine is Withering."

Every age has had its quacks and charlatans, and they still exist in our modern society. However, the eighteenth century produced more than its share of them and some of the world's most notorious quacks flourished during this period.

One of the most unusual and remarkable of them was "Crazy Sally of Epsom." Sarah Wallin Mapp was an enormously fat, drunken woman who had learned the art of bone-setting from her father. For centuries in England it was commonly believed that bone-setting could be transmitted from a father to his offspring through the combination of his communication of its secrets and skills, plus an inherited dexterity.

A flamboyant character, Sally roamed about the countryside, frequenting fairs, where she boasted and screamed of her powers as a bone-setter and healer. Calling herself Crazy Sally, she soon achieved fame and became so highly esteemed for her skill and art, that the town of Epsom offered her one hundred pounds to reside there.

She had a short and unsuccessful marriage to an Epsom "ne'er-to-do-well" named Mapp, who was attracted by her success. Following his desertion she found consolation in the fact that patients of high rank and great wealth flocked to her. She soon became a person of great fame and notoriety. Almost constantly, interesting facts about her would appear in the public press. An example of this reads as follows:

> The cures of the woman bone-setter of Epsom are too many to be enumerated; her bandages are extraordinary neat, and her dexterity in reducing dislocations and setting fractured bones wonderful. She has cured persons who have been twenty-five years disabled, and has given incredible relief in the most difficult cases. The lame come to her daily, and she gets a great deal of money, persons of quality who attend her operations making her presents.

As her practice grew, Crazy Sally visited London weekly, making the journey in an ornate chariot drawn by four white horses and attended by servants garbed in spectacular liveries. Her headquarters in London were at the Grecian Coffee House. Sir Hans Sloane, the famous eighteenth century physician, founder and president of the Royal Society, frequently witnessed her operations. In fact, he was so favorably impressed by her methods that he placed his niece under her care for treatment of a spinal affliction.

Crazy Sally's success was undoubtedly due to the strength of her hands and arms and she is said to have been able to reduce a dislocated shoulder unaided. Unfortunately, as time went on she became addicted to alcohol and her patients and friends fell from her. Her death was reported in the Grubb Street Journal, December 22, 1737, in the following item: "Died last week, at her lodgings, near Seven Dials, the much-talked-of Mrs. Mapp, the bone-setter, so miserably poor that the parish was obliged to bury her."

Scrofula or tuberculosis of the glands of the neck was a common affliction which was especially prevalent among children. It was called the "king's evil" because of the firm belief that the "king's touch" or the "laying on" of royal hands could cure the condition. This supposedly miraculous type of cure undoubtedly stemmed from an ancient belief in the "divine gifts and rights of kings." The "royal touch" is said to have originated with Edward the Confessor in England, however it was also practiced by the kings of France and other countries as well.

It was the custom for the assembled patients to be examined by the king's physician and those considered unsuited for treatment were turned away, while those chosen had to testify that they had not been "touched" before. The patients sores were then touched by the King and a gold piece was hung about their necks. Queen Anne was the last of English Royalty to carry on this practice and "royal touching" was terminated in France only shortly before the French Revolution.

It is reported that Dr. Samuel Johnson, the great lexicographer, had scrofula and that in 1712 at the age of three he was taken by his parents to London in a futile attempt to be healed of the "king's evil" by the royal touch of Queen Anne. From Boswell's account we know that Johnson was not healed and that he continued to suffer from scrofula all of his life.

Perhaps the "most successful of swindlers," "king of liars" and "arch quack" of all times was the notorious Count Cagliostro. Thomas Carlyle wrote a biography of him entitled *The Arch Quack* and Dumas used him for a central character in his *Memoirs of a Physician*. Cagliostro used mysticism and alchemy as the trappings of his cures. He treated nobles all over Europe for diseases that the physicians of those days could not cure. He sold beds that provided painless childbirth, chairs that cured rheumatism, and, for those who could afford it, he supplied an elixir of life.

Born in Palermo, Sicily, Cagliostro became notorious in childhood for trickery, theft and forgery, and while yet a youth was forced to flee from his native town. Then began his astonishing career of travel and deception. He went to Egypt, where with a little knowledge of chemistry he made much money by pretending to change baser fabrics into silk. Returning to Europe, he married a wife who quickly fell into his ways. They traveled over Europe with a coach and four horses, visiting nearly every capital and often finding access to the highest social circles. They sold potions and charms and pretended to heal the sick and restore youth to the aged. They carried a wine of Egypt which they sold in drops to restore youth and beauty to the old and wrinkled. Both were young and handsome, but they declared that they were past sixty, had a son in the Dutch army, and had been restored to youth by their own medicine. Their dupes numbered thousands, some of whom were among the nobility. One rich cardinal yielded himself wholly into the power of Cagliostro.

But now and then their dupes, whose eyes were opened to the trickery, became troublesome; hence, the charlatan and his wife suffered imprisonment in London, Paris, and other cities. In Paris they spent nine months in the Bastille. At length Cagliostro, having wandered to Rome, met his final downfall. The Church authorities had long had their eyes upon him. He was arrested, tried, and condemned to spend the remainder of his life in prison, where he died a few years later (1795).

James Graham, a clever Scotsman, opened a Temple of Health in London in 1779. He revived the miraculous beds of Cagliostro and exploited them further with a different approach. He rented his "Royal Patagonian Bed" to couples both young and old who wanted to be assured of conception. If used during coitus this bed was guaranteed to produce "male offspring as virile as Mars and daughters as beautiful as the Goddess of Love."

It was described as being a sumptous bed of brocaded damask, which was supported by four spiral crystal pillars and was trimmed in gold and festooned with flowers. Regardless of which side a person got into the "celestial bed," it started playing heavenly and angelic organ music.

One of Graham's assistants was Emma Lyon, the future Lady Hamilton, whose name was later associated with that of Lord Nelson. Graham also developed a fasting cure that was guaranteed to assure life for a century. However, he himself died before he was fifty.

To further illustrate the general credulity of the times, the English government passed a special Act of Parliament during the eighteenth century to acquire from Jane Stevens, for the sum of 5,000 pounds, the formula for her "powder recipe." This was a supposed "sure cure" for stone in the bladder. The preparation of this remedy would have required the maintenance of an almost complete zoological collection. Needless to say her remedy was finally analyzed and found to be entirely worthless.

The flourishing success of quackery during the eighteenth century can be ascribed to the colossal ignorance of both the physicians and patients of that period. Contributing in no small measure was the unsympathetic and tactless attitudes and methods of the medical profession.

Chapter 18

THE STORY OF SMALLPOX AND
THE BIRTH OF PREVENTIVE MEDICINE

F̲OR UNTOLD CENTURIES, smallpox was the greatest of scourges, exterminating tribes, ravaging nations and depopulating cities. A hideous, disfiguring and death-dealing disease, it was the most feared and hated of the many contagions that afflicted mankind.

The great Arabian physician, Rhazes, in about 900 A.D. provided the first authentic description of smallpox. Referring to it as being widespread throughout the East, he differentiated it from measles and was the first to describe it as a separate clinical entity. His description of smallpox and its eruption is so accurate that few if any changes would be needed to bring it up to date.

Prior to the time of Rhazes, various equivocal references extend the existence of smallpox back into the remote past. Although conclusive proof is lacking, there is almost certain evidence in the early records of Ancient China and Egypt to indicate that the disease existed in Asia and Africa from the beginning of recorded history.

Smallpox is known to have existed in China as early as 1700 B.C. and can be traced back to Egyptian mummies more than 3000 years ago. Hippocrates (460-361 B.C.) probably knew of smallpox. Mettler in her *History of Medicine* states that, "it has been imagined that the third book of the 'Epidemics of the Corpus Hippocracticum' and more particularly the 'Coan Praenotiones' contain references to smallpox, since, in both of these works, inflamed pustules (phlyzacia) are mentioned."

Thomas Bateman in his book, *A Practical Synopsis of Cutaneous Diseases,* published in 1818, thought that smallpox could be discerned in a description written by a Roman physician named Herodatus during the reign of Trajan in about 100 A.D. This account appears in the Tetrabiblion.

Some medical historians believe that the "Plague of Antoninus" which afflicted Rome in 189 A.D. may have been smallpox instead of bubonic plague. A Syrian epidemic which is believed to have been smallpox was described by Eusebius in 302 A.D. Another notable reference to the disease is that of Procopius (c. 490-562).

Smallpox was a disease well known and established in the East and Near East as early as the sixth century. It became epidemic in Arabia toward the end of that century and spread throughout the Mediterranean area on into Europe. Epidemics were reported in Italy and France in 570 A.D. by Marius, the Bishop of Avenches. Marius is said to have been the first to call the disease "variola," a term which is believed to have been coined by the Latin-speaking monks from the word "varus" which designated a pimple, papule or pustule.

Bishop Gregory of Tours in 582 wrote of another epidemic which undoubtedly was smallpox. He described this epidemic disease as beginning with a fever and backache which was soon followed by a pustular eruption.

Smallpox was well described by the Arabic writers from the time of Rhazes onward and was one of the commonest eruptive fevers of the Islamic World. In all likelihood, the most powerful agent responsible for diffusing this disease throughout Europe was the Crusades. The Crusaders during the eleventh, twelfth and thirteenth centuries brought smallpox home with them from the Holy Land where it was common. Later the disease was again brought from the East to the West by the Mohammedan Conquerors of Southern Europe.

Although poorly understood and frequently confused with other diseases, there is no doubt that smallpox not only existed, but became more prevalent in Europe during and shortly after the Middle Ages. Many diseases now recognized as distinct entities were at that time not differentiated.

The term, "variola," which had first been used to designate smallpox by the Bishop Marius in 570 A.D. continued to remain in use. It was also used in the eleventh century by Constantinus Africanus at the School of Salerno. The French called the disease "veriole," a term derived directly from the Latin "variola." In England, the disease was descriptively called "the pox" or "pocks." This word which was spelled both ways is derived from the Anglo-saxon word "poc" and is related to the Dutch word "pocke" designating a pustule or bubble. Also related is the German word "pocke" which originally meant a bag or pouch. The term "pox" included many of the eruptive fevers and the disease we now know as smallpox was commonly confused with measles, scarlet fever, chickenpox and later on, with syphilis.

At the end of the fifteenth century in the French medical literature, we quite suddenly find the comparative terms "la petite veriole" and "la grosse veriole" being used. Early in the sixteenth century the counterpart of these terms began to appear in the English literature as "the smallpox" and "the greatpox."

These terms came into use shortly after the introduction of syphilis into Europe. Apparently the European physicians at first were unable to distinguish smallpox from syphilis. The confusion and similarity between the two diseases centered around the common element of the pustular eruption. Hence, the terms "small" and "large" recognize the beginning awareness of a difference between the two diseases. The larger lesions of syphilis led to that disease being designated as "the great pox" while the disease formerly known simply as the "pox" became known as "the smallpox."

In the thirteenth century Gilbert, an Anglo-Norman, was the first to consider the disease contagious. Fracastoro in 1546, in his book *De Contagione,* treated smallpox rather lightly as a disease to which everyone is subject. He did, however, note that immunity ensues after an attack of smallpox or measles. Paré, the great French surgeon, referred to the disease and described cases he had seen in 1586, as well as at other times. In the seventeenth century, Sydenham diffrentiated and recognized smallpox as well as describing a number of epidemics. Later Boerhaave of Leyden proved that smallpox is spread exclusively by contagion.

Treatment was not only ineffective, but frequently foolish and based upon superstition. It commonly included directions on how to prevent or reduce the disfiguring scars of smallpox. For example, John of Gaddesden (c. 1280-1361) treated Prince John's smallpox by wrapping him in red cloths and hanging red curtains around the bed and sickroom. This procedure not only was used in an attempt to cure the disease, but also was supposed to reduce the pockmarks.

Kenelm Digby, pirate for his Britannic Majesty, commentator upon poetry and gentleman of fortune, in 1658 wrote a popular discourse upon *Powders of Sympathy*. He claimed that a Carmelite friar had given him a prescription for a miraculous powder, which would "cure according to the law of contagion." To effect a cure, it was only necessary to dissolve this "powder of sympathy" in water and to dip an article of the patient's clothing, or in the case of wounds, a blood smeared bandage into the solution. Digby's work enjoyed a tremendous popularity and went through many editions.

In 1688, three years after his death, Digby's chief steward, George Hartman, edited a work entitled *Choice and Experimental Receipts in Physick and Cirurgery, as also Cordial and Distilled Waters and Spirit Perfumes and other Curiosities, collected by the Honorable and Truly Learned Sir Kenelm Digby*. In this work, the reader is advised that, "To prevent marking in the Smallpox, as soon as ever the pocks appear, oyle of Sweet Almonds is to be painted all over the face. Then beaten gold leaf is to be carefully placed all over leaving no intervals and this will prevent any marking."

As time went on treatment became more rational, although it still remained highly ineffective. During the eighteenth century the generally accepted treatment of smallpox consisted of local application of cold to the skin, the administration of cooling drinks, and when convulsions appeared, the administration of opium.

From early descriptions it appears that smallpox was at first relatively mild and infrequently fatal in Europe. However, as the centuries passed, the disease not only increased in prevalence, but became more virulent. Smallpox is a disease subject to mutations with strains varying in virulence from the nonfatal to the highly malignant. Clinically the disease ranges from the deadly hemorrhagic type that kills in forty-eight hours to mild nonfatal cases having only a half-dozen papules.

In England toward the end of the Elizabethan period, the smallpox began to receive increasing recognition as a common and deadly disease. In 1629, the first printed bills of mortality for London listed smallpox as a separate disease and from then on it remained as a regular entry from year to year. There were frequent references

to the disease throughout the Stuart period and its increasing severity
was reflected in the rising figures of the London bills of mortality.

Smallpox is the most contagious disease the world has ever known.
It spared no country, nation or community and prior to Jenner's
time was the world's outstanding epidemic disease. Once as common
as measles and much more fatal, it made no distinction as to age,
afflicting all from tiny babes to the very aged. It spared neither the
good nor the bad, the wise nor the foolish, the clean nor the dirty, the
rich nor the poor.

Sparing neither the high nor the low, deadly disfiguring smallpox
not only struck the toiler on his cot of straw, but also penetrated behind
the royal purple drapes surrounding the beds of kings and queens.
In 1694, smallpox tumbled Queen Mary II of England from her
throne and in 1774, it rolled Louis XV of France from his royal bed
into the grave.

Macauley, in his account of the death of Queen Mary II, from
smallpox, wrote that it was

> . . . the most terrible of all the ministers of death. The havoc of the
> plague had been far more rapid, but the plague had visited our shores
> only once or twice within living memory; and smallpox was always
> present, filling the churchyard with corpses, tormenting with constant
> fears all whom it had not yet stricken, leaving those whose lives it spared
> the hideous traces of its powers, turning the babe into a changeling at
> which the mother shuddered, making the eyes and cheeks of the be-
> trothed maiden objects of horror to the lover.

In effect, he was pointing out the fact that plague was only an
occasional visitor to England while smallpox was always there, smouldering endemically and then periodically flaring up into epidemics.
Thus, although smallpox never possessed the immediate full-fledged
terror of the plague, it was in the end responsible for more deaths
and suffering than the Black Death because it was always present.

During the seventeenth and eighteenth centuries, smallpox not only
became epidemic, but at times was pandemic, both upon the European Continent and in England. In some of these epidemics as much
as half of the population died. Very few persons escaped and rare
indeed was the adult who did not bear the telltale scars of this deadly
disfiguring disease.

By the end of the seventeenth century, smallpox had come to be regarded as an inevitable part of childhood. Infants and young children were reported as having the disease in a milder form, while it was more often fatal to older children and adults. In Germany smallpox was so commonly regarded as a children's disease that it was called "Kinderblattern" or literally "children's pox." However, the disease was far from benign; William Douglas in 1760 noted that it was a chief cause of the high infant mortality rate of Europe, and Rosen von Rosenstein in 1765 stated that each year the disease carried off one-tenth of all of the Swedish children.

In Berlin from 1758 to 1774, there were 6,705 deaths from smallpox and of these, 5,876 occurred in children during the first five years of life. The London bills of mortality showed that 50 percent of all deaths were in children younger than five years of age. At the end of the eighteenth century, thirty-three out of every one hundred children who died before they were ten years of age died from smallpox and 10 percent of all deaths were from this disease.

In China the disease so terribly afflicted children that there was a proverb stating that "A mother does not number among her children those who have not yet had the smallpox, because she well knows how uncertain will be their stay in the family." Because infants and children were so commonly the victims of smallpox, the disease in England was cynically referred to as "the friend of the poor man who happens to be burdened with a large family."

Up until the time of Edward Jenner, smallpox was a leading cause of death and it is said to have killed 60 million Europeans during the eighteenth century. At the beginning of the century, 14,000 died in one year in Paris alone and it is said that 30,000 died annually in Germany. Early in the eighteenth century, an epidemic in Iceland was fatal to nearly 40 percent of the population. In the decade from 1760 to 1770 in London there were 24,234 deaths from smallpox and 234,412 deaths from all causes. As London's population during that time was about 650,000, this means that approximately 4 percent of the entire population died from smallpox in this decade.

Epidemics swept over Europe again and again and more than 80 percent of the inhabitants of any European country could count on being stricken with smallpox at one time or another. Approximately a quarter of those who took the disease died while those who escaped death were usually horribly disfigured, blinded or mutilated.

Persons who were not pockmarked were so uncommon that in the eighteenth century we find the London police using the description "not pock marked" as a means by which a "wanted criminal" could be identified. Pock-marked faces were so common and disfiguring that a woman was considered to be beautiful merely if she was fortunate enough to have escaped the ravages of smallpox and to have a smooth unpitted skin. The poet Ben Jonson voiced a pathetic and hopeless protest against the inevitable and disfiguring effects of smallpox in an epigram, as follows:

> Envious and foul disease, could there not be
> One beauty in an age, and free from thee?

It was from smallpox that the first clear concept of immunity arose. Just how long mankind knew that one attack of this disease conferred immunity is unknown. It had long been common knowledge that persons fortunate enough to recover from one attack were unlikely to get it again. For untold centuries it had been the custom among many ancient people to deliberately expose a person to a mild case of smallpox at a time when he was in a robust state of health in the hope and expectation that he would acquire a benign infection, recover and henceforth be immune. Parents frequently exposed their children to smallpox in this way in order to get the disease over with.

Averroes, an Arabian physician in Cordoba during the twelfth century, was the first to note medically that one attack of smallpox confers immunity. In 1546 Fracastoro in his book *De Contagione* also noted the immunity which is conferred after an attack of smallpox.

For thousands of years it had been known that people could be artificially infected with smallpox by rubbing them with the scabs obtained from an active case. Centuries before Christ the ancient Chinese practiced inoculation by introducing such crusts into the nose of a candidate for immunity. The early Hindus, Persians and many other ancient Oriental and African people knew of this principle of conveying infection and producing immunity. For untold centuries they protected themselves by practicing inoculation in a variety of forms, such as snuffing the crusts into the nose, injecting pustular material into the veins, or binding the scabs of smallpox onto a scratch or incision made in the skin.

Through the Arabian literature the practice of inoculation had found its way into the writings of the School of Salerno; however, it failed at that time to gain acceptance by the physicians of the Western World. Widely practiced in the Far East, inoculation traveled westward and was introduced into Turkey in 1647. It was from Turkey that Europe finally learned of the procedure.

The idea was introduced into England in 1713 through the correspondence of Emmanuel Timoni, a Greek physician living in Constantinople. His description entitled "An account of history of the procuring of the smallpox by incision or inoculation; as it has for some time been practised at Constantinople" appeared in a volume of the *Philosophical Transactions of the Royal Society* (1714-1716). The same small volume also contained another description of inoculation by Giacomo Pylarini of Venice, Italy.

Peter Kennedy, an English surgeon who had lived in Turkey, in his work "An Essay on External Remedies" (London, 1715) also described inoculation, writing as follows:

> . . . the common way now used in Turkey, and more particularly at Constantinople, is thus: they first take a fresh and kindly Pock from someone ill of this distemper and having made scarifications upon the forehead, wrists, and legs, or extremities, the matter of the Pock is laid upon the foresaid incision, being bound on there for eight to ten days together; at the end of which time the usual symptoms begin to appear, and the distemper comes foreward as if naturally taken ill, though in a more kindly manner and not near the number of Pox.

Apparently Kennedy's description attracted little or no attention.

Jacob De Castro, in his "A Dissertation on the Method of Inoculating the Smallpox" (London 1721), not only took cognizance of the earlier customs of inoculation, but recommended the use of virus from an artificially induced case, rather than from naturally occurring cases. He noted that such cases are of a "milder disposition." He was perhaps the first to recommend the "arm to arm" method of inoculation which was later to become popular and widespread.

However it was not through conventional medical literary channels that inoculation was introduced into Western Civilization. Knowledge of inoculation or variolation actually stemmed from the great reservoir of common medical folklore. Its subsequent adoption, popularization and diffusion into England and Europe was due to Lady Mary Wortley Montagu, the wife of the British Ambassador to Turkey.

A fascinating figure of history, Lady Mary was born in 1689, a daughter of the noble and socially prominent Pierpont family. Described as a pretty and precocious child, "carelessly brought up in a library," she frequently accompanied her proud father to numerous social, political and literary functions. The story is told that at the age of eight she was placed on a table and toasted by his cronies at the Kit Kat Club. She grew up to become a famous beauty and wit who achieved distinction in literature.

As a high-spirited girl of nineteen she eloped with and married Wortley Montagu, who later became one of England's richest men. In 1716 Montagu was appointed Ambassador to Turkey and along with his wife and son embarked upon the long and dangerous journey to the "Sublime Porte." Soon after their arrival the vivacious Lady Mary who loved both gaiety and excitement made it a habit to disguise herself and visit parts of Constantinople where no proper Ambassadress had any right to go. She achieved literary fame through her letters home which recounted her escapades and travels in an interesting and lively fashion.

Observing the successful practice of inoculation in Turkey, Lady Mary had her three-year-old son inoculated in March of 1717 at Pera. On April 1, 1717 she took smallpox as her theme and wrote a letter from Constantinople to her friend Miss Sara Chiswell in England.

The portion of the letter dealing with inoculation reads as follows:

Apropos of distempers I am going to tell you a thing that I am sure will make you wish yourself here. The smallpox, so fatal, and so general amongst us, is here entirely harmless by the invention of "ingrafting," which is the name they give it. There is a set of old women who make it their business to perform the operation every autumn in the month of September, when the great heat is abated. People send to one another to know if any of their family has a mind to have the smallpox; they make parties for this purpose and when they are met (commonly fifteen or sixteen together) the old woman comes with a nut-shell full of the matter of the best small-pox and asks what veins you please to have opened. She immediately rips open that you offer her with a large needle (which gives you no more pain that a common scratch) and puts into the vein as much venom as can be upon the head of her needle, and after binds up the little wound with a hollow bit of shell; and in this way opens four or five veins . . . The children or young patients play together all the rest of the day, and are in perfect health to the eighth. Then the fever begins to seize them, and they keep their beds two days, very seldom three. They have very rarly above twenty or thirty (pocks) in their faces, which never mark; and in eight days' time they are as well as before their illness. . . . I am patriot enough to take pain to bring this useful invention into fashion in England; and I should not fail to write to some of our doctors very particularly about it, if I knew any one of them that I thought had virtue enough to destroy such a considerable branch of their revenue for the good of mankind.

The Montagus returned to England in June of 1718 and Lady Mary immediately set about advocating inoculation. She promptly ran into all of the difficulties that crusaders usually meet when they attempt to introduce new medical procedures. Both the practice of inoculation and its sponsor were violently denounced. The majority of the medical men became greatly alarmed and forecast the most disastrous consequences that would result from such a barbarious practice being put to use in England. The clergy were equally aroused and cried out against the impiety of trying to wrest from the "Hands of Providence" the right to inflict smallpox upon the people. The papers expressed strong disapproval of parents who were willing to risk the lives of their children by submitting them to such a hazardous procedure.

However, Dr. Maitland, the physician who had been attached to the Montagus' mission in Turkey, began to inoculate under Lady Montagu's patronage and the custom grew in spite of the opposition. In the Spring of 1721, three years after the Montagus return from Constantinople, a severe epidemic of smallpox broke out in England. Lady Mary then had her five-year-old daughter inoculated in the presence of several physicians. The practice thus gained the support of several of the foremost physicians of the day, notably Sir Hans Sloane and Dr. Richard Mead who was then physician to His Majesty the King.

Lady Mary then thought of a brilliant scheme to further advance the cause of inoculation. She persuaded the authorities of the Court to allow her to try inoculation on seven criminals who were under sentences of death in Newgate Prison. Offered the chance of a pardon if they would submit to the procedure, the seven naturally accepted. They gladly left the shadow of the gallows and were inoculated on August 9th, 1721 by Dr. Maitland, Sir Hans Sloane and Dr. Mead. Six were inoculated by needle in the manner described by Lady Mary and one by the Chinese method of placing dried pocks into the nostrils. All seven contracted a mild form of smallpox and recovered, although the one on whom the Chinese method was used suffered more than the rest.

This successful demonstration greatly furthered the cause of inoculation and Lady Mary was successful in persuading the Princess of Wales to try inoculation on the children in the royal nursery. In April of 1722 the royal children were successfully inoculated. From then on inoculation or variolation became popular and was practiced widely.

Because smallpox was a universal disease and everyone from prince to pauper could expect to get it, most people were eager to accept any reasonably safe method of protecting themselves from this scourge. Therefore the practice of inoculation spread widely not only in England but also in France, as well as the other Continental countries. There was never a time when control of a disease was more needed than during the eighteenth century, because Europe was in an almost continuous state of epidemic.

Inoculation was soon brought to France and Voltaire became one of its most ardent exponents; however, it did not become a general practice until after 1750. Louis XVI of France was inoculated in 1774, the same year that his father Louis XV died of the smallpox.

In 1724, Dr. Maitland brought the procedure from England to Germany; however, the practice did not spread immediately throughout all of the German States. For example, it was not disseminated in Prussia until 1775 when Frederick II arranged to have the practice of inoculation taught to fourteen provincial physicians. The practice spread to Holland, Denmark, Sweden, Switzerland, Italy and Spain.

Many inoculators established excellent reputations and became quite famous. Among them was a Mr. Robert Sutton who practiced medicine and pharmacy in Suffolk. He devised a new technique which consisted of taking the person to be inoculated into the room of a patient sick with smallpox and removing some matter from one of the pocks and inserting it with a lancet under the skin of the candidate to be inoculated. Later in the century this technique became quite popular and variolation became known as "Suttonian inoculation" to distinguish it from its rival and ultimate successor "Jennerian vaccination."

Undoubtedly the person who achieved the greatest fame and fortune from the practice of inoculation was Dr. Thomas Dimsdale of London. Dimsdale's most famous act was his expedition in 1768 to Russia at the invitation of the Empress Catherine the Great for the purpose of introducing inoculation into that country.

An enlightened ruler, Catherine had been a pupil of Voltaire who was an ardent exponent of inoculation. Because Russia was experiencing a series of severe smallpox epidemics at this time, the Empress was desirous of following the example of other European countries who were successfully practicing inoculation. Catherine also had personal reasons for dreading the smallpox. Her husband's face had been badly pitted and hideously disfigured by an attack of this disease. In addition, she feared her fourteen-year-old son, the Grand Duke Paul, would die of smallpox before reaching the throne.

Catherine the Great was at the zenith of her prosperity and power at this time. Her husband had died or been killed by her lover eight years before. Her brilliant Court was a mixture of barbaric splendor and French refinement, over which she regally presided, along with her favorite advisor and lover, Count Gregory Orlov. It was to this glittering Court that Dr. Dimsdale was summoned to inoculate the Empress and her son

Fully aware of the possible dangers of inoculation, the Empress had relays of post horses prepared from St. Petersburg to the border to insure Dimsdale's escape, if the procedure went awry. The English doctor was warned by Count Parrin, the Prime Minister that, "To your skill and integrity will probably be submitted no less than the precious lives of two of the greatest personages in Europe." Dimsdale then suggested that the Empress should first observe the performance of the procedure on some lesser personages. Catherine replied "My life is my own and

I shall with the utmost cheerfulness and confidence rely on your care alone."

Nevertheless two military Cadets volunteered or were ordered to be inoculated first. Following the sucessful completion of the procedure on them, Catherine the Great was inoculated on Sunday, October 12, 1768. She had a mild case of smallpox with one pustule on her face and two on her wrist. She returned to her activities and appeared in Court on October 28th, where she received the congratulations of the assembled nobility. Her son the Grand Duke Paul was inoculated November 1st and recovered by November 22. However as history later proved, he was hardly worth saving from the smallpox, because his reign was that of a frenzied madman until it was finally terminated by his assassination in 1801.

Dr. Thomas Dimsdale received one of the finest fees ever paid to a physician. He was given an honorarium of 10,000 pounds, was paid 2,000 pounds for his expenses and was awarded a lifetime annuity of 500 pounds. In addition, he was honored by being made a Baron of the Empire, a Councilor of State and was appointed Body Physician to the Empress. He remained in Russia for some months and inoculated many members of the nobility, including Count Gregory Orlov. Following Dimsdale's return to England inoculation went forward in Russia at a rapid pace.

As the practice of inoculation gradually became accepted in England and then spread over Continental Europe, a parallel drama was being enacted in the New World.

Wherever mankind goes he carries with him much from his old environment, his culture, his language, his beliefs, and his diseases. During the fifthteenth, sixteenth and seventeenth century, wherever the white man went, smallpox followed. Hence, smallpox was introduced into the New World by the Spaniards shortly after its discovery.

Early records picture the Western Hemisphere as being relatively healthful and free from smallpox as well as most of the other major epidemic diseases of the Old World. The Indians who populated the land from the cold of the Arctic and Antarctic down through the temperate zones and into the Tropics were an isolated racial group of uncertain origin. They varied in culture from the fierce stone age savages of the north temperate zones and the friendly, gentle, naked natives of the West Indies, to the cultured and highly civilized Aztecs, Incas, and Mayans of Central and South America.

The conquest of the native population of half a world by a relatively small number of European explorers, adventurers and settlers was an amazing feat. It has been said that the Indians were defeated because they had no horses, no iron, and no firearms; however, more important than this was the fact that they had no immunity to the "white man's" diseases. The true facts are that the New World was conquered by disease and the White Man was an easy victor because he had smallpox and alcohol.

Wherever the European trod, death followed in his footsteps. The blight of disease descended upon the natives everywhere the European went, not by intent, but through ignorance and accident. With horrifying swiftness his diseases destroyed the Indians and smallpox led the list, killing more than firearms.

Although there was no coordinated plan or high command for the invasion of the New World, it proceeded as though by design. The invasion fell into three great segments of attack, each allotted to one powerful European nation. At the North came the French, aiming down the great waterway of the St. Lawrence, following it through to the Great Lakes and then south down the Mississippi to the Gulf and the sea. At the Center came the British aiming inland all along what is now the Eastern Seaboard of the United States, extending from New England down south past Virginia to Florida. To the South came the powerful Spaniards, striking at the West Indies, Mexico, Central and South America.

Very shortly after Columbus and his contemporaries had established Spain's advance base at Santo Domingo on the Island of Hispaniola (now known as Haiti), smallpox was introduced. The Spaniards with their insatiable greed for riches enslaved the Indians, cruelly overworking and starving them. This brutal treatment, together with the occurrence of severe epidemics of smallpox and other pestilential diseases soon depopulated the Island. The Indians diminished rapidly, dying off in such enormous numbers, that in a relatively short time the West Indian Islands knew them no more. As the native Indians died off the Spaniards were faced with the need of replenishing their supply of slave labor. Their solution was to replace the Red Man with the Black Man and hence slavery was introduced into the West Indies in 1501 or even earlier. A royal edict permitted Negro slaves born in slavery among Christians to be transported to Hispaniola and the direct importation of slaves from Africa was begun in about 1502.

Thus the Black Man was introduced into the New World struggle between the Red Man and the White Man. The Negro slave became a new actor in the drama of disease and served as the bearer of new and terrible diseases which were fatal to both Reds and Whites. The "Black Tragedy" of the slave traffic was to last for three centuries and it not only helped to disseminate smallpox but also introduced malaria and yellow fever to the New World.

Bernal Diaz del Castillo in his *History of the Conquest of New Spain* relates that Narváez, who landed in Mexico in May 1519 hoping to supersede Cortez, had with him a Negro slave who was sick with the smallpox. This Negro had contracted the disease in Cuba from whence Narváez had sailed. Smallpox had probably been brought to Cuba from Santo Domingo where a terrible outbreak raged during 1518 and 1519.

Narváez's Negro slave communicated his disease to the Indians who lived in a house they had at Cempoallen. These Indians in turn communicated the disease from one to another and being a disease new to them, it spread with inconceivable rapidity. As it spread all through the land, the Indians died by the thousands. Smallpox did not kill the Spaniards because probably every Spaniard in the New World had had the disease in childhood and hence was immune.

Thus the introduction of smallpox into Mexico proved to be far more potent as a factor in the conquest of that country than was the armed might of the Conquistadors. In many districts, one half or more of the native population had died and so the invading Spaniards frequently found the towns and countryside deserted and all resistance to an end.

Diaz described the condition of the last portion of Mexico City held by the Indians at the time of their surrender in August of 1521 as follows: "The streets, the square, the houses and the courts of Talteluco were covered with dead bodies, we could not step without treading on them and the stench was intolerable." All in all, it is estimated that smallpox killed approximately 3½ million Indians in Mexico.

The French settlements in Canada were started in 1535 under Cartier; the Indians began to diminish from then on. Numerous historical references as to the severe ravages of smallpox are found from 1635 onward, and the disease severely decimated the Iroqouis in 1684.

Smallpox also visited the English Colonies and the Reverend Increase Mather wrote: "About this time (1631) the Indians began to be quarrelsome touching the Bounds of the Land which they had sold to the English, but God ended the controversy by sending the Smallpox amongst the Indians to Saugust, who were before that time exceedingly numerous. Whole Towns of them were swept away, in some, not so much as one soul escaping the Destruction."

Governor William Bradford wrote in regard to the Indians about the Connecticut River Settlement in 1634:

> This spring, also, those Indians that lived about the trading houses there, fell sick of ye smallpoxe, and died most miserably.
>
> A sorer disease cannot befall them. . . . They that have this disease have them in abundance and for wants of bedding and linen and other helps they fall into a lamentable condition as they lye on their hard matts; ye poxe breaking the mattering and running one into another, their skin cleaving to the matts they lye on when they turn them a whole side will flea off at once and they will be all of a gore blood, most fearful to behold and they being very sore. . . . They dye like rotten sheep. For very few of them escaped. . . . But by ye marvellous goodness and providence of God not one of ye English was so much as sicke.

The ease of dissemination of the smallpox virus together with its deadliness made it an ideal disease to transfer by malicious intent. The fact that this disease could be used as an invaluable ally by a relatively immune invading force against a highly susceptible and nonimmune enemy was quickly grasped. Records show that this type of germ warfare was used during the Indian uprisings that attempted to destroy the British outposts west of the Allegheny Mountains.

Sir Jeffrey Amherst, commander of the British garrison, because of his limited resources and harassed by the seriousness of the outbreak, issued the following company orders: "You will do well to try and inoculate the Indians by means of blankets as well as to try every other method that can serve to extirpate this execrable race."

In response, Bouquet, stationed at Fort Pitt, stated: - "I will try to inoculate . . . with some blankets that may fall into their hands and take care not to get the disease myself." It was further stated: "Out of regard for them (i.e. two Indian Chiefs) we gave them two blankets and a handkerchief out of the smallpox hospital. I hope it will have the desired effect." That it apparently did was shown by the fact that a few months later smallpox raged among the tribes in Ohio and Delaware.

Later as the European settlers pushed westward and dispossessed the North American Indians of their hunting grounds, the Indians' resistance was completely undermined by the triple alliance of smallpox, tuberculosis and alcoholism.

Thus smallpox heavily hit the natives of the New World and reduced them to miserable remnants of their once powerful selves. Exact figures are lacking, but it has been estimated that of 12 million American Indians, 6 million fell victims to the smallpox.

Once introduced, smallpox continued to recur in repeated outbreaks throughout the New World. Although the disease continued to ravage the Indians of North and South America, it also became a serious problem to the English settlers of the North American Colonies. In fact it became the outstanding epidemic disease of the Colonies during the seventeenth century. It struck again and again in periodic epidemic waves and decimated the new Colonies. In Europe smallpox was always present and hence was a common disease of childhood. However the isolation of the Colonies prevented continuous or frequent exposure and hence the infection would be postponed for a generation and then it would strike an almost entirely nonimmune population with terrific force.

Smallpox epidemics struck the Massachusetts Bay Colony in 1633, the New Netherlands in 1663 and the Virginia Colony in 1667. In 1677 a severe epidemic struck Boston and brought forth the first medical publication in North America. This was Thomas Thacker's "A Brief Rule to guide the Common People of New England, How to order themselves and theirs in Small Pocks, or Measles." Thacker was a minister at the Old South Meeting House and ministered to the physical as well as the spiritual needs of his people. He obtained the information contained in his "Brief Rule" from Sydenham's works and his broadside gave good advice and great comfort to his people.

Inoculation against smallpox was introduced into the American Colonies by the Reverend Cotton Mather of Boston. This great Puritan preacher was a strange paradox in that he believed in both witchcraft and the germ theory of disease. Famed as a witch discoverer and author of the book *Memorable Providences,* which was the standard textbook on witches, Mather was also an astute student of medicine and the contagious diseases.

It is hard to believe that the same man who said "Go tell Mankind that there are Devils and Witches," knew of and believed in the protective value of inoculation against smallpox even before the European physicians did. In 1706 Cotton Mather had been given a Negro slave. This man servant, named Onesimus was a member of the Guramantee, an African tribe that practiced inoculation. In a letter to Dr. Woodward, Mather wrote as follows: "Enquiring of my Negro-man Onesimus, who is a pretty Intelligent Fellow, Whether he ever had ye Small-Pox; he answered both, yes, and no; and then told me, that he had undergone an Operation which had given him something of ye Small-Pox, and would forever Praeserve him from it." Mather further quoted Onesimus as describing the procedure as follows: "People take Juice of Small-Pox, and Cutty- Skin, and putt in a Drop; then by'nd by a little sicky, sicky; then very few little Things like Small-Pox; and no body dy of it; and no body have Small-Pox anymore."

When in 1714 Mather read in the *Philosophical Transactions of the Royal Society,* Timoni's account of inoculation, he resolved to try the procedure when the next epidemic came. His opportunity came on May 4, 1721 when the ship "Seahorse" arriving from Tortuga sailed into Boston harbor.

Eight days after the arrival of the "Seahorse" small pox appeared in Boston and in three weeks there were eighty cases and within a month over a hundred deaths. Mather then appealed to the physicians of Boston and was completely ignored by them. However one physician, Zabdiel Boylston, did listen and was convinced. Boylston

then took the first courageous step by inoculating his six-year-old son
and two Negro slaves on June 26, 1721, completely unaware that
Lady Montagu had introduced inoculation into England only a
short time before. Mather then had his own son Sammy inoculated
with excellent results.

Fierce resistance against inoculation was encountered and the
public outcry against Mather and Boylston was tremendous. The
townspeople distrusted the procedure and were fearful of the contagiousness of the inoculated. When a minister who was a kinsman
came to Mathers' home to be inoculated on November 14, a home-
made grenade was thrown into the house. Fortunately it failed to
explode, but attached to it was the message: "Cotton Mather: you
Dog, Damn you, I'll inoculate you with this, and a Pox to you."

The practice went on despite the opposition of the public, the
press and the physicians. When the epidemic was over the figures
revealed a victory for inoculation. Out of 8,000 victims, 844 had
died of small pox, or one in nine; while of the 286 inoculated by
Boylston and his helpers, only six had died, or one in forty-eight.

Inoculation gradually gained acceptance in the Colonies and Dr.
Zabdiel Boylston's pioneering efforts finally won him recognition and
membership in the Royal Society. However the inoculation controversy was to rage for many more years.

Benjamin Franklin became an advocate of inoculation after the
smallpox had killed his younger son. George Washington too, was an
ardent advocate of inoculation. He had contracted smallpox while in
the West Indies and the disease not only left him pockmarked, but
also with a healthy respect and fear of its dangers. He therefore
had his entire household inoculated. Later in 1776 when smallpox
became epidemic, he ordered every man in the fledgling American
Army to be protected by the "arm to arm" method of inoculation.

Because the procedure was still regarded with almost as much
fear as it had been fifty-five years earlier when Cotton Mather and
Zabdiel Boylston had performed their first inoculations, the Army
inoculations were carried out secretly. Fortunately everything went
well and Washington was able to announce that the inoculation program had been an "amazing success."

Inoculation was one of the most important and interesting episodes in the development of preventive medicine. The use of infective material of variola crusts for the transmission of smallpox marks the first attempt at the planned transmission of a disease with a view towards its control. In addition, the procedure clearly illustrated the fundamental phenomena of infection, susceptibility and immunity.

Although inoculations became widely accepted and did much good, it was a rather heroic method of protection. It never gained complete acceptance and continued to be regarded with apprehension and dread. The fact remained that it was an uncertain and dangerous procedure. In some instances the disease transmitted was fully as severe as naturally occurring smallpox. In other instances, plain suppurative infections occurred at the site of inoculation and were mistaken for "takes" and the person erroneously believed himself protected, but later contracted smallpox.

A not inconsiderable danger was in its possible fatal outcome; statistically the overall mortality rate of inoculation was shown to be approximately 3 percent. However, its greatest disadvantage lay in the fact that the inoculated individual contracted true smallpox and could transmit the disease to others and thus start an epidemic. Therefore while inoculation protected the individual, it endangered the community.

These difficulties were all swept away when inoculation became obsolete and was supplanted by Jenner's great discovery of vaccination. Thus, although inoculation passed from the medical scene, it can be said to have prepared the way for vaccination.

However, strange as it may seem the practice of inoculation persisted and continued to be used in England until 1840 when it was finally declared to be a felony by an act of Parliament.

So deeply imbedded in the medical folklore of primitive peoples was the practice of inoculation that authorities state that the procedure is still practiced to this day by tribes in North and Central Africa. Rosenau stated that he ran across it in an Arab village in Palestine in 1922.

The discovery of vaccination was one of medicine's greatest triumphs. It at long last gave to the world an effective weapon against one of its most terrible diseases. Jenner's successful demonstration of the effectiveness of cowpox vaccine against smallpox closed a "gate of death" and saved untold millions of lives. However, his discovery was more than the discovery of vaccination against smallpox, it was a basic medical discovery that changed the course of the world by introducing it to the concept of disease prevention.

Great as was Jenner's victory over smallpox, greater still was to be the impact of the extension of his principle of vaccination as a major weapon in mankind's fight against disease. His discovery formed the foundation stone upon which the science of preventive medicine was to be built.

Edward Jenner was born May 17, 1749, the son of the Reverend Stephen Jenner, vicar of Berkeley, in Gloucestershire, England. When he was five, his father died and he was raised by his elder brother who was a clergyman. During his early years, he apparently was an average youngster and exhibited no especial talents that would have led anyone to believe that he would rise to future greatness. He did, however, display an extraordinary interest in nature and nature studies.

At the early age of thirteen he was apprenticed to Daniel Ludlow, a surgeon and apothecary of Sudbury. In 1770 at the age of twenty-one he came to London to further his study of medicine at St. George's Hospital. A pleasant, sociable, but rather unambitious young man from the English countryside, he was privileged to become a house pupil of the famous English surgeon and naturalist, John Hunter. He resided with Hunter for two years and became one of his favorite pupils. This relationship carried over into a lifelong friendship and correspondence between the two men. Jenner's interest and abilities as a naturalist led to his being employed to help arrange and classify the zoological specimens brought back by Captain Cook on his famous first voyage to the Pacific. After graduation, Jenner received an offer to accompany Captain Cook on his next expedition. However, he turned down this and other tempting offers in order to return to his native Berkeley and practice medicine.

Jenner has been described as having the appearance of a typical English squire. Blond and blue-eyed, he was a rather handsome man of stocky build who loved to dress well. An extremely able and skillful physician, he was beloved for his congenial and kindly personality. In wide demand, he spent a great deal of time on horseback and later in a carriage going about the countryside in all kinds of weather to visit his patients.

Jenner not only was a competent physician, but also was interested in music and poetry. He played both the flute and the violin and was a minor poet of some distinction. That his interests were varied is shown by the fact that in 1783 he launched England's first hydrogen balloon.

Throughout his life, Jenner continued to pursue his nature studies and was encouraged and prodded on with these by his friend and correspondent, John Hunter. Hunter frequently wrote to Jenner in Gloucestershire asking for specimens for his collection. For example, he wrote, "Cannot you get me a large porpoise?" and "Have you any eves where the bats go at night?" In an another letter he wrote, "I want a nest with cuckoo's eggs in it; also one with a young cuckoo; also an old cuckoo. I hear you saying that there is no end to your wants." In turn, Hunter gave his friend and former pupil helpful advice. Jenner was interested in the phenomenon of hibernation and wrote to Hunter for some information. In reply, Hunter wrote, "but why do you ask me a question by way of solving it? I think your solution just; but why think, why not try an experiment?" The last phrase in the excerpt of this letter is frequently quoted as being the famous bit of advice that inspired Jenner to continue with his experimentation.

Jenner achieved scientific fame and recognition for his work as a naturalist long before he wrote on vaccination. His work on the migration of birds and his observations of the habits of the cuckoo won for him a much coveted Fellowship in the Royal Society.

Edward Jenner was not the first to recognize the fact that a localized cowpox infection conferred immunity against the smallpox. This belief was a legendary bit of medical folklore, prevalent for many years throughout the dairy regions of England. Almost a century before Jenner's time during the reign of Charles II, Court gossip told of this type of protection. The Duchess of Cleveland, whose beauty and debauchery had made her the mistress of the King and the scandal of Europe, was cursed by a courtier who wished that she would be stricken with the smallpox and robbed of her beauty. She supposedly replied that she could not get the smallpox because she had once had the cowpox.

Jenner was thoroughly familiar with smallpox and the procedure of inoculation as a means of preventing this disease. As a country doctor he had performed many inoculations upon his patients. In addition he carried with him the painful and vivid memory of the severity of his own reaction following inoculation when he was but a boy. The story is related that in 1768 at the age of nineteen, while still a medical apprentice to Dr. Ludlow at Sudbury, Jenner first learned of the legend that dairymaids who had been infected with the cowpox were immune to the smallpox. While interviewing a patient who was a milkmaid he questioned her about any possible history of smallpox and she is said to have replied: "I cannot take that disease for I have had the cowpox." Jenner was intrigued by the dairymaid's chance remark and the incident left an indelible impression upon him.

Thus Jenner early in his career encountered the common belief of the country people of Gloucestershire that there was a simple harmless preventive for smallpox. Although his medical contemporaries believed this to be but an old country legend without any foundation of fact, Jenner believed that there was truth to the tale. However, his progress in proving his belief was extremely slow. Three decades were to lapse between the time of the Gloucestershire milkmaid's remarks in 1768 and the publication of his classic work on vaccination in 1798.

As he gained medical experience over the years, Jenner's memory was continuously stimulated by his frequent encounters with the widespread notion that persons who had had the cowpox enjoyed an immunity against smallpox. He methodically began to collect examples of persons who had had the cowpox and afterwards had escaped smallpox, or who, having had cowpox did not react successfully to smallpox inoculation. His observations extended over a quarter of a century and he became obsessed with the idea that cowpox produced a complete and permanent protection against smallpox.

Finally, in 1796 Edward Jenner performed the first controlled experiment which scientifically proved the effectiveness of vaccination.

Greatly enthused by the results of his experiment and studies, he applied to the Royal Society for permission to present his findings before them and to have his paper published in the *Transactions*.

His request was refused with the advice that he "should be cautious and prudent . . . and ought not to risk his reputation by presenting to the learned body anything which appeared so much at variance with established knowledge, and withal so incredible." The members of the Society felt that the contents of his paper might spoil his good name and ruin the scientific reputation that he had gained by his previous researches on the nesting habits of the cuckoo. Undaunted, Jenner in 1798 privately published his now famous paper which was entitled: "An Inquiry into the Causes and Effects of the Variolae Vaccinae, a disease discovered in some of the Western counties of England, particularly Gloucestershire, and known by the name of the Cowpox."

In this monumental seventy-five page booklet which changed the history of the world, Jenner carefully documented his findings. On pages two and three of the "Inquiry" he states the origin of this disease to be as follows:

> There is a disease to which the Horse, from his state of domestication, is frequently subject. The Farriers have termed it "the Grease." It is an inflammation and swelling in the heel, from which issues matter possessing properties of a very peculiar kind, which seems capable of generating a disease in the Human Body (after it has undergone the modification which I shall presently speak of), which bears so strong a resemblance to the Small Pox, that I think it highly probable it may be the source of that disease.
>
> In this Dairy Country a great number of Cows are kept, and the office of milking is performed indiscriminately by Men and Maid Servants. One of the former having been appointed to apply dressings to the heels of a Horse affected with "the Grease" and not paying due attention to cleanliness, incautiously bears his part in milking the Cows, with some particles of the infectious matter adhering to his fingers. When this is the case, it commonly happens that a disease is communicated to the Cows, and from the Cows to the Dairy-maids, which spreads through the farm until most of the cattle and domestics feel its unpleasant consequences. This disease has obtained the name of the Cow Pox. It appears on the nipples of the Cows in the form of irregular pustules.

Summing up these findings Jenner concludes on page six, as follows: "Thus the disease makes its progress from the Horse to the nipple of the Cow, and from the Cow to the Human Subject."

To prove his thesis that cowpox protects against smallpox, Jenner collected and recorded twenty-three cases in his "Inquiry." His most important and crucial experimental work is set forth in cases XVI and XVII. Excerpts from Case XVI are as follows:

> Sarah Nelms, a dairymaid at a Farmer's near this place was infected with Cow Pox from her master's Cows in May 1796. She received the infection on a part of the hand which had been previously in a slight degree injured by a scratch from a thorn. A large pustulous sore and the usual symptoms accompanying the disease were produced in consequence. The pustule was so expressive of the true character of the Cow Pox, as it commonly appears upon the hand, that I have given a representation of it in the annexed plate.

At this point in his booklet Jenner included a full page drawing of the hand of Sarah Nelms depicting the cowpox lesions that she had acquired. He also added an illustration of a small pustule on her forefinger which he stated: "did not actually appear on the hand of this young woman, but was taken from that of another and is annexed for the purpose of representing the malady after it has newly appeared."

In his "Inquiry" on page thirty-two he then proceeds with Case XVII as follows:

> The more accurately to observe the progress of the infection, I selected a healthy boy, about eight years old, for the purpose of inoculation for the Cow Pox. The matter was taken from a sore on the hand of a dairymaid, who was infected by her master's Cows, and it was inserted, on the 14th of May 1796, into the arm of the boy by means of two superficial incisions, barely penetrating the cutis, each about half an inch long.
>
> On the seventh day he complained of uneasiness in the axilla, and on the ninth he became a little chilly, lost his appetite, and had a slight head-ache. During the whole of this day he was perceptibly indisposed, and spent the night with some degree of restlessness, but on the day following he was perfectly well.

Jenner then proceeded to test the protection afforded by his historic first vaccination and on page thirty-four he stated:

> In order to ascertain whether the boy, after feeling so slight an affection of the system from the Cow Pox virus, was secure from the contagion of the Small-pox, he was inoculated the 1st of July following with variolous matter, immediately taken from a pustule. Several slight punctures and incisions were made on both his arms, and the matter was carefully inserted, but no disease followed. The same appearances were observable

on the arms as we commonly see when a patient has had variolous matter applied, after having either the Cow-pox or the Small-pox. Several months afterwards he was again inoculated with variolus matter, but no sensible effect was produced on the constitution.

Thus, in simple straight-forward language, Edward Jenner announced to the world his great discovery of vaccination. He thereby not only immortalized his own name, but along with it, the names of Sarah Nelms, the dairymaid who gave the cowpox virus and the boy James Phipps who received it. The "Inquiry" was undoubtedly one of the most significant works ever to be published in the entire realm of medical literature.

Jenner had concluded his "Inquiry" with the words: "I shall myself continue to prosecute this inquiry, encouraged by the hope of its becoming essentially beneficial to mankind." True to these words, Jenner began to wage a long, hard battle for recognition of his discovery. He went to London for a period of three months in 1798, but failed to arouse any great interest in vaccination, among either his fellow physicians or the public at large.

The effect of Jenner's publication was at first similar to that of many other great announcements of science. Some authorities completely accepted his work, others vigorously denounced it, while the great majority seemed unconcerned.

The first break for the advancement of vaccination came when Henry Cline, a surgeon, used a quill of dried cowpox serum, which Jenner had left with him, as a counterirritant in treating another disease, and found later that his patient had become immune to smallpox inoculation. From interest created by Cline's report of this incident the practice of vaccination began to spread.

As vaccination became popular, there was no lack of detractors, nor of persons seeking spurious credit for its discovery. However, Jenner's work was based on sound experimental data and he had made his chain of evidence complete. He himself said, "I placed it on a rock where I knew it would be immovable before I invited the public to take a look at it."

Jenner continued to live and practice in Berkeley and wrote two additional pamphlets on vaccination. In 1799 he published, "Further Observations on the Variolae Vaccinae or Cowpox" and in 1800 he published "A Continuation of Facts and Observations Relative to the Variolae Vaccinae, or Cowpox."

The results of vaccinations were so excellent and so convincing and the need for this sure, safe prophylaxis against smallpox was so great that Jenner received official recognition and achieved world-wide fame earlier in life than is usually the case. In 1802 the English Parliament voted him a grant of 10,000 pounds for his discovery and a few years later in 1806 granted him an additional 20,000 pounds. In 1813, Oxford conferred upon him the degree of Doctor of Physic. As his fame continued to grow he was honored by almost every country in the world.

On the other hand, opposition to vaccination grew. Ministers denounced it from their pulpits as man's interference with the ways of God. Antivaccinationist societies were formed (some remain even today) and even poets denounced vaccination in verses which warned the people that they would "grow furry ears and have a bovine tail."

Shortly after Jenner's publication appeared, a number of people attempted to claim priority to the discovery of vaccination. One of these was Benjamin Jesty, a yeoman farmer of Dorset. It was established that this bold and enterprising farmer who was familiar with the commonly accepted belief of the countryside that cowpox protects against the smallpox, preceeded Jenner by twenty years in performing vaccination.

In order to protect his family against the dread smallpox, this strong-minded farmer in 1774 had taken a stocking needle and boldly scratched cowpox material into the skins of his wife and two sons. It was claimed that he even followed up on this family vaccination by later inoculating them with material from a smallpox case in order to check their immunity.

Following this crude uncontrolled family experiment, Jesty apparently lost all interest in preventive medicine and devoted himself to farming for the next twenty years. However, upon hearing that Dr. Jenner had been awarded 10,000 pounds by Parliament he attempted to establish his priority and become recognized as the discoverer of vaccination. Jesty enlisted the aid of the village clergyman and his local member of Parliament. Letters claiming his priority were sent to Parliament and to the Jennerian Society in London.

As a result he was invited to London. But all that came of his claim was that he had his portrait painted and he was presented with a pair of gold-mounted needles as a souvenir of his bold excursion into the realm of medicine.

A letter from a Mr. Banks was introduced into the House of Commons, concerning the justice of naming any particular person as the discoverer of vaccination. He pointed out that the technique was a matter of common knowledge in the following words: ·"There was, I am sure, abundant proof of the disorder being known, and of its preventive power, long before Dr. Jenner's name was heard."

Despite these attempts to detract from Jenner's fame, the fact remained that he had performed the first scientifically controlled experiment on vaccination. He was also the first to attempt to put it into practice and in his "A Continuation of Facts and Observations" published in 1800, he stated that vaccination was ". . . an antidote that is capable of extirpating from the earth a disease which is every hour devouring its victims; a disease that has ever been considered as the severest scourge of the human race!"

A report of Jenner's work reached America in 1799 in the current newspapers and in the Medical Repository. Dr. Benjamin Waterhouse, the first professor of theory and practice of physic at Harvard Medical School, becoming convinced of the value of Jenner's work wrote to him and obtained some dried vaccine impregnated on a silk thread. On July 8, 1800 he vaccinated his five-year-old son, Daniel Oliver Waterhouse, who thus became the first person to be vaccinated in America. Waterhouse also vaccinated two slaves and afterwards inoculated them with smallpox with negative results.

Vaccination spread rapidly in America and Thomas Jefferson vaccinated his own family and thereby materially helped to spread the new doctrine. On October 21, 1801, Jefferson wrote to Dr. Henry Rose, "I received from Dr. Waterhouse of Boston some vaccine matter of his own taking and some from Dr. Jenner of England just then came to hand. Both of them took well, and exhibited the same identical appearance in the persons into whom they were inserted. I inoculated about 70 or 80 of my own family, my two sons in laws as many." He then goes on to state, ". . . from the trials I made, the cowpox can hardly be called a disease. It produces no more inconvenience than a burn or blister of a quarter of an inch in diameter."

Later Jefferson paid tribute to Jenner and wrote to him saying, "Future nations will know by history only that the loathsome smallpox has existed, and by you has been extirpated."

Many other tributes were paid to Jenner. In 1812 a tribe of American Indians sent him a belt and a string of wampum and thanked him by saying, "In token of our acceptance of your precious gift, we beseech the Great Spirit to take care of you in this world, and in the land of spirits." In far-off Japan the natives of a fishing village erected a statute to him. The Dowager Empress of Russia sent him a ring and gave the name "Vaccinoff" to the first child to be vaccinated in Russia, along with the provision that this child be educated at public expense.

Even though France and England were at war, Napoleon paid Jenner a supreme compliment, when in 1805 he ordered universal vaccination for all of his troops. In 1813 when a relative of Jenner's was captured, Jenner wrote to Napoleon asking for his release. Napoleon on reading the letter said, "Ah, it's Jenner! I can refuse Jenner nothing," and ordered the prisoner released.

Noting that Napoleon and Jenner were contemporary figures in history, James Simpson in 1847 paid tribute to Jenner by commenting that, "The lancet of Jenner has saved far more human lives than the sword of Napoleon destroyed."

Largely unaffected by his great fame and the many honors accorded to him, Jenner continued to reside for the rest of his life in Chantry Cottage, his beloved home in Berkeley. He died of a cerebral hemorrhage on January 26, 1823 at the age of seventy-four and was buried in the Chancel of Berkeley Church.

Chapter 19

THE CONQUEST OF SCURVY
AND THE ADVANCE OF
NAVAL AND MILITARY HYGIENE

ANOTHER NOTABLE VICTORY in the newly born field of preventive medicine was secured during the eighteenth century with the conquest of scurvy by the British naval surgeon, Dr. James Lind.

Scurvy has been known since the earliest of times and it is quite possible that Job was a victim of it when he complained: "My bones are pierced in me in the night season and my sinews take no rest. . . . My skin is black upon me and my bones are burned with heat."

However this may be, there is no doubt about the fact that the Crusaders suffered badly from this disease. The first concise account of scurvy came from the pen of Jacques de Vitry, who in the thirteenth century described its ravages at the siege of Damietta during the Fifth Crusade. Educated for the priesthood, de Vitry was called by Pope Innocent the Third to preach the Crusade against the Albigenses. He became a Bishop and spent several years in Palestine; later he was elevated to the rank of Cardinal. During his stay in the Holy Land he wrote *Histoire des Croisades* in which he described scurvy as follows:

> A large number of men in our army were attacked also by a certain pestilence, against which the doctors could not find any remedy in their art. A sudden pain seized the feet and legs; immediately afterwards the gums and teeth were attacked by a sort of gangrene, and the patient could not eat any more. Then the bones of the legs became horribly black, and so, after having suffered continued pain, during which they showed the greatest patience, a large number of Christians went to rest on the bosom of the Lord.

Another graphic description of scurvy was given by Jean, Sire de Joinville. He had accompanied King Louis the Ninth on the Seventh Crusade and in his history of "St. Louis" he gave the following vivid eye witness account:

> . . . we were attacked with the army sickness, which was such that our legs shrivelled up and became covered with black spots, and spots the colour of earth, like an old boot; and in such of us as fell sick the gums became putrid with sores, and no man recovered of that sickness, but all had to die. It was a sure sign of death when the nose began to bleed: . . . The sickness became much more severe throughout the camp, and the proud flesh in our men's mouths grew to such excess that the barber-surgeons were obliged to cut it off, to give them a chance of chewing their food or swallowing anything.

The term "scurvy" was first applied to this disease during the Middle Ages and apparently was an English folk word, phonetically allied to the French "skorbut" the Spanish "escorbuto" and the German "shorbut." The term probably stems from the early low German "shoren" (to lacerate) and "buk" (belly), while the scientific term "scorbutus" is a Latinized artificial implant.

There are many more early accounts of scruvy written by adventurers who while exploring or waging war in strange and far-off lands encountered this disease as a result of severely restricted diets and near-starvation. However, scurvy did not assume calamitous proportions until sailing ships replaced oared galleys and long ocean voyages became possible. Prior to the time of Columbus, ships had seldom ventured far from land, but with the growth of exploration, colonization and trade, sailing voyages extended from months to years. As oceanic travel grew and the European nations sent their ever-expanding fleets of sailing ships on long and arduous journeys, they were faced with the difficult problems of the recruitment of seamen, provisioning and preservation of the ships' stores as well as the health maintenance of their crews.

Because the world has long been thrilled with the fictional glamour of the countless tales of adventure surrounding the men who sailed the seven seas, few people today realize the privations, hardships and diseases they endured. The sailor's lot was a hard and brutal one and he worked and lived under the most terrible of conditions. Despite their stately and picturesque appearance the full-rigged ships of the "age of sail" were actually miserable, unsanitary "floating hells." Constantly water soaked, their wooden hulls and holds were slowly and continuously rotting away. The entire ship and especially the crews quarters were overcrowded and dirty, as well as being rat and vermin infested. Overall hung the permeating and terrible odor of foul bilgewater, dead rats, stale cooking and unwashed humanity.

The ships' stores including the food were subject to mold, putrefaction and infestation with vermin. The food rations consisted mainly of salt pork, salt beef, and ship's biscuits. The salted beef was frequently so hard that it could be cut and carved and used for making models, while the biscuits were so rotten that they had to be tapped on the table or eaten at night because they were so full of maggots and weevils. The drinking water was usually inadequate and so poorly stored that it soon became foul and contaminated. The sailors were poorly and scantily clad, and their clothing which was nearly always wet seldom dried out and soon became ragged, filthy and verminous.

Because of these well-known hardships and the hazards of "a life at sea" it was almost impossible to voluntarily recruit a crew and hence men were "prest" into service. Frequently the prisoners from a local jail or debtor's prison could elect to go to sea, rather than to serve their sentences. It was also a common practice for "press gangs" from ships needing crews to go out after dark and forcibly seize able-bodied men from out of the taverns or off of the streets.

The combination of all these factors served to make scurvy "the scourge of the sea." It has been said that in the three centuries from 1500 to 1800 scurvy killed more sailors than all other diseases, disasters, naval engagements, shipwrecks and accidents combined. It has also been estimated that in the 200 years from 1600 to 1800 over a million lives were lost from this disease. In practically every famous voyage the historical records relate that large numbers of men died or were laid low by this malignant form of avitaminosis. Admiral Hawkins estimated that he had lost over 10,000 men from scurvy during his twenty years at sea. A vivid example of the ghastly mortality from scurvy was demonstrated during Commodore Anson's voyage around the world in 1740-44. Of the seven ships in Lord

Anson's squadron only one returned. Of the 1,955 men who sailed from England, 1,051 died, practically all of them from scurvy.

One of the most interesting and graphic early accounts of scurvy is found in the description of its occurrence among the sailors of Jacques Cartier's exploratory expedition to the New World in the sixteenth century. This account is remarkable also for the fact that it relates how his men learned of a cure for this malady from the Indians. The account is related in Richard Haklyut's *Collection of Voyages,* which was published in about 1600.

Jacques Cartier sailed from St. Malo in May 1535 with a crew of 110 men, for the purpose of exploring the coast of New Foundland and the St. Lawrence River. Scurvy soon struck his crew and spread so rapidly that in six weeks' time only ten men remained unaffected. "Then," writes Cartier, "it pleased God to cast his pitifull eye upon us and send us the knowledge of remedie of our healthes and recoverie." Cartier was fortunate enough to learn from a native "that the juice and sappe of the leaves of a certain tree" cured this complaint from which the native himself had previously suffered. The curative effect of the native's remedy upon the stricken crew was soon very apparent. "If all the physicians of Montpellier and Louvaine had been there," continues Cartier, "with all the drugs of Alexandria they would not have done so much good in one year as that it did in six days; for it did prevail, that as many as used of it by the grace of God recovered their health."

Cartier's account is one of the earliest references to the use of a vegetable substance for the treatment of scurvy. He described the use of an infusion made from the bark of a tree which the Indians called the "Ameda." Haklyut believed this to be the sassafras tree but Lind, who later carefully studied Cartier's voyages, stated in his *Treatise on Scurvy* that it was the "large swampy American spruce tree." It is of interest to note that although Cartier had described an effective cure for scurvy, his discovery attracted little or no attention and was soon lost to the world. As has so often been the case in medical history, valuable knowledge and discoveries have been lost or forgotten and have had to be rediscovered at a later date before they could effectively be put to use.

The credit for conclusively demonstrating that scurvy was a deficiency disease that could be prevented or cured by the addition of fresh fruits and vegetables to the diet belongs to Dr. James Lind. He proved beyond a doubt that it was not a contagious or occupational disease, but a nutritional disorder resulting not from the excessive consumption of certain articles of diet but from the insufficient intake of others. It was Lind who gave the first scientific account of scurvy and its treatment with lemon juice. He must also be credited with having brought the matter to the attention of the authorities and giving them precise instructions as to what must be done to prevent the disease. His work ultimately convinced the governmental authorities to take decisive remedial and preventive actions which in turn eliminated this terrible "scourge of the sea," thereby changing the destinies of nations and altering the course of history.

Coming from an upper middle class family, James Lind was born in Edinburgh, Scotland, October 4, 1716. At the rather early age of fifteen he was apprenticed to George Longlands, a well known Edinburgh physician. In 1739 when the war between England and Spain began, Lind entered the Royal Navy as a surgeon's mate.

During his ten years of service, Lind had a great deal of personal experience of "life at sea" and saw many men ill with scurvy. He had ample opportunity to observe that after a few weeks at sea, the ordinary seaman's restricted and deficient diet, together with overwork, fatigue, wetness and cold produced the signs and symptoms of scurvy with appalling frequency.

On May 20, 1747 James Lind, aboard H.M.S. Salisbury in the English Channel, started his experimental work on scurvy. He inaugurated a series of simple scientific tests and conducted what was probably the first controlled clinical trial ever undertaken. He later confirmed his observations and published his findings in 1753 in his great medical classic *A Treatise on the Scurvy.* In his introduction he wrote: "I shall propose nothing merely dictated by theory; but shall confirm all by experience and facts. . . . The world has now almost dispaired of finding out a method of preventing this dreadful disease at sea; and it has become a received opinion that it is altogether impossible either to prevent or cure it."

Lind studied twelve patients with scurvy and he reported as follows:

I took twelve patients in the scurvy, on board the Salisbury at sea. Their cases were as similar as I could have them . . . They lay together in one place in the forehold; and had one common diet, water-gruel sweetened with sugar in the morning; fresh mutton-broth often times for dinner; and for supper, barley and raisins, rice and currants, sago and wine, or the like. Two others took twenty-five gutts (drops) of elixir vitriol three time a-day, upon an empty stomach . . . Two others took two spoonfuls of vinegar three time a-day, upon an empty stomach. . . . Two of the worst patients . . . were put under a course of sea-water. Of this they drank half a pint every day . . . Two others had each two oranges and one lemon given them every day. These they eat with greediness, at different times, upon an empty stomach. They continued but six days under this course, having consumed the quantity that could be spared. The two remaining patients took the bigness of a nutmeg three times a-day, of an electuary recommended by a hospital surgeon, made of garlic, mustard-seed, horse-radish, balsam of Peru, and gum myrrh.

The consequence was, that the most sudden and visible good effects were perceived from the use of the oranges and lemons; one of those who had taken them, being at the end of six days fit for duty . . . The other was the best recovered of any in his condition; and being now deemed pretty well, was appointed nurse to the rest of the sick." Lind further concluded that:—"The results of all my experiments was that oranges and lemons were the most effectual remedies for this distemper at sea. I am apt to think oranges preferable to lemons, though perhaps both given together will be found the most serviceable.

Leaving the Royal Navy in 1748, Lind returned to Edinburgh to obtain his degree in medicine. He was licensed by the Royal College of Physicians of that city and in 1750 was elected to Fellowship. In 1757 Lind published his second great volume on nautical medicine entitled *An Essay on the Most Effectual Means of Preserving the Health of Seamen in the Royal Navy.* This, together with his classic work on scurvy, attracted the interest and admiration of Lord Anson, then First Lord of the Admiralty. This undoubtedly influenced the appointment of Lind in 1758 to the post of Chief Physician at Haslar Hospital. A new Royal Naval Hospital near Portsmouth, Haslar was one of the largest hospitals in Europe, capable of caring for approximately 2,200 patients.

Lind served for twenty-five years at Haslar and during his long service there continued his studies on scurvy. He also availed himself of the ample opportunities which were present at this large hospital to study many sick seamen. These men were afflicted with a wide variety of diseases, acquired not only in European waters, but in all parts of the world. From these studies came his third book, *An Essay on Diseases Incidental to Europeans in Hot Climates,* published in 1768.

Lind's three books: on scurvy, on the care of sailors' health, and on tropical diseases, formed a trilogy which served as the foundation stones for modern nautical medicine. All three of his books were well accepted and over the years went through many editions. Lind is frequently referred to as "the conqueror of scurvy" and "the father of nautical medicine and naval hygiene."

In summing up the achievements which may be credited to Lind, Louis H. Roddis in his book *James Lind, Founder of Nautical Medicine* cites the following points:

1. The classic experiment proving the importance of citrus fruits or their juices in prevention of and in treatment for scurvy. Application of these principles late in the seventeenth century and early in the eighteenth century led to virtual elimination of scurvy in men of the Royal Navy.

2. Recommendation that new recruits be brought first to receiving ships for quarantine, and that they be bathed and issued clean clothing. This did more to eliminate shipboard typhus fever than any other measure.

3. The suggestion that special ships be run between England and naval blockading squadrons to supply fighting ships with fresh provisions, fruits, and green vegetables. Adoption of this suggestion for maintaining ships' crews in fighting trim is believed to have been a definite deciding factor in favor of the British in their wars with Napoleon.

4. Demonstration of a practical method of obtaining fresh water from sea water by simple distillation, adapting utensils normally found on shipboard.

5. Recommendations for physical examination of naval recruits with maintenance of records thereof.

6. Suggestion of issuance of naval uniforms to seamen, a measure favorably affecting both health and morale of these men.

7. Insistence on physical exercise and on cold baths as "toughening-up" processes.

8. Use of cinchona bark for prevention of malaria.

9. Recommendations that in the tropics ships be anchored well off shore, and that crews not be given work details or liberty ashore at night. This did much to reduce the incidence of malaria.

Although Lind's book on scurvy was published in 1753, it was not until 1795, a year after his death, that the Admiralty made the use of lime or lemon juice compulsory for the Royal Navy. Gilbert Blane, one of Lind's former pupils who became Commissioner of the "Board of the Care of Sick and Wounded Seamen," finally succeeded in persuading the Admiralty to adopt Lind's recommendations for the prevention of scurvy. Thus by the addition of lime juice and other fresh citrus fruits to the diets of seamen, scurvy was forever banished from the Royal Navy and British sailors were soon nicknamed "Limeys."

Death finally closed Dr. James Lind's remarkable career at the age of 78 on July 18, 1794.

Another important factor contributing to the conquest of scurvy was the famous experiment of Captain James Cook. This famous English naval captain and explorer, who undoubtedly was familiar with Lind's work on scurvy, conclusively demonstrated that if sailors had fresh foods, scurvy would be prevented. On his long second voyage of exploration to the South Seas in the ships Resolute and Adventure, he did not lose a single sailor from scurvy. During this voyage which lasted for three years and sixteen days, from July 13, 1772 to July 29, 1775, he enforced orders to have his men eat the fresh foods with which he supplied the ships' larders. He fed his men liberal rations of "sweetwort and sauerkraut," as well as supplying fresh meat, onions, and fresh citrus and other fresh fruits and vegetables whenever possible.

In 1776 the Royal Society presented him with a gold medal and made him a Fellow in recognition of his achievements against scurvy.

During the same period of time that Lind was reforming naval hygiene, Dr. John Pringle was working on the improvement of military medicine. A practical physician and an outstanding scientist, Pringle in 1752 wrote a book entitled *Observations on Diseases of the Army*. His work proved to be a best seller and ran through seven editions. It was responsible for reforming military hygiene and raising the standards of military medicine.

John Pringle (1707-1782) was a Scot who became surgeon general of the English Army and served in that capacity from 1742 until 1758. He helped introduce the ideas and teachings of Boerhaave into England, and was a friend of Benjamin Franklin, with whom he corresponded in regard to the use of electricity for the treatment of "palsies." He was not only a noted physician and hygienist, but also served as president of the Royal Society.

In his studies on military medicine Pringle analyzed the questions of diet, water supply, camp sanitation and personal cleanliness. As a result of his recommendations, army life was revolutionized. The men were provided with suitable clothing, good boots, and adequate food, along with proper rest and exercise. Camp sanitation was well planned, and good water supplies and adequate drainage was provided, along with better housing and well-ventilated sleeping quarters. As a result of these improvements and reforms, sickness and infection were reduced and the health and morale of the army was greatly improved.

Pringle was also a pioneer and advocate of the "Red Cross idea" and worked tirelessly to have hospitals recognized as sanctuaries.

The outstanding work of both Pringle and Lind gradually gained acceptance and the authorities began to recognize the important preventive aspects of good hygiene and proper diet. Sir Gilbert Blaine wrote: "The means of prevention are more within our power than those of cure; for it is more in human art to remove contagion, to alter man's food and clothing, to command what exercises he is to use, and what air he is to breathe, than it is to produce any given change in the internal operation of the body."

Despite all this, hygienic reforms were slow in being put into actual practice and unhygienic conditions lingered for a long time in both the army and the navy.

Chapter 20

LATE EIGHTEENTH AND EARLY NINETEENTH CENTURY: FOUNDATION STONES FOR MODERN PUBLIC HEALTH AND PREVENTIVE MEDICINE

P<small>RIOR TO THE EIGHTEENTH CENTURY</small> it was generally believed that the microscopic creatures first discovered by Van Leeuwenhoek were produced from lifeless matter by spontaneous generation. However, during the eighteenth century considerable controversy arose as to whether these minute creatures were spontaneously generated or whether they arose from pre-existing seeds. Most investigators noted that they were intimately associated with the process of fermentation and putrefaction. They found them present in sour milk, rotting meat, spoiled boullion and wherever decay and fermentation took place. Furthermore, they found that all that was necessary to produce swarms of these organisms where they had not previously existed was to place easily spoilable organic matter in a warm place for a short time. In view of these observations the idea was readily accepted that these microscopic creatures were spontaneously generated from lifeless matter. The great Italian scientist Spallanzani disagreed with this concept and proceeded to prove it false.

Although not a physician, the Abbé Lazzaro Spallanzani (1729-1799) made a number of important contributions to medical science. This versatile Italian priest and natural scientist conducted a variety of brilliant investigations and experiments in the fields of biology, physiology and geology.

He made a number of important observations on the physiology of digestion and established the fact that digestion was not after all another form of putrefaction, as was commonly believed. By obtaining specimens from the living by means of a sponge attached to a cord, he confirmed previous findings that food was digested by the gastric juices.

Spallanzani extensively employed the microscope, which was then a relatively new tool in biologic research, to study many forms of life. From his investigations he concluded that microorganisms were carried into infusions of organic matter by the air and that when flasks containing organic matter were hermetically sealed, the air excluded, and heat applied long enough, no organisms appeared.

After his refutation of the theory of spontaneous generation, Spallanzani demonstrated that spermatic fluid was necessary for fertilization of the ovum. Despite his work, the theory of spontaneous generation continued to be widely held and debated until well into the nineteenth century.

A practical application of Spallanzani's work was the discovery of the process of canning by Nicolas Appert. In 1795, Revolutionary France was at war with several hostile nations and the problems of securing adequate food supplies was an acute one. The French Directory therefore offered a prize of 12,000 francs to anyone who would develop a new and successful method for the preservation of food. Appert, an obscure Parisian confectioner and distiller, entered the competition and won the award in 1809. In 1810, he published the first treatise on Canning entitled *The Art of Preserving All Kinds of Animal and Vegetable Substances*. The first English translation of his work appeared in the following year.

Appert apparently had no technical training or scientific experience, yet it is evident that he was a capable experimenter and close observer. At the time of his work, the scientific causes of food spoilage were not known and in fact were not to be discovered until the work of Louis Pasteur half a century later. Therefore, in view of the existing knowledge of the times and Appert's limited background, his discovery of the process of canning was truly a remarkable accomplishment.

In his process, Appert used wide-mouthed glass bottles which he filled with food. After carefully corking and sealing them, they were thoroughly heated by immersing them in boiling water. His early text described the procedures for the preservation of more than fifty foods. Although he did not know the scientific reasons why, Appert recognized the necessity of thoroughly sealing his containers and the need for complete cleanliness and strict sanitation in his operations. The use of metal containers instead of glass came later and the term "can" is an abbreviation of the term "tin cannister."

Appert died in 1841 at the age of ninety-one without ever receiving the recognition that he deserved. The discovery of how to preserve foods by the process of canning was an important forward step in preventive medicine because it provided a more adequate food supply and thereby made better nutrition possible. Strange as it may seem, this experience in food preservation remained restricted to the food industry and had no immediate effect upon the scientific world.

An admirable instance of "sanitary sleuthing" that was a forerunner of modern public health methods occurred during the eighteenth century. Between September 1762 and July 1767, almost 300 cases of a mysterious ailment called the "Devonshire Colic" were admitted to the Exeter Hospitals. Dr. George Baker noted that all of the cases were associated with the drinking of cider made in Devonshire. He also noticed that the symptoms of colic and palsy which afflicted the victims of the Devonshire Colic were similar to the symptoms suffered by painters with lead colic.

Baker solved the mystery of the Devonshire Colic and prevented further cases by the simple procedure of performing a chemical analysis. His analysis showed that Devonshire cider contained a high percentage of lead. Further investigation revealed that this came from the lead lining of the cider presses, a type that was used only in Devon.

During the latter part of the eighteenth century there was a growth of the concept that governments were responsible for the health of their people. In 1789, Jeremy Bentham, an English philosopher and jurist, published a work entitled *Introduction to Principles of Morals and Legislation*. In it he advocated numerous governmental, social, welfare and health reforms.

He pioneered in prison reform and thoroughly studied the poor laws. He set forth the "principle of utility" and stated that the object of all legislation must be "the greatest happiness for the greatest number." Because health was an essential requirement for the happiness of many, Bentham advocated the improvement of everything pertaining to health. In his "Constitutional Code" he proposed a cabinet of fourteen members, among whom would be a minister for health, who would deal with environmental sanitation, communicable diseases, and the administration of medical care.

Bentham's ideas not only influenced thought and legislation in his own country, but in other European countries as well. While much of his work did not come to fruition during his lifetime, it foreshadowed the future and exerted a tremendous influence in bringing about the sanitary reforms of the nineteenth century that helped create the modern public health movement.

In France during this same period of time, Mirabeau and other Revolutionary leaders preached the idea that "the health of the people was the responsibility of the State." However, it remained for Johann Peter Frank at the end of the eighteenth century, to crystalize these various concepts of governmental responsibility for health into a clearly defined function of the State.

The foundations for modern public health and hygiene were laid down by Frank in a six-volume treatise entitled *A Complete System of Medical Policy*. This was a complete system of medical police measures, aiming to teach not so much physicians, but rather the governmental authorities how to keep people healthy. It set forth a complete and comprehensive program for public health protection and founded a new concept of State Hygiene. Frank maintained that governments should not only take charge when the public health was threatened and endangered by epidemic and contagious diseases, but should be responsible for the public's health at all times.

Johann Peter Frank was born in 1745 at Rodalben and grew up in this borderland between French and German civilization. His early education was received from the Piarists and Jesuits in various church schools. He later studied philosophy and science and received his Ph.D. from Pont-a-Mousan. His father wanted him to be a businessman and his mother wanted him to enter the church. However, Frank was attracted to medicine and went on to study at Strasbourg and Heidelberg. He received his M.D. from the latter university in 1766 at the early age of twenty-one.

In his autobiography Frank states that when he graduated the dean asked him what his plans for the future were and he informed him that he wanted to study the life of man in his physical and social environment from conception to the grave. He further informed him that he wanted to devise the best means of making this life a healthy and happy one and would like to teach rulers how to keep their subjects in good health, to write a comprehensive book on this subject and draft laws to protect the people's health.

Frank had an adventuresome medical career, spanning a period of fifty-three years. He moved about a great deal, holding a variety of public health appointments and practicing medicine in half a dozen different places. Although he knew what he wanted to do early in life, the necessity of earning a livelihood forced him into private medical practice.

However, after practicing medicine in France for some time, he obtained his first position in public health by becoming the state medical officer for Baden. He soon advanced to become "physician-in-ordinary" to the Margrave of Baden-Baden and was attached to the Court at Rastatt. A short time later he was offered a better position in the service of the Prince-Bishop of Spires, whose "body physician" he became in 1775.

In 1779 at the age of thirty-four, he published the first volume of his book. However, the completion of his monumental six-volume work on public health was to span a period of forty years, and his last volume was published in 1819 at the age of seventy-four. Over the years, as the various volumes appeared, they attracted a great deal of attention and established Frank's reputation as a great teacher and hygienist. Because his writings were both widely praised and attacked, he frequently encountered opposition in the position he currently held, while at the same time receiving attractive offers to go elsewhere.

After the publication of his third volume in 1784, Frank was offered professorships in Mainz, Goettingen and Pavia. He accepted the offer at Goettingen, but after one year decided to go to Pavia where he arrived in 1785.

At this time Pavia was a center of medical education and Frank found a cordial welcome there. He was appointed "Protophysicus" or director general of public health for Austrian Lombardy and the Duchy of Mantua. He was also professor of clinical medicine and dean of the medical school at the University of Pavia. He immediately surveyed the entire region, visiting all of the hospitals and pharmacies, interviewing physicians, surgeons and midwives. He also studied the living and working conditions of the people in great detail. He began a series of reforms and reorganized the hospitals and the Board of Health. At the University he doubled the number of courses, created new chairs, and raised salaries. He founded a pathological museum, established a model pharmacy and had a new pharmacopiea compiled.

However, in all of his work Frank encountered an insurmountable barrier in the dire poverty of the people. He found that they were rotten with poverty, ignorance and disease in a land of plenty. They were starving because the land did not belong to them, but was owned by a small group of patrician families. He recognized that poverty was the chief cause of disease, and he called public attention to this in a lecture he delivered in 1790 to the graduating class of the Medical School at Pavia. The title of his address was *"De populorum miseria: morborum genitrice"* or "The Peoples Misery: Mother of Diseases." In this oration he pictured conditions as they were and made a passionate plea for social and economic reforms. Although he was a social reformer, Frank was not a revolutionary, but was a firm believer in an enlightened monarchy. He believed that a monarch should be to his people what a father is to his family. He advocated that a good monarch, like a good father, should do everything he could to improve the health and welfare of his people.

As a result of these progressive views and his outspoken advocacy of sanitary, social and economic reforms, Frank encountered a great deal of opposition. Therefore in 1795 when he was offered the directorship of the Vienna General Hospital he promptly accepted the appointment. At Vienna he continued his work as a hygienist and teacher. He improved administration, established strict discipline, built a new autopsy room and founded a museum of pathological anatomy. He made more beds available for teaching purposes and set up special rooms for the isolation of patients sick with contagious diseases.

Opposition is inevitably encountered by all reformers and Frank once again met up with it at Vienna. Becoming tired of these pressures he accepted a call to go to Russia where he served as physician-in-ordinary to the Czar and director of the Medico-Surgical Academy.

After three years he returned to Vienna in 1809 just as Napoleon and his army were marching into the city after the Battle of Wagram. Because of Frank's worldwide reputation in Public Health, Napoleon invited him to France. However, Frank distrusted the Emperor and feared the jealousy of his physician Corvisart. Therefore he decided to retire to Freiburg and devote his time to writing. However, in 1811 he returned to Vienna and remained there until his death in 1821.

Johan Peter Frank not only pioneered in public health, but also in the field of social medicine. He studied the social conditions under which men lived and recommended social means of improving them. He had the basic idea that government can accomplish a great deal for the health of people that is beyond an individual physician's power.

He proposed numerous forward-looking social and economic reforms, among which were the providing of free meals for children and a proposed tax on bachelors. He also was the first to propose a family allowance so that children should not suffer through the poverty of their parents. In his writings on marriage, reproduction and child birth, he postulated the requirement: "that persons with exceptionally severe and disadvantageous hereditary diseases should not be allowed to marry."

During the eighteenth century prostitution was universally accepted and the venereal diseases were extremely widespread and taken lightly. Frank advocated the segregation and regulation of prostitutes and aimed his attack against the venereal diseases at clandestine prostitution. He insisted that all venereally infected persons both male and female be restrained from sexual intercourse until it was ascertained that they were safe and restored to health.

Frank entitled his comprehensive six-volume work a *System einer vollständigen medizinischen Polizey* which is probably best translated as a *System of a Complete Medical Policy*. However, the German word "polizey" also means police, and hence it implies that Frank meant that anyone who did not abide by the rules of hygiene should be forced to do so.

In the introduction to his book he explains his meaning as follows:

"The internal security of the State is the aim of the general science of police. A very important part thereof is the science which will enable us to further the health of human beings living in society." He further states: "Medical police therefore, like the science of police in general, is a defensive art, is a doctrine whereby human beings and their animal assistants can be protected against the disadvantageous consequences of crowding too thickly upon the ground."

Frank served under so-called enlightened monarchs whose attitudes toward their peoples were purely paternalistic. The monarch ordered measures to keep his people healthy and forbade what was harmful. Frank was a firm believer and staunch supporter of this system and philosophy. His aim was to promote health through good legislation and enforce the health laws through the power of the State. Frank realized that while it was possible to promote personal hygiene by appealing to the individual much more was needed. He knew that the power and wealth of the State was needed to relieve poverty, supply more and better medical facilities and personnel, as well as to build water supplies and sewage disposal systems.

Because the impending Industrial Revolution was soon to bring great political, economic and social changes to Europe, Frank's work was almost antiquated at the time of his death. However, his book exerted a tremendous influence over a considerable period of time. It served to lay the foundations of modern public health by setting standards and setting forth a broad approach to the problems of health and disease.

Chapter 21

THE LADY WITH THE LAMP

Modern methods of nursing were born during the first half of the nineteenth century and began with the revival of the Deaconnesses of the early church. The Institute of Protestant Deaconnesses at Kaiserwerth, founded by Pastor Theodore Fliedner and his dedicated wife Friederike, set the stage for the world wide development of modern nursing education.

In 1833 Pastor Fliedner and his wife opened a tiny refuge for the care of discharged prisoners. In 1836 the need for the care of the sick poor impelled them to open a little hospital. Here Pastor Fliedner taught his Deaconnesses ethics and religious doctrine, while his wife taught them sound practical nursing methods. As the hospital grew, the Kaiserwerth Motherhouse developed many "Daughterhouses" which extended their doctrines and nursing methods. Nursing's great heroine, Florence Nightingale, received her administrative training and practical nursing experience at Kaiserwerth. Thus modern nursing schools can trace very definite lines back to Kaiserwerth and the Fliedners.

In ancient times wives, mothers and "wise old women" acted as nurses. In the Pagan world, women played a limited part by serving as "Priestesses" to an assortment of gods and goddesses of health and healing. With the rise of Christianity and the monastic hospitals, nursing, such as it was, passed into the hands of the religious orders. Many of the monastic hospitals delegated nursing care to so-called monastic women, whose origins are to be found in the early orders of widows and virgins. In 1212 the Bishops of France drew up rules and regulations for church hospitals and their nursing staffs. They decreed that all nursing orders were to take the vows of poverty, chastity and obedience and wear a religious garb.

The upbuilding of modern nursing began in the seventeenth century

with the work of St. Vincent de Paul and the French women associated with him as the "Sisters of Charity." St. Vincent brought young
country girls to live in the homes of the "Dames de Charité" and to
go with them to work in hospitals under their supervision. In addition
to hospital work he sent his Sisters to distant parishes to do visiting
nursing. Interestingly enough, he counseled them to take no more
than eight cases daily, which is approximately the same work load that
modern visiting nurse associations use.

St. Vincent advised his Sisters as follows: "My daughters, you
are not religious in the technical sense," and he then went on to
admonish them not to become nuns, because, "Nuns must have a
cloister, but the Sister of Charity must needs go everywhere."

As the Protestant Movement grew and drove out the religious
orders, hospital care and nursing deteriorated. This was especially
true in England where under the violence of Henry the Eighth the
dissolution of the monasteries was carried out in a very drastic manner.
The loss of this system left English nursing to the incompetent care
of "secular servant nurses." In general, the English retained the form
of the monastic nursing hierarchy. A matron continued to be at the
head of the nursing staff even though she was only an untrained
housekeeper and the title of Sister was given, as before, to the head
nurse of a ward. An ordinance of 1699 specified that only the
wives of "freemen" could hold the position of Sister, hence all of
the under-nurses were of an inferior social status.

With the suppression of the monastic orders, the responsibility
for hospital care and nursing services was transferred to the secular
authorities. Characteristically society as a whole extended little en-
couragement and less money to those whose function it was to care for
the sick and the poor. Consequently, most hospitals degenerated into
gloomy, unaired, dirty places. "Hospital smell," the result of dirt and a
lack of sanitation, was considered unavoidable and nauseated all who
entered.

The sick came into the hospitals filthy and remained filthy. It
was common practice to put a new patient into the same sheets used
by the last occupant of the bed and the mattresses were soiled and
sodden. The wards were so crammed with beds that even simple

decency was impossible. Overcrowding was so great that patients were frequently housed two or more to a bed.

Nursing was such an ill-paid, thankless and degrading a task that it attracted only the coarsest and most ignorant of women. Nurses were commonly recruited from "women who had lost their characters" and they were notorious for their immorality. Gin and brandy were smuggled into the wards and drink was the curse of both nurses and patients.

Hospital nursing consisted of a continuous round of dreary back-breaking drudgery, with one untrained nurse being assigned to care for twenty or more sick people at a time. At night conditions were even worse and one nurse was left to care for at least one hundred helpless and hopelessly ill patients. Due to this lack of care, the patients were forced to care for themselves and each other and had to empty their own bed pans and slops.

Those who could not or would not enter a hospital fared as badly, or even worse, at the hands of ignorant servant nurses of the type which was immortalized by Charles Dickens in the person of Sairy Gamp.

The time was ripe for reform and society needed desperately to be rescued from the appalling services of the coarse, ignorant women to whom the business of nursing had fallen. It remained only for the pen of Charles Dickens to banish them with satire and laughter while Florence Nightingale reformed them out of existence.

In *Martin Chuzzelwit,* Dickens portrayed the nurse of his times as follows:

> She was a fat old woman, this Mrs. Gamp, with a husky voice and a moist eye, . . . she wore a very rusty black gown, rather the worse for snuff, and a shawl and bonnet to correspond. The face of Mrs. Gamp—the nose in particular—was somewhat red and swollen, and it was difficult to enjoy her society without becoming conscious of a smell of spirits. Like most persons who have attained to great eminence in their profession, she took to hers very kindly; . . . she went to a lying-in or a laying-out with equal zest and relish.

To supplement her uncertain income Sairy Gamp had a lady-like arrangement with Mr. Mould, the prosperous undertaker, whereby for a small commission she would readily recommend potential customers.

Dickens reveals the callous type of care given in the following scene, where Sairy Gamp has her supper interrupted by the nervous agitation of an elderly patient.

> "Why, highty tighty, sir!" cried Mrs. Gamp, "is these your manners? You want a pitcher of cold water throw'd over you to bring you round; that's my belief." When she had finished the last crumb, Mrs. Gamp took him by the collar of his coat, and gave him some dozen or two of hearty shakes backward and forward in his chair; that exercise being considered by the disciples of the Prig school of nursing (who are very numerous among professional ladies) as exceedingly conducive to repose, and highly beneficial to the performance of the nervous functions. Its effect in this instance was to render the patient so giddy and addle-headed, that he could say nothing more; which Mrs. Gamp regarded as the triumph of her art.

Florence Nightingale's drive, genius and extraordinary personality created the respected profession of nursing as we know it today. The most important outcome of the Crimean War was the fight she waged for the decent care of the sick and wounded soldiers of the overcrowded army hospital at Scutari. Her revolutionary reforms in the treatment and nursing care of the sick and wounded marked the beginning of a drive for higher standards. Her struggle was not only against disease, but against bureaucracy, inefficiency and the traditionally callous attitude of society toward people in need of care.

Florence Nightingale became the very symbol of hope and mercy to thousands of sick and wounded soldiers of the Crimean War. Nightly, she had walked down the endless rows of the wounded, carrying her lamp, nodding and smiling, as she comforted the sick and dying during the endless hours of the dark and fearful night. She emerged from the Crimean War a heroic and legendary figure, famed throughout the world as "The Lady With The Lamp." Out of the misery of the Crimean War she created the modern nurse, stamping and molding her in the heroic image of an "Angel of Mercy." Never again was the professional nurse to be pictured as a callous, slovenly, drunken harlot.

Wealthy and wellborn, Florence Nightingale was a lonely and somewhat neurotic crusader who believed that "God had called her to His service." With an almost fanatic zeal she braved family disapproval, sacrificed her health to hardship and spurned romance, marriage and social eminence to accomplish her mission.

She was named for the city of her birth, Florence, Italy, where her parents had gone on one of their periodic visits to the Continent. Florence received her elementary education in the usual fundamental subjects from her father, who was a country gentleman of wealth and culture. As a young girl she doctored sick pets and was especially fond of babies. She displayed an unusual interest in the sick and was accustomed to visit hospitals in her immediate environs as well as in London.

Nursing was a menial occupation and was not considered a suitable calling for an educated lady of high social standing when Florence Nightingale sought training in this field in 1850. However, she had learned of the excellent reputation of the Institute of Protestant Deaconnesses at Kaiserwerth on the Rhine and decided to go there for her training. She remained in Kaiserwerth for an extensive tour of training and upon her return to England was appointed superintendent of the Hospital for Invalid Gentlewomen in London.

In 1854 the British Army was fighting in the Crimea and the initial engagements exposed the deplorable lack of suitable food, hygiene, and sanitation in the British army, as well as the neglect of the wounded and inadequate nursing of the sick. The need for radical reform was evident, and Florence Nightingale, through her friendship with Sidney Herbert, the secretary of war, was commissioned to care for the sick and wounded soldiers in the Crimea. Under her direction, a small group of nurses was recruited and proceeded to Turkey. The staff assembled consisted of representatives from the Roman Catholic Church, Sisters of Mercy of the Church of England and nurses from various London hospitals.

The barracks hospital at Scutari, a makeshift structure, grossly inadequate, infected, and filthy, was her assignment in the Crimea. It lacked a kitchen, plumbing, central heating, utensils, garments for the patients, soap and towels. Most of the food was spoiled. One pint of water per patient was allotted for drinking and washing. The day they arrived 500 British soldiers were brought in. The men had been wounded at the battle of Balaklava ten days before, but their wounds had not yet been washed or bandaged. Florence Nightingale organized her nurses into round-the-clock squads, scrubbing floors, making mattresses, and washing the wounded. Within a few months, Miss Nightingale and her associates transformed the barracks into a military hospital with clean wards, a laundry, a suitable kitchen, reading and recreation rooms, and a banking service for the soldiers to send money home. She established an enviable pattern in overcoming ancient regulations and substituted efficient administration and effectual nursing care. A phenomenal decrease in mortality followed.

The work Florence Nightingale began under the emergency of war was continued in peacetime and she added the training of civilian nurses to her interests. With money provided by friends and admirers, the Nightingale School and Home for Nurses was established at St. Thomas' Hospital. This training school not only served as a model for other schools, but its graduates became the heads of other schools in England and the United States. Religious training was no longer considered essential, but good character was insisted upon; and thousands of women began to take up a career which had been raised from the level of domestic work to the status of a profession.

Florence Nightingale not only reformed nursing, but also reformed hospital practices and procedures. In addition to effective nursing, she insisted upon light, warmth, well-cooked meals and, above all, scrupulous cleanliness. She further advocated the recording of vital statistics, including admissions, discharges and the incidence of disease and death.

Three years after Florence Nightingale's return from the Crimea the conscience of the world was further aroused to take action to provide proper medical care for the wounded of war. In 1859 the Swiss investment banker and philanthropist, Jean Henri Dunant, was present at the bloody battle of Solferino in Italy and was shocked and horrified at the lack of available medical care. To meet the emergency he organized a volunteer nursing service and called upon the local civilian population for bandages, food and care.

Adopting the motto *"sono fratelli"* (we are all brothers), Dunant called for the establishment of a permanent international society for the relief of suffering from war. He proposed that neutral zones for hospitals, doctors and nurses be set up on battlegrounds under the protection of an emblem of mercy that would be recognized by all. Some years later, in 1864, his efforts finally culminated in the holding of an international convention in Geneva which gave birth to the International Red Cross. Twelve nations signed agreements of participation and the emblem adopted by the convention was the reversal of the Swiss flag, which is now the well known red cross on a white field.

The successful efforts of Florence Nightingale, Dunant and others for the betterment of medical and nursing care was one of the most important contributions of the nineteenth century.

Chapter 22

DOCTORS! WASH YOUR HANDS

OCCASIONALLY, THE CAUSE of preventive medicine has been advanced by a sound, self-evident observation that could be summed up in a simple edict, which, if carried out, could save countless lives. Such an observation was made in 1847 by Ignaz Philipp Semmelweis when he discovered that the common obstetrical practice of examining parturient women without the simple precaution of washing the hands was the cause of puerperal sepsis. Strange as it may seem, his simple edict of "Doctors! Wash your Hands" met with violent opposition. His crusade to prevent childbed fever resulted in his being reviled, ridiculed and persecuted by his contemporaries. As a result he died broken hearted in an insane asylum at the early age of forty-seven, a martyr to his cause.

During the seventeenth, eighteenth and nineteenth centuries childbed fever became the scourge of motherhood and the terror of the lying-in hospitals. Killing thousands of mothers and often their newborn babies, it swept through the maternity wards with frightful regularity frequently killing one mother out of every six.

We now know that childbed fever is a form of septicemia due to the dread streptococcus. The "strep" germs reach the uterus via dirty hands during examination or on dirty instruments during difficult deliveries. Although the disease had been known since ancient times, it only occurred then as an occasional complication of childbirth. Primitive women had little childbed fever, because when all was normal, birth was spontaneous, while abnormal cases ended in death. Although the ancient Greeks had developed obstetrics to the point where they actively aided deliveries, they had little infection because they used wine as an antiseptic.

During the Dark and Middle Ages women were delivered in their homes with little or no interference and hence had few infections.

However, in the sixteenth century Paré rediscovered podalic version and the Chamberlain Family's secret of the forceps became known. These advances ushered in the era of medical obstetrics and the "man-midwives." Although saving many lives, these techniques entailed active interference in the birth process and thus frequently introduced infection.

With the growth of cities and the establishment of large charity hospitals where the poor could bear their children, puerperal sepsis grew to pestilential proportions. Physicians, medical students and midwives, ignorant of antisepsis, unwittingly carried death on their hands and instruments as they went from patient to patient. Thus childbed fever was actually a product of medical advancement and civilization.

Many theories were advanced to explain its cause and in general all of them postulated two influences or factors, one external and the other internal. Most observers took both factors into account but usually weighted one more than the other. The external factors were dependent upon an adverse condition of the weather or atmosphere and were classified as miasmic, cosmic or telluric. The internal factors were dependent upon the peculiar conditions attending pregnancy. They explained childbed fever on the basis of (a) lochial suppression, (b) "milk fever" due to a suppression of the mother's milk, (c) a crasis or dissolution of the blood or (d) a "gastric-bilious" condition.

It was not until well into the eighteenth century that infection and contagion came under suspicion as to being the cause of puerperal fever, and, occasionally obstetricians recognized it for what it was. John Burton of England in 1751 was the first to suggest that it was brought to the patient by the carelessness of physicians and midwives. Dr. Charles White of Manchester in 1773 observed that the incidence of puerperal sepsis varied greatly among different segments of the population. He inferred that this was related to the degree of cleanliness present and might be due to exogenous matter carried to the patient by the midwives.

The first clear-cut statement on the contagious nature of childbed fever was given by Dr. Alexander Gordon of Aberdeen in 1795. In his *Treatise on the Epidemic Puerperal Fever* he stated that he had unquestionable proof that the cause was a specific contagion or infection. He went on to say that "This disease seized such women only, as were visited, or delivered, by a practioner or taken care of by a nurse, who previously attended patients affected with the disease. Every person, who had been with a patient in the puerperal fever, became charged with an atmosphere of infection, which was communicated to every pregnant woman, who happened to come within its sphere." Gordon further recommended the burning of the bedclothes and apparel of infected patients and advised thorough washing by the attendant doctors and nurses. Finally, Robert Collins who was "Master" of the Rotunda, the famous Lying-In Hospital of Dublin, instituted chlorine disinfection of the hands to suppress the dread disease.

In America childbed fever was far from unknown, but because hospitals had not reached the high degree of development that they had in Europe, the disease did not assume epidemic proportions. However, the situation was serious enough to come to the attention of Oliver Wendell Holmes and cause him to "take his pen in hand" and become a "protector of motherhood."

Better known historically as a poet and a man of letters, Holmes was also a physician and an outstanding medical thinker. Being a prodigious reader he was familiar with the literature on obstetrics and puerperal fever in England. Judging from these reports and from an imposing array of statistics gathered from other physicians he produced his best known and only contribution to clinical medicine.

Holmes read his famous essay on "The Contagiousness of Puerperal Fever" to the Boston Society for Medical Improvement in 1843. He cited a formidable list of cases in which puerperal fever had followed treatment by physicians who, before going to the delivery had performed postmortem examinations upon cases of gangrene, erysipelas or peritonitis; or had treated other cases of puerperal infection. He correctly and bluntly concluded that, "the disease known as puerperal fever is so far contagious as to be frequently carried from patient to patient by physicians and nurses."

Holmes' eloquence brought down upon him a storm of abuse and controversy. The obstetricians and practioners of his day were not yet ready to admit that they were the cause of puerperal fever.

Although his work preceded that of Semmelweiss by four years, Holmes was not an obstetrician and his conclusions were not based on original clinical observations. In addition to not having the full facts, Holmes also lacked the fanatic zeal and crusading spirit of Semmelweiss. Turning more and more to poetry, literature and teaching, Holmes let his fight against puerperal fever lapse.

Ignaz Philipp Semmelweis was born July 1, 1818 in Buda, Hungary before it was united with its sister city of Pest. He was the fourth of seven children and apparently had a relatively normal and happy childhood. However, due to a faulty preliminary bilingual education, he had some difficulty with speaking and writing, which in later years handicapped him in clearly expressing his ideas to the medical world. His father, who was a merchant, wanted him to become a lawyer and Semmelweis spent two years at the University of Pest before going to Vienna to complete his legal education. He found the law to be a dull subject and through his contacts with medical students in the Vienna Coffeehouses he soon turned to the study of medicine.

The transition from law to medicine was easily accomplished by Semmelweis and he was able to pass all of his courses creditably. He received his Doctorate in Medicine from the University of Vienna in April of 1844 at the age of twenty-six. Apparently his interest in obstetrics had developed before graduation and by taking special courses in obstetrics he received the postgraduate degree of Master of Midwivery six months after graduation.

While waiting for an appointment as assistant in the Obstetric Clinic of the Allegemeines Krankenhaus, Semmelweis took volunteer courses at the clinic. He also faithfully attended the autopsies performed by Carl von Rokitansky, the professor of pathological anatomy, upon women who had died of gynecologic or obstetrical disorders, thereby laying the foundation for his superior knowledge in this field.

When Semmelweis secured his appointment as assistant in the First Obstetrical Clinic, a curious state of affairs existed that intrigued his eager, questioning mind. The startling fact was that ten times as many mothers died in the First Division Clinic, where the medical students worked, than in the Second Division, which was devoted to the training of midwives. No published statistics were needed for the poor of Vienna to know that if they entered the First Clinic to have their babies they might not return home alive. Many women on admission to the hospital begged to be assigned to the midwives in the Second Clinic, where for some unknown reason, their chances for survival were greater. Others sought to avoid the hospital altogether and many girls with illegitimate pregnancies delivered spontaneously in the streets near the hospital and then were admitted for after-care. Still others were delivered by midwives and then driven to the hospital. Strange as it may seem, most of these mothers did not develop childbed fever despite the dirt and filth which attended these so-called street births.

Disturbed and puzzled by these deaths, Semmelweis tabulated and compared the morbidity of the two Divisions. Between 1841 and 1846 there were almost 2,000 deaths among 20,000 cases in the First Division; in the Second Division there were less than 700 deaths in a slightly smaller number of cases admitted. The comparable percentages were 9.9 and 3.4. In 1846, the mortality was 11.4 per cent in the First Division and 2.7 per cent in the Second Division. He studied and examined again and again the accepted theories of the cause of childbed fever, but none of these satisfactorily explained either the cause of this deadly disease or why more women died in the First Clinic than in the Second.

Semmelweis found no answer to this puzzle, until the death of his pathologist friend Kolletschka in 1847 provided him with the necessary clue. Kolletschka had died from a small scalpel wound incurred during autopsy which led to his death from a fulminating blood poisoning. Semmelweis noted that the necropsy performed upon Kolletschka revealed pathological changes identical with those found upon women dying from puerperal fever. He then recognized that the deadly "cadaveric poison" that had killed Kolletschka was being carried to mothers on the hands of medical students and doctors.

It was customary for medical students to receive obstetrical instruction directly from cadavers, and the bodies of dead mothers and babies were used for demonstration and practice. The students and doctors moved freely, without the benefit of hand-washing, from the morgue and from infected patients to examine and deliver parturient women. The terrible truth came to Semmelweis that the reason mothers sickened and died in rows of beds on the obstetrical wards of the First Clinic was that they were examined in rows. Death came less often to the Second Clinic because the midwives did not visit the morgue and also because they examined their patients less frequently.

Semmelweis checked his records and they seemed to bear out his theory that the women of the First Obstetrical Clinic were being inoculated by the unwashed hands of the accoucheurs themselves. In order to test his thesis he required every one of his students and assistants to thoroughly wash his hands in an aqueous solution of chloride of lime, before examing or delivering a woman. As might be expected, this procedure was resented by both his students and collegues, who failed to understand or refused to accept the reasons for these precautions. However, the results were dramatic and the death rate from puerperal fever fell from 18 per cent in April 1847 to 1.2 per cent in July 1848.

It would seem that a discovery so momentous, and one that brought about such an immediate reduction in mortality, would be fully accepted and acclaimed. However, the doctors and students refused to believe that their own ignorant and careless practices were killing innocent mothers.

Some of Semmelweis' University friends were convinced that he had found the answer to the cause of puerperal fever and they urged him to publish his findings and to speak before medical groups. However, for reasons not entirely clear, Semmelweis neither published his results nor presented his findings to any organized medical society.

Although his medical associates, Hebra, Skoda and Rokitansky spoke or wrote in his behalf, his fellow obstetricians failed to recognize his discovery. Instead of adopting his methods, they not only scorned and belittled him, but actively fought his reforms. Among the leaders of the opposition was his own chief of obstetrics, Professor Klein, who vented his resentment by refusing to appoint Semmelweis as Privat-Docent of Midwifery at the Allegemeines Krankenhaus.

Gravely disappointed, Semmelweis returned to Hungary where

he accepted the directorship of Obstetrics at St. Rochus Hospital at Pest. This gave him the opportunity to prepare his only treatise on his subject, which was published in German in 1861 and was entitled *The Etiology, Concept and Prophylaxis of Childbed Fever.*

His book was largely ignored and drew unfavorable comments from many of the leading obstetricians of the times. Wounded to the quick, Semmelweis became bitter and wrote several scathing open letters to his critics. To Scanzoni of Würzburg he wrote: "Your teaching, Herr Hofrath is based upon the dead bodies of lying-in women, slaughtered through ignorance. If . . . you go on to write . . . to teach your students the doctrine of epidemic puerperal fever, I denounce you before God and the world as a murderer."

Denounced as a crazy Hungarian and a man to be laughed at and ignored, Semmelweis became increasingly embittered and angry. Haunted by the cries of dying mothers, he continued his lonely struggle to protect motherhood. The strain finally became too much for him and in July of 1865 at the age of forty-seven he showed serious signs of insanity. His wife and friends had to place him in a sanitarium at Vienna. However, ironic as it may seem, he did not die of his insanity, but died from blood poisoning received from a small finger wound incurred during one of his last operations.

On the day before Semmelweis died on August 12, 1865, Joseph Lister announced his principals of antiseptic surgery. There is no question but that Semmelweis practiced antisepsis fully fifteen years before Lister did.

The final justification of Semmelweis' work came with the discovery by Louis Pasteur of the causative organism of puerperal fever. Had Semmelweis lived, he might have said as did Oliver Wendell Holmes in 1883 to Dr. Chadwick: "I shrieked my warning louder and longer than any of them and I am pleased to remember that I took my ground on the existing evidence, before the little army of microbes was marched up to support my position."

Semmelweis is one of the tragic figures of medical history and had he lived a little longer, he would have seen his work fully accepted and his prophylactic methods used throughout the world.

Chapter 23

PASTEUR AND
THE BIRTH OF BACTERIOLOGY

No MAN HAS EVER made a greater contribution to the health and
and welfare of humanity than Louis Pasteur. He is one of the few
men of science whose name has become a household word and
whose work, directly or indirectly, has touched the lives of everyone. By refuting the theory of spontaneous generation and proving
the germ theory of disease, he ushered in the "Golden Age of Bacteriology." His discoveries transformed medicine, revolutionized surgery, and launched the science of preventive medicine.

Prior to the discoveries of Pasteur, medical men knew little more
than the Ancients about the actual causes of plague, pestilence, and
the host of other devastating diseases that scourged the human race.
Medical science was burdened with many false beliefs concerning
the causes of disease and the means of treating them. Superstition,
sorcery, and magic still held sway.

Pasteur's great grandfather was a serf of the soil, who for four
pieces of gold obtained his freedom and became a tanner. This
occupation was to become the family trade and was followed by
Pasteur's father, Jean Joseph Pasteur. Jean married Jeanine Etien-
nette Roqui, a village girl of Dole, France, and four children were
born of this union. Louis Pasteur was born in Dole on December
27, 1822, their second child and only son. In 1827 the family moved
to the nearby city of Arbois where the father established a tannery.
Despite modest circumstances and their own meager education, the
family gave their children all the educational advantages that were
available.

Louis grew up in Arbois and after completing his primary school-
ing attended the little College of Arbois. From there he went on to
the Royal College of Besancon which was located only thirty miles

from his home. Here, in 1842, he received his baccalaureate degree in science. Although his scholastic work was creditable, it was not brilliant and ironically enough, he was rated "mediocre" in chemistry.

After graduation, Pasteur was ready to realize his long cherished ambition of studying at the Ecole Normale in Paris. In the fall of 1842 he went to Paris where he tutored to finance his studies until he passed his entrance examinations in October 1843. At the Ecole Normale Pasteur plunged into his work with feverish energy. He was appointed assistant to the Chemist A. J. Balard in 1846 and attended courses at the Sorbonne given by Jean-Baptiste Dumas, France's most celebrated chemist. In 1847 he presented and defended two theses, one in chemistry and one in physics, thereby fulfilling the requirements for his doctorate degree.

The Revolution of 1848 caused a temporary interruption in Pasteur's career. He joined the National Guard and participated in the Revolution. When peace was restored, he returned to his studies in crystallography. In his twenty-sixth year he achieved his first scientific triumph by presenting to the Academy of Sciences his "Report on the Relationship Between the Crystalline Form, the Chemical Composition, and the Direction of Rotary Polarization." Therein he reported having found that tartaric acid crystallizes in two chemically identical but physically different forms, and that these right-faceted crystals in solution consistently rotate rays passing through a polarimeter to the right, or to the left, in accordance with their physical character. Met with skepticism, Pasteur won the friendship of a number of leading French scientists, including Jean-Baptiste Biot, when at their insistence he presented them with carefully worked out proof.

In September 1848, Pasteur was appointed professor of physics at the lyceum in Dijon but in December he accepted the position of assistant professor of chemistry at the University of Strasbourg. Pasteur found Strasbourg to be a favorable place in more ways than one. He enjoyed his lectures in chemistry and was still able to find time to continue his research work in crystallography. Here he met and married, Marie Laurent, the daughter of the rector of the Academy at Strasbourg. This proved to be a happy marriage and throughout his career his wife assisted him with his notes and records, as well as looking after his physical well-being.

Pasteur's academic career progressed favorably and in 1852 he was made a full professor of chemistry at Strasbourg. In 1854 he was appointed to the chair of chemistry of the Faculty of Sciences in Lille, as well as dean of the university. His work on crystals had launched a new branch of science, stereochemistry; and in Lille, in the heart of the sugar beet country, Pasteur began his studies on the fermentation of sugar to form alcohol.

With the help of his microscope, Pasteur found that microorganisms were responsible for alcoholic fermentation; and that faulty fermentation resulted from contamination by unwanted types of organisms. This work was of especial importance for his future career in that it took him across the boundary that separated chemistry and biology. Henceforth, it was the microorganisms that were to become the chief object of his research. Thus did Pasteur, the chemist, begin his transformation into Pasteur, the microbiologist.

Returning to Paris in October 1857 he joined the faculty of the Ecole Normale, thus becoming a professor at the institution where he had once been a pupil. Despite his many administrative and teaching duties, he set up a laboratory and resumed his research. The only available space for his laboratory consisted of two small dark attic rooms that were unbearably hot in the summer and cold in the winter. Years later his associate, Emile Duclaux said, "From this wretched garret, which nowadays would hardly be considered fit for a rabbit's cage, radiated the movement that has revolutionized all aspects of science."

During the year of 1859 while studying fermentation, he met with a great sorrow, for in September he lost his eldest daughter from typhoid fever. However, he continued his research on fermentation and these studies led him to his greatest and most revolutionary scientific discoveries. From these studies came his refutation of the theory of spontaneous generation and the undisputable proof of the existence of germs, their modes of reproduction, and their causation of specific diseases.

Pasteur's fermentation studies inevitably brought him face to face with the problem of the origin of the microorganisms that caused fermentation. Beginning with the study of the atmosphere, his microscope soon confirmed his belief that germs were invariably present and suspended in the air. His next question was: Do germs enter putrescible substances due to exposure to air, or are they generated within the substance? Pasteur conducted exhaustive experiments, in the laboratory, on mountain tops, and under every conceivable condition. When his flasks were heated to boiling and sealed to air, no growths appeared. When opened in the laboratory, contamination followed. Flasks opened, exposed, and resealed in the comparatively pure air of mountain heights remained clear. When reopened at lower levels, growths appeared.

The outstanding proponent of spontaneous generation and Pasteur's most noteworthy opponent was Professor F. A. Pouchet, director of the Museum of Natural History at Rouen. He and other supporters of spontaneous generation denounced and derided Pasteur and publicly challenged him with purported contrary evidence.

Pasteur's most effective demonstrations to refute these charges were with his swan's neck flasks. Broth was placed in the flask, the neck of which was heated and drawn out to form a swan's neck shape. When the broth in the flask was heated to boiling, air was forced out; on cooling, air pressure outside forced air to reenter the flask. Due to the small tubular swan's neck, if entering air were permitted to flow into the flask slowly, air-borne particles would fall by gravity to the surface of the lower curve of the neck, and, as long as the flask was not tipped or agitated, no microbial growth occurred. If, however, the flask were tilted until broth touched the lower curve of the neck, or, if air were drawn in rapidly by violent agitation, growth appeared.

Summarizing his findings in a treatise entitled: "Organic Corpuscles Which Exist in the Atmosphere," Pasteur received a prize from the Academy of Science for his work. The years devoted to the problems of spontaneous generation were years of growing fame. The controversies in which Pasteur engaged reached beyond the walls of the Academy and the subject was discussed in the popular press and became a favorite topic of chatter in polite society.

To clarify his position and to confound his opponents, Pasteur requested that a commission be appointed to settle the debates. On

April 7, 1864, he held a symposium on spontaneous generation at the Sorbonne before a large audience which included leading scientists of the day. After describing his experiments in detail Pasteur summed up his findings with these words: "There is now no circumstance known in which it can be confirmed that microscopic beings have come into the world without germs, without parents similar to themselves. Those who maintain this view are victims of illusions, of ill-conducted experiments, blighted with errors that they have either been unable to perceive or unable to avoid." Thus was spontaneous generation laid to rest and the "germ theory" officially introduced.

Pasteur was able to apply his growing knowledge of microbes and fermentation toward the solution of practical problems. The city of Orléans in France was a great center for the production of vinegar and those engaged in its manufacture were suffering losses from faulty fermentation. After devoting nearly a year of study to this problem, he was able to show the Orléans vinegar manufacturers how to improve their yield and thus saved them millions of francs annually. He introduced several improvements in the methods of production and demonstrated that if vinegar is heated, thus killing its organic life, it may be kept clear and pure for a long period of time.

Pasteur's studies on vinegar afforded a natural introduction to his study of the maladies of wine. France's important wine industry was sick and suffering great financial losses. The Emperor Napoleon III, who had followed Pasteur's career with interest, called upon him for aid.

Entering upon this investigation with his accustomed energy, Pasteur soon demonstrated that proper fermentation resulted from the action of wild yeasts that were deposited upon the ripening fruit. He further found that the "diseases" of wine which affected their flavor and keeping qualities, resulted from other parasitic germs which had either fallen on the fruit or had been accidentally introduced into the vats or presses.

The remedy was quite simple and after trying antiseptics without much success, Pasteur tried heat. He found that the vintners could protect their product, without injury, by heating the bottled wine for several minutes at 55 degrees Centigrade. Thus the process which is now called Pasteurization was introduced to the world. The importance of the subsequent application of this process to the fields of public health and food preservation are well known. His studies on wine were summed up in a book dedicated to his royal patron, entitled *Studies on Wine.*

Napoleon III, as well as the Empress, conceived a personal liking for Pasteur and occasionally had him as a guest at the palace. Unfortunately the triumphs of this active period of his life were marred by the deaths of his father, in 1865, and three of his daughters: Jeanne, in 1859; Camille, in 1865; and Cécile, in 1866. Only his son, Jean-Baptiste, born in 1851, and his daughter, Marie-Louise, born in 1858, survived. In later years the son entered government service; and Marie married a young secretary, René Vallery-Radot, who became Pasteur's confidant and biographer.

In 1865 while still at work on the diseases of wine, Pasteur received an urgent appeal from his old friend and teacher, Dumas, to investigate the diseases of silkworms. These diseases were devastating the silkworm industry to such an extent that France was producing but a small fraction of her previous yield. Dumas was a Senator from a silk-producing region in the south of France that was badly infested and faced financial ruin. He picked Pasteur as the one man most likely to bring relief to the silk industry by finding a scientific solution for its problems.

After careful study Pasteur found that two separate diseases were responsible for the devastation of the nation's silk industry. He not only discovered the causative agents, but devised means of detecting them and measures for eliminating the passage of these parasitic diseases from one generation of silkworms to another. Thus after six years of labor, Pasteur conquered the diseases of silkworms and the silk industry of France was saved.

During the years spent upon the diseases of silkworms, Pasteur was also occupied with a number of other matters. A series of disturbing incidents at the Ecole Normale resulted in his being relieved of his administrative duties and he accepted a chair at the Sorbonne. The Emperor had authorized the establishment of a research laboratory for Pasteur and construction had been started.

Unfortunately the intense and arduous life which Pasteur had been leading brought on a paralytic stroke that seriously threatened his life. Thus in 1868, at the relatively early age of forty-six, it seemed as though Pasteur's great scientific genius was to be lost to the world. The attack began during the day with a tingling of the left side, followed by a chill. However, this did not deter him from reading a paper before the Academy. That evening he suffered a more severe attack that temporarily deprived him of his speech. Although the best medical aid of Paris was summoned his condition remained critical for many days. He suffered intermittent states of paralysis, speech dysfunction, and mental confusion, which alternated with periods of improvement and mental clarity. The entire scientific world watched his condition with great concern and the Emperor and Empress dispatched a footman daily to obtain news of his health.

Recovery was slow and Pasteur was left with a mild partial paralysis of his left arm and leg. When his strength returned the Prince Imperial invited him and his family to stay at his estate, the Villa Vincentina near Trieste. Here Pasteur superintended the culture of silkworms from healthy eggs. The result was that the Villa yielded a net profit of 22,000 francs, thus marking the first time it had paid anything in ten years. Pasteur remained at the Villa for eight months and completed his book, *Studies on the Diseases of Silkworms,* which he dedicated to the Princess Mathilde.

Upon his return to Paris he was greatly disturbed by the rumors of the approaching war with Prussia. His patriotism was so intense that when the University of Bonn in 1868 had conferred upon him the honorary degree of Doctor of Medicine, he had rejected the diploma because the German Emperor's name appeared upon it. Thus when the Franco-Prussian War broke out in 1870 it not only interrupted Pasteur's work, but also gave him a grave dual concern for the welfare of his country and the safety of his only son who was then in the army.

At the close of the war, Pasteur wrote to his old friend and collaborator Duclaux, "My head is full of the most beautiful projects for research. The war has compelled my brain to lie fallow. Now I am ready for new productive labors; . . . Oh, that I might begin a new life of study and work. Poor France, dear country, what would I not do to relieve your distress!"

Pasteur conceived the idea of perfecting the French brewing industry so that France would no longer have to pay tribute to her enemy by importing German beers. Beers like wines were subject to several diseases, and frequently became ropy, sour, or putrid. Pasteur found that the diseases of beer were due to contaminating microorganisms that were introduced through the use of impure yeasts. He found that through the selection of pure yeasts which could be tested microscopically the contamination of beer could be prevented. He also introduced the process of heating or "pasteurizing" bottled beer thus killing off the unwanted ferments and preventing spoilage. He brought his researches and studies on this subject together in a volume entitled *Studies on Beer*.

In 1873 Pasteur was elected a member of the Academy of Medicine by a margin of one vote. This was a great tribute to him and he valued this connection because it afforded him an opportunity to create interest in the germ theory of disease. Unfortunately, it also precipitated him into an almost endless fight with official medicine. Many medical men regarded him as a "mere Chemist" meddling in the affairs of medicine.

In 1874 the National Assembly rewarded Pasteur by granting him a lifetime pension of 12,000 francs annually. This was acceptable to Pasteur because ill health had forced him to give up his chair at the Sorbonne.

Although Pasteur had already made many important basic discoveries, the years from 1877 to 1886 were filled with more new discoveries which were of great significance to medical progress.

For many years Pasteur had pondered over the possible relation and application of his researches to the cause, spread, and prevention of human dseases. Medicine had already received its first dividend from Pasteur's work through Lister's introduction of antiseptic surgery.

Joseph Lister, a professor of surgery at Edinburgh, had followed Pasteur's work on fermentation and putrefaction with great interest. He became convinced that the deadly surgical infections that occurred so frequently were due to microorganisms that gained access to the wounds from the outside. He reasoned that if this were true then surgical techniques must be developed to get rid of these offending organisms. Hence Lister disinfected everything in an operation, the instruments, the bandages, and the surgeon's hands were all washed in a solution of carbolic acid. In addition, a mist of carbolic acid was sprayed above the operative site to kill any germs that might be floating in the air.

Pasteur was not alone in his belief that certain diseases were caused by microorganisms. A number of physicians and veterinarians were carrying on experiments with the idea of proving that this was the case. However, their experiments were often so loosely contrived and so defective that Pasteur felt that they were "more likely to compromise the good cause than to serve it." Therefore, he started to work on the problem of infectious diseases and chose anthrax for his experiment.

The subject of anthrax is one of those focal points in the history of medicine at which a number of different lines of research flow together. A great many scientists had been interested in anthrax long before Pasteur's attention was directed toward it. In 1850 two French workers, Davaine and Royer, found large numbers of microscopic straight motionless rods in the blood and spleens of cattle that had died of anthrax. However, they were unaware of the significance of their observations. These findings were confirmed ten years later by another microscopist named Pollender, who suggested that these rods were the contagious element of the disease. Unfortunately, all of these early workers had failed to establish their thesis conclusively and the whole problem of anthrax was in a state of confusion.

Pasteur did not know that he had been forestalled in his research on anthrax by the brilliant German investigator, Robert Koch, who was then just beginning his famous career. In 1875, Koch grew anthrax bacilli in a pure culture; this was the first organism to be so grown. In 1877 he definitely proved that the anthrax bacillus was the specific etiologic agent of this disease. Pasteur acknowledged Koch's experiments and made additional experiments of his own to confirm the causative role of the anthrax bacillus.

Having proved that a great many diseases were caused by microorganisms, the next and much more formidable problem was to discover some means of protecting both men and animals from infection. Pasteur was well aware of the fact that there were many diseases from which people suffer only once because they acquire an immunity from them. He had been deeply impressed by Jenner's success in vaccinating against smallpox and wondered if this method of prevention could be used for other diseases.

As sometimes happens when a man is seriously studying a problem, a fortunate accident occurs that helps him to find the answer. In 1879 Pasteur was carrying out experiments on chicken cholera and his work had been interrupted so that the cultures of the bacillus of cholera he had previously prepared in his laboratory became rather too old for inoculation purposes. Because he had failed to produce cholera after injecting this old culture into fowls he was forced to wait until he could obtain a fresh and virulent growth from a new outbreak of fowl cholera. But when he inoculated his former chickens again with this fresh culture he found to his great surprise that they remained entirely free from signs of cholera. Yet when other chickens, never previously inoculated, were injected with it, they promptly succumbed to the disease, thereby proving that the new culture was a virulent one. Pasteur immediately saw in this occurrence an analogy with what happened after cowpox inoculation, that is to say that the inoculated person does not acquire smallpox. Further experiments which were made served to confirm the conclusion that by proper culture the chicken cholera germ could be weakened so that when it was inoculated into healthy fowl it would not only do them no harm, but would protect them against the disease. Pasteur had made his great discovery—the attenuated virus.

Pasteur now set out to attenuate the anthrax bacillus and to prepare a protective vaccine. His experiments were successful and he announced his discovery to the Academy of Sciences. Some received it with enthusiasm while others regarded it with distrust. One of the skeptics was Rossignol, who was an editor of the Veterinary Press. Rossignol challenged Pasteur to a public test of the vaccine and raised funds for the purpose of purchasing animals for the experiment.

Accepting the challenge, Pasteur prepared his attenuated vaccine and made the preliminary inoculations at the farm Pouilly le Fort on May 5, 1881. A large crowd of doctors, veterinarians, and farmers turned out to witness the tests. It was specified that twenty-five sheep were to be inoculated with anthrax vaccine and afterwards inoculated with anthrax. Twenty-five unvaccinated sheep were to be inoculated with anthrax alone. Six cattle were to be inoculated and four others kept as controls. Two weeks after vaccination the sheep and cattle vaccinated and unvaccinated alike were to be given an injection of virulent germs of anthrax and three days later the meeting was to be called to witness the results.

Pasteur and his assistants, Chamberland, Roux and Thullier, returned again on June 2 to witness the results of what they had done. As Pasteur's party drew near to the pens they heard the sound of loud cheering. The results of the great experiment had surpassed all expectations. All the vaccinated sheep were well. Twenty-one of the control sheep and the single goat were dead of anthrax, two other control sheep died in front of the spectators, and the last unprotected sheep died at the end of the day. The six vaccinated cows were well and showed no symptoms, whereas the four control cows had extensive swellings at the site of the inoculations and also febrile reactions. It was an immense triumph for Pasteur and his vaccination methods.

In 1880 Pasteur in collaboration with his former pupil Emille Roux began his studies on rabies. Pasteur had long pondered over this mysterious and dreadful disease. He had retained vivid childhood memories of when a mad wolf had charged through the Jura, biting men and animals as it ran its terrifying course. He also recalled when as a small boy he had watched the wounds of one of the wolf's victims being cauterized with red hot irons at a blacksmith's shop. Therefore, when the veterinarian Bourrel contacted him and sent him two rabid animals for experimentation, in the hope that a means of prevention and cure could be found, Pasteur accepted the challenge.

Rabies is a disease of great antiquity and is one of the oldest diseases known to mankind. A documented reference to it occurs in the Pre-Mosaic Eshunna Code of Ancient Mesopotamia as far back as the twentieth century B.C. In this Code the following passage occurs:

"If a dog is mad and the authorities have brought the fact to the knowledge of its owner; if he does not keep it in, it bites a man and causes his death, then the owner of the dog shall pay two-thirds of a mina (40 shekels) of silver. If he bites a slave and causes his death, he shall pay 15 shekels of silver."

The disease in animals was described with amazing accuracy by Democritus in the fifth century B.C. Aristotle in the third century B.C. wrote "Dogs suffer from madness which puts them in a state of fury and all animals which they bite when in this condition become also attacked with madness." Celsus in about 30 A.D. gave a good description of the disease and advocated that the wounds be washed in water and burned with a hot iron to prevent the disease. He also knew that the disease was bite transmitted and called it hydrophobia, a term which was used by the early Greeks. This term literally means "fear of water" and comes from the Greek "hudor" or water and "phobos" or fear. The term refers to the commonest symptom of human rabies, the so-called, fear of water phenomenon which is due to the painful spasms of the swallowing muscles. Later Roman physicians descriptively named the disease "rabies" which is a Latin word literally meaning madness and comes from "rabo" meaning to rave.

In the Ancient world rabies was believed to be due to extraterrestial forces. It was noted that dogs were especially subject to seizures during the hot weeks of late summer. These were known as "dog days," when Sirius, the Great Dog, brightest star in the heavens, rose in the morning and supposedly added its heat to that of the sun.

A popular though worthless treatment for rabies was the application to the wound of a so-called madstone. Madstones were rounded porous stones which supposedly possessed the magic ability of absorbing venum from a bite. Another type of madstone was the "ammonite," which was named after the God Jupiter-Ammon. Ammonites were curved fossil shells found in limestone formations, whose shape resembled the sacred ram's horn of Ammon.

In 1804 Zinke was the first to demonstrate rabies in the saliva. He successfully transmitted rabies by rubbing the saliva of a rabid dog into freshly made wounds on rabbits and dogs. The first positive demonstration that the agent of rabies in man and dogs was the same occurred in 1813 when Magendie and Breschet were able to infect dogs with saliva from a human patient. This, then, in essence, was the existing knowledge on rabies until 1880, when Pasteur's classical work opened up new vistas.

Pasteur at first attempted to discover the causative organism of rabies, however because of its ultramicroscopic nature, these experiments failed. It was obvious, however, that the infecting organisms, whatever they might be, were present in the central nervous systems of the persons or animals attacked, for other animals could be infected by injecting into their brains fragments taken from the central nervous system of those that had died of rabies.

Pasteur's assistant Roux had suspended the spinal cord of a rabbit previously dead from rabies, in order that he might discover how long the infective agent managed to survive the process of drying. While gazing at the flask containing the rabbit's shrivelling cord, the idea was born in Pasteur's mind of protecting dogs from rabies by inoculating them with a series of emulsions of dried cord.

He found that by drying the cord aseptically, the virulence of the causative factor of rabies decreased to the point of avirulence in fourteen days. Since the incubation period (from time of bite to onset of disease) for rabies was several weeks, Pasteur found that he could successfully treat an animal, already bitten by a rabid animal, if treatment were begun within a few days after the injury. Treatment consisted of injecting daily an emulsion of cord, beginning with the least virulent material (dried for fourteen days) and progressing to the most virulent (dried for one or two days). Thus, rabies could be prevented. Although these experiments were successfully repeated again and again in animals, Pasteur hesitated to try his vaccine on human beings.

Pasteur wrote to his friend Jules Vercel; "I have not yet dared to treat human beings after bites from rabid dogs; but the time is not far off, and I am much inclined to begin by inoculating myself with rabies and then arresting the consequences; I am beginning to feel very sure of myself."

Fortunately fate decided the issue for him. A little nine-year-old Alsatian boy, Joseph Meister, was brought to Pasteur's laboratory by his mother. Two days previously the boy, while on his way to school, had been furiously attacked by a mad dog and severely bitten about the face and hands. The dog was shot and an examination showed that its stomach was filled with hay and bits of wood that had been devoured in its mania for biting. The fourteen severe bite wounds that the boy had suffered were covered by saliva. A Doctor Weber who was consulted, washed, cauterized, and dressed the boy's wounds and advised the parents to take him to Paris and consult with Pasteur.

Pasteur secured quarters for the mother and child and consulted with Doctors Vulpian and Grancher, in whose careful judgment he had great confidence. After a careful review of the case and examination of the bites, the decision was made to start the inoculations as soon as possible. Treatment was started on July 7, 1885 and Joseph Meister was given thirteen successive inoculations of progressively stronger emulsions of infected spinal cord.

Vallery-Radot, Pasteur's son-in-law, gives us an account of him at the time of this first test of the vaccine on a human being. "Pasteur was going through a succession of hopes and fears and an ardent longing to snatch little Meister from death. He could no longer work. At nights feverish visions came to him of this child, whom he had seen in the gardens, suffocating in the mad struggles of hydrophobia like the dying child he had seen in 1880." His restlessness and his anxieties rose as stronger and stronger emulsions of cord were being used, but the child did not die. He recovered and thus was the first to be delivered from the dreadful death of rabies. Joseph Meister returned safely to Alsace and many years later, as a grown man, he became gate-keeper of the Pasteur Institute in Paris. It is told that in 1940 he committed suicide rather than open Pasteur's burial crypt for the German invaders.

The second case to be treated was a shepherd from the Jura who, while protecting some children from a mad dog, was himself bitten. He also survived and his heroic deed is commemorated in a statue which stands in front of the Pasteur Institute. A few weeks later Pasteur presented to the Academy of Sciences his famous report, "Method of Preventing Rabies After a Bite." Publication of this report brought pilgrims to his laboratory for rabies treatment from all over the world. On March 1, 1886 Pasteur submitted to the Academy of Sciences his further report: Of 350 persons who had received treatment following bites of rabid animals, there had been but one death—a girl brought to him thirty-seven days after she had been bitten by a rabid animal.

Nineteen Russians who had been bitten by rabid wolves were brought to Pasteur's laboratory. A number of them were in very serious condition because of the severity of their bites. The percentage developing rabies after being bitten by rabid wolves was known to be very high, averaging about eighty-two out of a hundred cases. Two weeks had elapsed since the Russians had been bitten and hence it was considered very doubtful that they could be saved. Therefore, it was decided to give two inoculations daily in order to speed up the protective process. Greatly to Pasteur's grief, three of the Russians soon died but the rest recovered and returned to Russia. In behalf of these and other Russians who had been saved, the Tsar presented Pasteur with the Diamond Cross of the Order of St. Anne. In addition, he donated a hundred thousand francs for the Pasteur Institute for which funds were then being collected.

Physicians and scientists from all over now flocked to Pasteur's laboratories to learn about the prophylactic treatment against rabies and about other of Pasteur's doctrines which were rapidly revolutionizing the practice of medicine.

The conquest of rabies was the crowning achievement of Pasteur's career. On November 14, 1888, the Pasteur Institute was dedicated and offered unrivaled facilities for research. Unfortunately the great scientist's health was steadily declining and his work became limited to advising and consulting with the members of his devoted and efficient staff.

Pasteur's seventieth birthday on December 27, 1892 was the occasion for a fitting celebration in his honor. This ovation was held at the Sorbonne and was supported by the French Academy of Sciences and was presided over by the President of the Republic. It was attended by a brilliant assemblage of great scientists and political dignitaries from all over the world. Lord Lister, representing the Royal Societies of London and Edinburgh paid him a great tribute and said, "The great honor has been accorded me of bringing you the homage of the sciences of medicine and surgery. As a matter of fact, there is no one living in the entire world to whom the medical sciences owe so much as they do to you. . . . You have lifted the veil that for centuries has hidden the infectious diseases." At the close of the ceremonies, Pasteur was too moved to speak, and asked his son to read his acknowledgment.

Death came to Pasteur on September 27, 1895 at the age of seventy-three. At the request of the French Government, Pasteur's body was interred in a beautiful chapel at the base of the Pasteur Institute. Its marble walls bear the names of the chief investigations in which he had won renown, while in the laboratories above his tomb, his great work still goes on.

Chapter 24

THE GOLDEN AGE OF MEDICAL DISCOVERY

Pasteur's great work gave birth to the new science of bacteriology and thereby ushered in the "Golden Age of Medical Discovery." Hard and fast upon the heels of his work, the names of numerous scientists flashed across the scientific sky, illuminating it with one great bacteriological discovery after another.

The science of bacteriology developed rapidly from this time on. As discovery followed discovery, an ever-increasing number of bacteria were isolated and identified. The causative organisms of disease after disease became known as well as their manner and means of spread. Along with this came the discovery of various sera and vaccines that could cure or better yet, prevent many of these diseases. Thus, preventive medicine came into its own and for the first time in the history of civilization, mankind could "cure certain diseases by never letting them happen at all."

Although Pasteur was the father of bacteriology it was Robert Koch (1843-1910) who placed the infant science upon a firm experimental foundation. Between them, Pasteur and Koch changed the entire course of medical thinking.

Robert Koch was born December 11, 1843 in the small German town of Klausthal. He was the son of a mining engineer and came from a large family. Always precocious as a child, he showed an early interest in science. Under the guidance of his father he became quite knowledgeable in the fields of geology, botany, and zoology, and acquired an extensive collection of specimens. After completing his preliminary education at the local gymnasium he entered the University of Goettingen. Koch proved to be an able and outstanding medical student and was fortunate in having some of the great men of medicine as his teachers. He had the privilege of studying under the renowned anatomist, Jacob Henle, and the famous pathologist,

Krause. He thereby acquired some useful research experience, as well as a thorough knowledge of the techniques of microscopy.

Following graduation in 1866 he served his internship and held junior posts in hospitals at Hanover and Hamburg. He then married Emmy Fraatz, a sweetheart of his student days, and spent several years as a small town general practitioner. His career was interrupted by a short term of service as an army surgeon in the Franco-Prussian War. Dissatisfied with the life of a general practitioner, Koch obtained a diploma in public health, qualified for and received an appointment as the district physician of Wollstein in East Prussia. In this position, he combined the duties of a medical officer of health with that of a general practitioner.

Koch became a self-made bacteriologist and started on his road to fame approximately one year after his appointment as district physician. His experience was limited and his equipment was simple, with the exception of his microscope. His devoted wife, utilizing her household money, bought him a new microscope which she presented to him on his thirtieth birthday in 1873. Installing his laboratory next to his consulting room, Koch in between clinical cases started his bacteriological studies.

In Koch's remote corner of Prussia, anthrax was a common and ever-present disease, afflicting both men and animals. Patiently and precisely, the nearsighted young physician began examining the blood and tissues of infected animals.

He consistently found present the rod-shaped organisms which had first been noted by Pollender in 1849 and again described by the Frenchman Davaine, in 1864. Although unable to prove it, Davaine had considered it highly probable that anthrax was caused by these organisms.

Koch set out to prove that this was the case. Using mice, Koch inoculated them with the blood of sick animals and produced anthrax in them. He demonstrated that the disease was transmissible and reproducable in a series of mice for more than twenty generations.

Isolating and cultivating the organism, Koch succeeded in growing it outside of the body. For this purpose he devised the "hanging drop" preparation in which the organism could be grown and observed. He utilized the fluid humor from the eye of an ox as a medium for bacteriological growth. As Koch went on with his studies he discovered the spore stage of the anthrax bacillus. He demonstrated that under adverse conditions the rods entered into a dormant or resistant phase and that when conditions for growth became favorable the spores again developed into typical disease-producing rods.

By injecting his cultures into mice and other animals Koch was able to produce anthrax. He then recovered the organisms from his experimental animals, cultured them once again and used them over and over to produce the disease. Robert Koch thus charted the life cycle of a bacillus for the first time in medical history.

In the spring of 1876 Koch wrote to Ferdinand Cohn, the famous professor of botany and microscopy at the University of Breslau. He wrote as follows:

> After many vain attempts, I have finally been successful in discovering the process of development of the anthrax bacillus. After many experiments, I believe to be able to state the results of these researches with sufficient certainty. Before, however, I bring this into the open, I respectfully appeal to you, esteemed Herr Professor, as the foremost authority on bacteria, to give me your judgment regarding this discovery.

Cohn invited Koch to present his findings at his Botanical Institute at Breslau in April of 1876. Among the scientists invited to witness Koch's demonstration were: Carl Weigert, the first to stain bacteria; Leopold Auerbach, the famous anatomist; Frantz Traube, the pioneer of osmosis; and Julius Cohnheim, the famous pathologist.

Koch successfully demonstrated the life cycle of the anthrax bacillus and proved conclusively that this organism would produce the disease in susceptible animals. This epochal demonstration of the fact that specific diseases were caused by specific germs, was so dramatic that the pathologist, Julius Cohnheim, rushed to his laboratory and told his students: "Drop everything and go at once to Koch, I consider this the greatest discovery yet made in bacteriology."

The successful demonstration at Breslau started Koch on his rise to fame. Cohn and Cohnheim recognized that he had performed a great scientific feat in his small backroom laboratory in rural Wollstein. They began to bombard the Imperial Health Office with pleas to free him from his routine duties and to elevate him to a full time research position.

In the meantime, Koch continued his bacteriological studies and the next year published and described procedures for the examination, preservation, and photography of bacteria. He introduced and greatly improved the methods of staining bacteria. These staining procedures stemmed directly from Carl Weigert's work on tissue and cell staining. Other papers soon followed and firmly established Koch as an unsurpassed scientific investigator. Koch himself stated: "As soon as the right method was found, discoveries came as easily as ripe apples from a tree."

In 1880 Cohnheim's efforts bore fruit and Koch was transferred to Berlin as a member of the Imperial Sanitary Commission. He was subsequently appointed as an extraordinary associate of the Imperial Health Office and was given a laboratory and two associates.

One of Koch's greatest achievements occurred in 1881 when he devised a technique that made it possible to grow bacteria in pure culture. Known as the poured plate method, this consisted of spreading liquid gelatin mixed with meat infusion on a glass plate, and thereby producing a transparent solid medium. He soon replaced the gelatin with agar-agar and this eventually became the standard medium used in bacteriological culture technique. Koch demonstrated his first pure cultures of bacteria at the International Medical Congress in London that same year. After the lecture the great Pasteur rushed forward and exclaimed, "C'est un gran progris!"

It was on the 24th day of March, 1882, that Koch announced to the Berlin Physiological Society his discovery of the mycobacterium tuberculosis. He cultured the bacillus on blood serum slants and conclusively settled the controversy as to whether or not the disease was infectious and due to a bacillus. Koch simply stated, "I have succeeded in discovering the real cause of tuberculosis. It is the tubercle bacillus, a true parasite." His announcement received great public acclaim and his name became a household word and he was soon affectionately called the "father of the bacillus."

While isolating the tubercle bacillus Koch developed his famous "four postulates." These are the rules or steps necessary to prove that a specific organism caused a specific disease. These postulates possibly constitute Koch's single greatest contribution to bacteriology; because they became the guiding light for the army of microbe hunters that followed. In brief, the four postulates are as follows:

1. To prove that a specific organism causes a specific disease, the organism must exist in all cases of the disease.
2. The organism must be separated from the diseased body and grown outside in pure culture.
3. Inoculation of healthy animals with the pure culture must cause the disease.
4. With an organism from the inoculated animal, step two must be repeated.

From mid-August 1883 to May 1884, Koch and his assistant, Gaffky, investigated cholera in Egypt and India. Going first to Alexandria where cholera was epidemic, Koch soon succeeded in isolating the causative organism and announced his discovery upon his return to Berlin. Having traced the cholera explosion in Egypt back to India, Koch and Gaffky went to Calcutta where cholera was still raging. Here they succeeded in isolating the comma-shaped vibrio cholera bacillus from the dead bodies of every one of forty cholera victims. They not only isolated the organism but also demonstrated its manner of transmission and were able to cultivate it from drinking water, food and clothing. Upon his triumphal return home, Koch was honored by the German Emperor. He was awarded the "Order of the Crown with Star" and received a prize of 100,000 marks.

In 1885 Koch was offered and accepted the appointment of professor of hygiene at the University of Berlin. However, after a few years of teaching, he resigned to return to his beloved research work. A special post was created for him, and in 1891, he was appointed director of the Institute for Infectious Diseases.

In appearance Koch was a typical Prussian professor; he was a dignified and modest man of unceasing industry. No little of Koch's genius lay in his ability to teach others and to imbue them with his own patience and eagerness to learn. His two laboratory assistants, Löeffler and Gaffky, later became famous bacteriologists in their own right. Although many of Koch's pupils became famous, perhaps the most famous of these was the Japanese bacteriologist, Shibasaburo Kitasato. Kitasato, who became known as the Japanese Koch, cultured the tetanus bacillus and also isolated the bacillus pestis. Koch also was the teacher of the great Ehrlich and the famous American pathologist, William H. Welch.

Koch continued his research on tuberculosis, hopefully seeking to find a preventive vaccine or cure. In 1890 he announced his discovery of "tuberculin," which he believed to be such an agent.

However, his scientific record was marred by his refusal to reveal the nature of this substance. In addition to being secretive, he was prematurely enthusiastic and was severely criticized when his "tuberculin" was found to be useless, as either a cure or preventative. Fortunately, tuberculin was later found to be a valuable diagnostic agent.

Koch's conduct has been defended on the grounds that the preparation and use of tuberculin required a high degree of skill and he feared that accidents would occur if it were prepared and used indiscriminately. Other historians state that his policy of secrecy was dictated by the German Ministry of Health, who wanted to retain a monopoly on its manufacture.

In 1891 Koch established a landmark in epidemiology, when he pointed out the relationship between epidemics and polluted water, and demonstrated that water-borne epidemics could be prevented by filtration.

Koch's renown was now so great that he was called upon to study diseases and epidemics all over the world. In 1896, he studied "rinderpest" or cattle plague in Africa, and was able to identify the virus and prepare a vaccine. At the request of the British Government, he went to India and carried out important studies on bubonic plague. He studied the tsetse fly in German East Africa and went to Ceylon for research on malaria.

Domestic difficulties and divorce complicated Koch's later years. Subsequently, he married an attractive young art student named Hedwig Freiberg, who travelled everywhere with him and was able to cope with his various moods. This action was unpopular and resulted in a great deal of personal criticism. Reaction was so great that the inhabitants of Klausthal, his birthplace, tore down a tablet they had erected in his honor.

However, Koch's great scientific accomplishments overshadowed his personal problems and the German Ministry of Health built a research institute in Berlin which was completed in 1901 and named in his honor. In 1905, he was awarded the Nobel Prize for distinguished service to medicine. In 1908, the German government conferred upon him the title of "Civil Servant Extraordinary."

After an interrupted and uncompleted around-the-world trip in 1908, Koch returned to Berlin to rest and two years later, on May 27, 1910, at the age of sixty-seven, he died from a heart attack at a Baden-Baden sanitarium.

By his own wishes, Koch's body was cremated and his ashes were deposited in the walls of the Robert Koch Institute in Berlin.

The work of Pasteur and Koch stimulated intense activity in the new science of bacteriology. This research took two main directions and proceeded along different, but complementary lines. The Germans, under the leadership of Koch, sought to discover and to catalogue with characteristic thoroughness the infective agents of the different diseases, whilst the French continued along Pasteur's special line of research on the problems of immunity.

Chapter 25

MILK-BORNE DISEASES

SINCE TIME IMMEMORIAL the pastoral peoples of the world have used milk and milk products and have thrived upon them. There are many biblical references to milk, the best known of which is the one that refers to the Promised Land as "The Land of Milk and Honey."

The cow has frequently been called the "foster mother of the world" and is considered to be the most indispensable of all domestic animals. Milk is a cheap, valuable food and an article of universal consumption. It is the only substance in nature whose sole function is to serve as a complete food and from a nutritional point of view, it is our "most nearly perfect food."

Up until about the middle of the nineteenth century, no one believed that epidemic diseases could be spread through milk. The fact that milk spoils easily and sours readily was well known; hence, emphasis was always placed on getting freshly drawn milk and keeping it cool until used. Long before the bacteriological era, the need for cleanliness was recognized. However, this was from a standpoint of retarding spoilage rather than from any thought of preventing disease.

It was also common knowledge that the flavor of milk was affected by what the cows ate. Garlic, turnips, wild onions and mouldy hay and grain were all known to give milk a bad taste. It was especially noted that the practice of feeding cows on fermented distillery wastes produced a poor quality, off-flavor milk.

The first milk-borne disease to be recognized and reported was "milk sickness" or "trembles." This was a serious and often fatal disease that afflicted the early settlers of the United States. It was recognized as early as 1776 in North Carolina and was reported again in Illinois in 1797. Abraham Lincoln's mother, Nancy Hanks, is said to have died of "trembles" in the autumn of 1818 when that disease nearly exterminated the little community of Pigeon Creek. The disease occurred in areas where pasture was poor and was correctly suspected of being due to drinking milk from cows that had fed on poisonous plants.

In 1852 the pioneer American physician Daniel Drake headed a medical committee to investigate milk sickness and reported that it was due to cattle eating Rhus Toxicodendron. In 1861 evidence accumulated showing that the disease was due to cattle eating a plant known as white snake root. The problem was not fully solved until 1926, when Dr. James F. Couch of the Bureau of Animal Industry of the United States Department of Agriculture identified the poison responsible. He isolated from white snake root and rayless goldenrod a poisonous chemical substance which he named "tremetol."

Milk sickness can be prevented by making sure that cattle do not eat either of these poisonous plants. As a result of this knowledge, the disease has practically disappeared.

In a rural society, milk was handled on a simple, personal basis; the family cow or a neighbor's cow was the source and the supply. With the growth of towns and cities the family cow was replaced by the "friendly producer," a farmer with a few cows, who sold milk to the townspeople. As growth continued, practically all milk was brought to the city by producers' wagons and delivered direct to the customers. The milk was hauled loose in cans and ladled out to the customers, who furnished their own containers.

As industrial growth and urbanization progressed, the flow of milk coming into the cities grew from a mere trickle to a veritable river. Gone were the "good old days" of the family cow and the friendly producer. They were replaced by milk peddlers, whose methods were neither scientific nor sanitary.

As the distance between the city and country grew, producers had a longer haul to bring their milk into the city. In about 1840 milk began to be shipped by rail from the country to the city. As a result of increased distances and longer hauls, there was a considerable increase in the time required for getting milk from the cow to the consumer. This, plus a lack of proper refrigeration, unclean containers, dirty milk and careless handling, produced a hazardous milk supply.

Unscrupulous dairymen further complicated the problem by diluting and adulterating the milk. They removed cream by skimming and added water or lime water to increase their profits. They added various chemical preservatives, such as borax, boric acid, benzoic acid or formaldehyde to prevent and delay souring. As a result, various laws were passed both here and abroad to regulate against these practices. In 1854 Massachusetts passed a law prohibiting the adulteration of milk. In 1860 the first English law was passed prohibiting the watering of milk.

The first evidence that disease may be spread by milk was presented by Dr. Michael Taylor of Penrith, England in 1857. By a careful epidemiological study, Taylor was able to demonstrate that a case of typhoid fever occurring in the family of a milk producer resulted in an infected milk supply and was transmitted to fourteen other families who were consumers of this milk. This was done before the scientific establishment of the germ theory of disease. Again in 1868 Taylor demonstrated that an otbreak of scarlet fever in Penrith had been spread through the medium of infected milk.

At about the same time Professor Oswald Bell investigated an epidemic of scarlet fever and came to the same conclusion. In 1870 E. Ballard reported 170 cases of typhoid in Islington, England which were traced to a single source of milk. In 1877 E. G. Jacobs reported a milk-borne epidemic of diphtheria in Sutton, England. In 1881 Ernest Hart furnished convincing evidence of the relationship between milk and disease. At the International Medical Congress in London he presented a paper giving a record of fifty epidemics of typhoid, fifteen of scarlet fever and four of diphtheria, which were all due to milk.

The dangers of raw milk were becoming evident and recommendations for the heating and boiling of milk began to be made. The boiling of milk had long been customary in many parts of Europe and it was observed that these areas had little or no milk-borne disease. However, these were empiric observations that preceded the bacteriological era and further progress in milk sanitation was to stem from the discoveries of Pasteur.

Shortly after the discoveries of Pasteur gave birth to the science of bacteriology it was found that milk was an ideal culture media for bacteria. It was not only an ideal food for humans, but it also was an excellent food for bacteria. During the period of 1860 to 1864, Pasteur heated wine in glass bottles at temperatures ranging from 122 to 140 degrees Fahrenheit for a "few minutes" and succeeded in killing the bacteria and yeasts causing the souring of wine. In 1870, he similarly heated beer and destroyed the organisms which caused it to sour. It was only a matter of time until this process was successfully applied to milk and named "pasteurization" in his honor.

Up until the middle of the eighteenth century infant life was held cheap. It is reliably estimated that during this period four out of every ten babies born alive died during infancy. Infant feeding presented serious problems and in order to survive a baby had to be breast-fed, either by the mother or a wet nurse. Little or no knowledge existed concerning infant nutrition and artificial baby feeding with cow's milk was seldom practiced. In England, as well as in other parts of Europe, the unfortunate superstition prevailed that if an infant was given cow's milk it would develop cow-like characteristics.

During the nineteenth century physicians began to recognize the problems of infant feeding and hospital records frequently read that death resulted from "a want of breast milk." At the same time, nutritional studies began to stress the great nutritional value of cow's milk. Gradually, it was recognized that mothers who could not breast-feed their babies should be able to obtain a fresh, clean supply of cow's milk at reasonable prices.

Throughout mankind's existence on earth, his greatest risk of death at any one time has always been—and in many places still is—the first year of life. Because of an inadequate knowledge of infant feeding and a lack of basic sanitation and hygiene, babies used to "die like flies." For example, in New York City during 1870, 235 infants out of every 1,000 born alive died during the first year of life. The population of New York was doubling at that time and the combined problems of poverty, overcrowding and poor sanitation created an intolerable situation, especially for the nonbreast fed baby. These, then, were the conditions that existed when Abraham Jacobi, who was to become the "father of American pediatrics," practiced in that city.

Abraham Jacobi (1830-1919) was born in Germany and received

his medical education there. Shortly after receiving his degree from the University of Bonn in 1851, he immigrated to America. Establishing himself in New York City in 1853, he pioneered in the practice of pediatrics and in 1860 founded the first pediatric clinic in America. In the same year he was appointed professor of infantile pathology and therapeutics at the New York Medical College and thereby became America's first clinical professor of pediatrics.

Jacobi's practice extended over a span of more than sixty years. During this period, he virtually founded clinical pediatrics, bringing it from the neglect and ignorance of the nineteenth century into the scientific light of the twentieth. Although many "firsts" are attributed to Jacobi, his greatest contribution to clinical pediatrics was in the field of infant feeding.

A strong advocate of breast-feeding, Jacobi nevertheless recognized the great lifesaving need for improving the methods of artificial feeding. As early as 1873, he publicly advocated the boiling of milk as a sanitary measure. He further advised that the milk be diluted and sugar added, expressing a preference for cane sugar over milk sugar.

No greater contribution to preventive medicine has ever been made than that of Abraham Jacobi, who carried on a crusading campaign to "boil the milk until you see the bubbles." The carrying out of this simple procedure has probably saved more infant lives than any other single procedure prior to the discovery of antibiotics. An astute clinical observor, Jacobi's admonition to "boil the milk" evolved from practical experience. Knowledge in the field of bacteriology in his time was almost nonexistent, and the field of chemistry was too young to be meaningful in regard to solving the serious problem of death in infants due to improper feeding.

Not only was Jacobi a great and discerning clinician, but he also was a born crusader with a calling to "teach and preach." His advice to "boil the milk" was successful because it killed bacteria and made the tough curd of milk soft, so that the protein was readily digested. Moreover, his clinical astuteness made him aware that, by boiling milk for too long, babies developed scurvy. Thus, he became an active advocate of the use of fresh fruit juices for babies long before he or anyone else knew of such a thing as a vitamin.

In 1886, Franz von Soxhlet, a German chemist of Munich, recommended that all cow's milk fed to infants be boiled or sterilized to kill bacteria. He was the first to devise a small home apparatus for holding and heating baby bottles to sterilize milk by heating it to 212° Fahrenheit for forty minutes.

As a result of these developments and trends, programs for infant and child care began to appear in various countries during the 1890's. Milk depots, or stations, known as "gouttes de lait," were set up in France. The first of these was established by the Paris pediatrician J. Comby in 1890 and the program was greatly expanded in 1892 by Gaston Variot.

In 1893 Nathan Straus, a prominent New York business man and philanthropist who was greatly influenced by Jacobi's work, became convinced that the infant death rate could be greatly reduced by improving the milk supply. Especially concerned over the terrifically high death rate of New York City's tenement babies from "summer diarrhea" and "cholera infantum," he established America's first milk depot and infant feeding station.

From June to November of 1893 this first milk station distributed 34,400 bottles of pasteurized milk. The milk was prepared according to formula, and after being pasteurized it was dispensed in nursing bottles. The mothers who came with their babies were given instructions on infant care and feeding. So successful was this first demonstration in reducing infant mortality that in 1894 six more milk stations were established. The program continued to develop and expand, setting a pattern for infant care and infant feeding that was widely copied.

The Straus milk stations gave an impetus to governmental action along similar lines; in 1897 Rochester, New York established the first municipal milk station under health department auspices. Numerous governmental and charitable health agencies, both here and abroad, developed similar programs. They adequately demonstrated their effectiveness in promoting child health and reducing infant mortality. The three basic successful elements of these infant milk and welfare centers were, first, teaching mothers how to care for their babies; second, providing clinical facilities to weigh and examine babies; and third, providing a clean, safe milk supply.

Jacobi had advised Straus to use the Soxhlet method of heating milk for sterilization before dispensing it in his milk stations. The heat sterilization of infant milk was also being used in Europe and this procedure, both here and abroad, was reported as being effective in reducing infant deaths due to diarrheal disease. However, in 1894 the German professor Flugge opposed such heating of milk on the ground that after heating there remained organisms which would cause putrefaction and formation of toxins. His announcement retarded for several years any great extension of the process of heating milk for infants and did much to prevent the adoption of the heating process by the milk industry.

It was the discovery by a series of investigators that the high temperatures of Soxhlet sterilization were not necessary for infant milk that laid the foundation for present-day pasteurization. The low temperatures used by Pasteur for wine and beer were again tried for milk. The discovery that the milk-souring organisms and the pathogenic organisms of infected milk are killed at temperatures much below the temperature of boiling water caused a great revival of interest in the process of heating after the depression caused by Flugge's announcement. This revival took place from 1895 to 1906 and was accompanied by numerous laboratory investigations into the effect of heat on bacteria and on milk, and the development of new apparatus for heating milk at low temperatures in the home and by the milk industry. Low temperature pasteurization, for example at 160° F. or less, was accepted by many investigators as effective in destroying pathogenic bacteria.

In Denmark much experimenting had been done and by 1890 a form of continuous heater had been developed which became widely used. This machine momentarily heated milk and cream to 185° F. A few of these Danish heaters reached the United States between 1890 and 1900 and were used by some commercial concerns to heat large quantities of milk to prevent souring. Because of the rapidity this method became known as the flash method.

In 1895, Monrad, a Danish expert, recommended the holding of heated milk in tanks for thirty minutes or more as a means of increasing the efficiency of commercial pasteurization, but this suggestion passed unnoticed by the health authorities and the industry. Momentary heating of milk in large quantities by many forms of heaters was widely adopted by the milk industry between 1900 and 1905. The temperatures used ranged from 158° F. to 165° F. and the time of exposure from a few seconds to two minutes.

Although it was universally recognized that the milk front was of outstanding importance in the fight against infant mortality, physicians and others continued to oppose the use of heated milk. The idea still prevailed that only freshly drawn milk, untreated and untouched in any way, should be used for human consumption.

In 1853 Gail Borden of White Plains, New York, discovered that he could can and preserve milk by a process of condensation and sweetening. Whole milk was evaporated at low heat under a vacuum and cane sugar was added. This product, known as condensed milk, contains approximately 40 percent sugar and 27 percent water. Borden perfected and patented his process in 1856 and began the commercial manufacture and sale of condensed milk in that year.

Physicians were slow to make use of condensed milk in infant feeding. It was condemned because of the great quantity of sugar that it contained. In 1884 unsweetened evaporated milk was developed in Switzerland by John B. Meyenberg. Condensed milk began to be used quite widely following the introduction of the formula or percentage method of infant feeding by Dr. Thomas M. Rotch of Harvard in about 1890. As pediatricians and physicians began to use "formula feeding" and diluted the milk and adjusted the percentage of sugar, fat and protein, canned milk proved to be both successful and popular. Thus Borden's "Eagle Brand" and other condensed and evaporated milks proved to be a boon to mothers and saved the lives of thousands of babies.

In 1892 Dr. Henry L. Coit of Newark, New Jersey, needing a good milk supply for his own baby, formulated a plan for the production of a good clean, fresh milk supply under the auspices and supervision of a medical milk commission. He coined and applied the term "Certified Milk" to milk so produced. Certified milk was an unaltered raw milk of good quality and uniform composition. It had to come from tuberculin-free cows, could not contain more that 10,000 bacteria per cubic centimeter and could not be more than thirty-six hours old when delivered.

The idea of certified milk and the medical milk commissions spread.

The name "certified milk" was registered in the United States Patent Office in 1904. The American Association of Medical Milk Commissions was formed in 1907. It was believed that cleanliness and good dairy practices could produce safe raw milk and that the boiling, or pasteurization, of milk covered up poor dairy practices and disguised dirty milk. Although it hampered pasteurization, certified milk had a good effect on milk sanitation. It was a fine ideal and a noble experiment that helped raise the standards and quality of the entire milk supply. The difficulty with certified milk was that it was expensive and because it still was raw milk it could, and did, convey disease and hence was dangerous.

Milk is the chief vehicle for the conveyance of bovine tuberculosis from cow to man. The bacilli get into the milk, either directly as a result of tuberculosis of the udder, or indirectly from milk contaminated with cow manure. Cows ordinarily swallow their saliva and hence those with pulmonary tuberculosis infect their intestinal tracts and pass living tubercle bacilli in their feces. Bovine tuberculosis generally produces extra-pulmonary infection in man. It is the chief cause of scrofula or glandular tuberculosis, and tuberculosis of the bones and joints. It occurs chiefly among children in the preschool age group and to a lesser extent in older children and adults.

As early as 1847 Klencke stated that there was a positive connection between the milk of tuberculous cows and tuberculosis in children. However, the relationship of milk to tuberculosis was not thoroughly recognized until almost a generation after the discovery of the tubercle bacillus by Koch in 1882. For many years, Koch maintained that all tubercle bacilli were identical, regardless of their animal origin. This was disproved by Dr. Theobald Smith, who in 1896 and 1898 demonstrated that human and bovine tubercle bacilli were distinct species.

The establishment of this fact led to investigations as to whether the disease was transmissable from cattle to man. The subject was thoroughly studied by a number of independent groups—the Gesundheitsamt in Berlin, the British Commission on Tuberculosis in London, and the Research Laboratory of the New York City Health Department—and each came to the conclusion that bovine tuberculosis was transmissible to man.

Numerous studies both here and abroad succeeded in isolating living bovine tubercle bacilli from market milk. Hess in 1909 examined 107 samples of New York's market milk and found that 16 percent contained tubercle bacilli. A similar study in Chicago by Tonney in 1910 revealed that 10.5 percent of 144 samples of raw milk contained tubercle bacilli. In Great Britain 40 percent of the cattle were found to have tuberculosis and live bacilli were found in the milk of five out of every one thousand cows.

There are two ways of combating the spread of tuberculosis through milk. One is universal pasteurization and the other is the elimination of tuberculosis in cattle. Both of these avenues of control have been so widely and successfully used in our country that bovine tuberculosis has virtually been eliminated as a human public health problem.

In 1917, the United States Department of Agriculture, in cooperation with the respective states, inaugurated a concerted and militant plan for the eradication of tuberculosis in cattle. This consisted of the one sure way of eliminating bovine tuberculosis, which was to tuberculin test and to slaughter the positive reactors. On the basis of this "accredited herd" plan, local communities enacted legislation requiring all milk to come from tuberculin tested animals.

The firm application of this "test and slaughter" program entailed a long hard struggle and aroused much bitter opposition before it gained general acceptance. However, over the years it has proved to be highly successful and progressed to a point where for all practical purposes tuberculosis in cattle has been eradicated.

Another important milk-borne disease in brucellosis. Well known for over 150 years in various Mediterranean countries the disease was first described by Burnett in 1814.

It has been subject to much confusion and has been known by a variety of names, the most common being Malta fever, Mediterranean fever, remittant fever, febris sudoralis, Gibraltar fever, goat fever, Rio Grande fever, and most commonly undulant fever. In cattle, the disease is commonly called infectious abortion or Bang's Disease.

Brucellosis constituted a febrile illness which puzzled the medical personnel of the British Army and Navy stationed in the Mediterranean area during the later part of the nineteenth century. In 1863 Jeffry Allen Marston, a Royal Army surgeon, presented an accurate clinical report of his own illness. This detailed description of brucellosis differentiated the disease from malaria, typhoid and other fevers.

The etiological agent was described by David Bruce in 1887. Sir David Bruce (1855-1931) was a famous British pathologist and bacteriologist who became internationally known for his investigations into the causes of tropical diseases. He entered the Royal Army Medical Corps in 1883 and rose to the rank of Major-General. While stationed in Malta he succeeded in isolating the organism from the spleens of persons who had contracted the disease from drinking raw goat's milk. He cultured the organism and was able to transmit the disease to monkeys. Because he had discovered the organism on the Island of Malta, Bruce named it the micrococcus melitensis. He derived the term from the Latin word "melita" or honey, which was the name the ancient Romans had given to the island because of the fine honey bees found there.

In 1897 Wright and Semple described an agglutination test for undulant fever that distinctly advanced the diagnosis of the disease.

The first accurate knowledge of the epidemiology of the disease resulted from the studies of the British Commission for Investigation of Mediterranean fever. During the years of 1905-1907 they demonstrated that the drinking of unpasteurized goat's milk was the undisputed source of the infection in man on the Island of Malta. They found that 10 percent of the goats they examined excreted bacilli in their milk and that in some herds the infection rate was as high as 50 percent. As a result of the Commission's studies, the disease was eliminated from the military garrison on Malta by the simple procedure of prohibiting the use of raw goat's milk.

In 1896 Bang, a Danish veterinarian, assisted by Stribolt, isolated the organism causing contagious abortion in cattle. He named the organism the baccillus abortus; however, it soon became known as Bang's bacillus. In 1914, Jacob Traum of the United States Department of Agriculture isolated a suis strain of this organism from the aborted fetuses of swine.

One of the strange occurrences in the history of bacteriology was the failure, over a period of thirty years, to identify these organisms which are so closely related as to be almost indistinguishable. Not only was the relationship overlooked, but different generic names were used to designate them. The widely varied geographic distribution of the disease, the different animals primarily affected, and the fact that Bruce incorrectly called his organism a micrococcus, all served as barriers.

In 1917 Alice C. Evans, working in the Dairy Division of the United States Department of Agriculture, was making a study of the bacterial flora of cow's milk. The problem of infectious abortion was confronted and Dr. Eichhorn, the chief of pathology, suggested that she make a comparative study of Bang's bacillus and Bruce's melitensis organism. This was done with the astonishing results that the two organisms were indistinguishable, except by agglutinin absorption tests. Since the goat strain or melitensis organism could cause human disease, it seemed reasonable to her that the cattle or abortus strain could also do so. She called attention to this and advised physicians to look for it and they soon began to find and recognize the disease.

As a result of this knowledge, order came out of chaos and all of these organisms were called Brucella in honor of Sir David Bruce. It was now recognized that there are three common strains of the organism, as follows:

1. Brucella melitensis or the caprine strain, infecting goats.
2. Brucella abortus or the bovine strain, infecting cattle.
3. Brucella suis or the porcine strain, infecting swine.

All three strains can and do cause disease in humans. Primarily the disease is one of livestock, infecting the goat, cow, and hog. It is characterized by abortion in the female animal and a carrier state with excretion of the bacilli in the milk.

The control of brucellosis or undulant fever in man consists primarily of pasteurization of the milk supply. Another means of control is the elimination of infectious abortion from dairy herds. Since 1935 the United States Department of Agriculture has cooperated with individual states in carrying out a program embracing the testing of cattle, slaughtering those found infected and vaccinating calves against brucellosis.

As knowledge accumulated, it became apparent that milk is easily susceptible to bacterial contamination and constitutes one of our potentially most hazardous foods. It also became apparent that compulsory universal pasteurization was the only practical way of safeguarding our milk. Pasteurization makes possible a "germ-free" controlled milk supply.

Considerable opposition attended the development of pasteurization. A long, hard fight ensued and the bitter senseless opposition that was aroused against this sanitary measure was almost unbelievable. However, scientific evidence demonstrating the health hazards of raw milk was accumulating. In 1901 William H. Park of the New York City Health Department Laboratory showed that milk delivered to consumers in the summer was highly contaminated with bacteria and might contain more than 5 million organisms per cc. He published a paper that year entitled "The Great Bacterial Contamination of the Milk of Cities. Can it be lessened by the Action of Health Authorities?"

In 1902 L. Emmet Holt, a famous New York pediatrician, studied infant diarrhea or cholera infantum and demonstrated its relation to the bacteriology of the milk consumed. In 1903 Park and Holt in New York fed two groups of tenement house babies on raw milk and on the same milk pasteurized. The babies on the pasteurized milk diet showed a strikingly lower mortality from infant diarrhea, as well as from other causes. This conclusive demonstration was of marked influence in molding opinion on the merits of pasteurized milk. Adding to the weight of this evidence was the publication by the United States Public Health Service in 1909 of its famous "Bulletin 56" which listed five hundred outbreaks of milkborne disease between 1880 and 1907.

The work of Milton J. Rosenau in the Hygienic Laboratory of the United States Public Health Service in 1906 on the thermal death points of pathogenic bacteria, did much to settle the question as to the efficiency of low temperatures in the destruction of the species of pathogenic bacteria commonly carried by infected milk. His findings that 140° F. for twenty minutes was sufficient for their destruction for the first time inspired confidence in the use of such low temperatures for pasteurization.

In 1907 the first large scale commercial plant pasteurization apparatus was installed in New York City. The following year, in 1908, the City of Chicago adopted the first ordinance requiring the pasteurization of all milk, except that of the highest sanitary quality. New

York City passed a pasteurization requirement in 1910. Up until this time almost all milk supplies in the United States were raw; now community after community began to require pasteurization.

National standards of milk sanitation were established and the American Public Health Association published the first edition of its "Standard Methods" for the examination of milk in 1910. Health Departments throughout the nation began to pass and enforce milk sanitation regulations and pasteurization requirements. In order to secure uniformity of regulations and enforcement, the United States Public Health Service published its first "Standard Milk Ordinance and Code" in 1924.

The pasteurization of milk and good milk sanitation is now universally accepted and enforced. It represents a great sanitary victory for public health in a bitter struggle that extended over a period of more than thirty years. Never before in the history of the world has any food stuff been the subject of so much study, supervision and legislation as milk and its products.

Chapter 26

THE WATER-BORNE AND FECAL
DISCHARGE DISEASES

THE MOST IMPORTANT of the water-borne diseases are typhoid fever and cholera. However, various dysenteries, diarrheas, amoebiasis and intestinal parasites may also be disseminated by water. All are due to organisms from the fecal discharges of patients or carriers which gain entrance into drinking water. The causative organisms of these diseases do not reproduce in water and usually die rapidly within a few days. The actual number of disease-producing organisms in a polluted water supply is ordinarily quite small and the water is only a temporary habitat, but it serves as the medium of transfer from an infected person to others in the community. The control of this group of diseases is one of the most notable achievements of preventive medicine. The application of sanitary science to the proper disposal of human body wastes and the safeguarding and purification of water supplies has been the most important factor responsible for the dramatic decline in the disease and death rates of these diseases.

The Eberthella typhosa or Bacillus typhosus and the vibrio cholera or "comma bacillus" are the pathogenic organisms responsible for the greatest number of water-borne epidemics. The dramatic impact of the great water-borne epidemics of typhoid and cholera have overshadowed the other modes of transmission of these diseases.

In the past, water played a large role in the spread of typhoid and cholera; however, due to the sanitary disposal of human body wastes and the filtration and chlorination of water supplies these diseases have diminished almost to the vanishing point. In the last half of the nineteenth century and in the early twentieth century typhoid fever was rampant at various times and in many places and was primarily water-borne. It now occurs only sporadically and is seldom water-borne. Although cholera still occurs in Asia and other parts of the world, it has not occurred epidemically in the United States since 1873.

The history of preventive medicine is replete with the records of numerous epidemics due to polluted water supplies. Many of the facts of some of the water-borne epidemics that are related in this chapter were taken from Sedgwick's *Principles of Sanitary Science and Public Health;* and Rosenau's, *Preventive Medicine and Hygiene.*

One of the earliest instances, if not the first, in which water was proven to convey a specific disease was the "Case of the Broad Street Pump." In 1854 an epidemic of cholera occurred in London and prevailed with great intensity in the vicinity of a well located in Broad Street. Dr. John Snow made a classic and detailed epidemiologic study of this outbreak and published his findings in a monograph entitled "The Mode of Communication of Cholera." The detailed epidemiology presented in his report established beyond question the interrelationship of the disease to sewage and drinking water and that persons using other sources of drinking water were unaffected except as they may have become contact cases.

The epidemic was conspicuously circumscribed in area and was extremely virulent with a high fatality rate. Approximately 700 deaths occurred during the seventeen weeks that cholera raged and the death rate was 220 per 10,000. The disease broke out with especial intensity August 30 and declined sharply after September 10. At Snow's request the handle of the Broad Street pump was removed on September 8 after he had demonstrated that most of the victims had utilized water from this well. A study of seventy-three deaths occurring in the locality of the pump revealed that sixty-one of the cases constantly or occasionally used to drink water from the Broad Street well. In six instances, no information could be obtained and in six cases it was stated that the deceased persons did not drink from the pump.

On the other hand, Snow discovered that while a workhouse in Poland Street was three-fourths surrounded by houses in which cholera deaths occurred, out of 535 inmates of the workhouse only five cholera deaths occurred. The workhouse, however, had a well of its own in addition to the city supply, and never sent for water to the Broad Street pump. If the cholera mortality in the workhouse had been equal to that in its immediate vicinity it should have had 50 deaths.

A brewery in Broad Street employing seventy workers was entirely exempt from cholera. However, the brewery had its own well and also gave the employees a free allowance of beer; hence, they never used water from the Broad Street well.

It was quite a different story in a cartridge factory at 38 Broad Street where about two hundred people were employed. Here two tubs of drinking water were kept on the premises and always filled from the Broad Street well. Among these employees, eighteen died of cholera. Similar facts were elicited from other factories on the same street, all tending to show that in general those who drank water from the Broad Street well suffered from cholera, while those who did not drink that water escaped.

Snow conclusively forged the chain of evidence by his report of the following cases:

> A gentleman in delicate health was sent for from Brighton to see his brother at No. 6 Poland Street who was attacked with cholera and died in 12 hours, on the first of September. The gentleman arrived after his brother's death, and did not see the body. He only stayed about 20 minutes in the house, where he took a hasty and scanty luncheon of rump steak, taking with it a small tumbler of cold brandy and water, the water being from the Broad Street pump. He went to Pentonville, and was attacked with cholera on the evening of the following day, and died the next evening.
>
> The deaths of Mrs. E and her niece, who drank the water from Broad Street at the West End, Hampstead, deserve especially to be noticed. I was informed by Mrs. E.'s son that his mother had not been in the neighborhood of Broad Street for many months. A cart went from Broad Street to West End every day, and it was the custom to take out a large bottle of the water from the pump in Broad Street, as she preferred it. The water was taken out on Thursday, the 31st of August, and she drank of it in the evening and also on Friday. She was seized with cholera on the evening of the latter day, and died on Saturday. A niece who was on a visit to this lady also drank of the water. She returned to her residence, a high and healthy part of Islington, was attacked with cholera, and died also. There was no cholera at this time, either at West End or in the neighborhood where the niece died. Besides these two persons only one servant partook of the water at West End, Hampstead, and she did not suffer, or, at least, not severely. She had diarrhea.

John York, secretary and surveyor of the Cholera Inquiry Committee, surveyed the locality and examined the well, cesspool and drains at 40 Broad Street. His report revealed the following condition:

The well was circular in section, 28 feet 10 inches deep, 6 feet in diameter, lined with brick, and when examined contained 7 feet 6 inches of water. It was arched in at the top, dome fashion, and tightly closed at a level 3 feet 6 inches below the street by a cover occupying the crest of the dome. The bottom of the main drain of the house from No. 40 Broad Street lay 9 feet 2 inchs above the water level, and one of its sides was distant from the brick lining of the well only 2 feet 8 inches. This was an old-fashioned drain 12 inches wide, with brick sides; the top and bottom were made with old stone. It had a small fall to the main sewer. The mortar joints of the old stone bottom were found to be perished, as was also the jointing of the brick sides, which had brought the brickwork into the condition of a sieve, through which the house drainage must have percolated for a considerable period.

Snow found the cesspool intended for a trap, but misconstructed, and upon and over a part of the cesspool a common privy, without water supply, for the use of the house had been erected. The brickwork of the cesspool was found to be in the same decayed condition as the drain. Snow stated:

From the charged condition of the cesspool, the defective state of its brickwork, and also that of the drain, no doubt remains upon my mind that constant percolation, and for a considerable period, had been conveying fluid matter from the drains into the well. A washed appearance of the ground and gravel flow corroborated this assumption. The ground between the cesspool and the well was black, saturated, and in a swampy condition, clearly demonstrating the fact.

This evidence, although circumstantial, was sufficient to connect the cesspool with the well, and leaves little doubt, but that the water became contaminated with cholera germs through this channel. As far as could be determined, the contamination of the well came from an unrecognized case of cholera in the house at 40 Broad Street. It is interesting to note that this outbreak and epidemiologic study occurred before the days of bacteriology. Thus, through practical epidemiology and empiric public health practice, Dr. John Snow stopped a cholera epidemic by the simple expedient of removing the handle from the pump of the Broad Street well.

The first epidemic of typhoid fever traced to a water supply that attracted general attention occurred in Lausen, Switzerland in 1872. It is also of interest because of the remote and unusual method by which the infection reached the water supply. Lausen was a well kept village of ninety houses and 780 inhabitants. It had never, so far as known, suffered from a typhoid epidemic and for many years had not even had a single sporadic case. Suddenly, an epidemic exploded and between August and October of 1872, 130 of the 780 inhabitants were stricken with typhoid fever.

A short distance south of Lausen is a little valley, the Furlethal, separated from Lausen by a hill, the Stockhalden, and in this valley on June 19 upon an isolated farm, a peasant who had recently been away from home fell ill with a severe case of typhoid fever, which he had apparently contracted during his absence. In the next two months there occurred three other cases in the neighborhood—a girl, and the wife and son of the peasant.

No one in Lausen knew anything of these cases in the remote and lonely valley, when suddenly on August 7 typhoid fever appeared. The fever was distributed quite evenly throughout the town, with the exception of certain houses which derived their water from their own wells and not from the public water supply. Attention was thus fixed upon the latter, which was obtained from a well at the foot of the Stockhalden hill on the Lausen side. Only six houses used their own wells, and in these six there was not a single case of typhoid fever, while in almost all the other houses of the village, which depended upon the public water supply, cases of the disease existed.

There had long been a belief that the Lausen well had a subterranean connection with the Furler brook, in the neighboring valley. Since this brook ran near the peasant's house and was known to have been freely polluted by the excreta of the typhoid fever patients, absolute proofs of the connection between the well of Lausen and the Furler brook could not fail to be highly suggestive and important. Fortunately, such proofs were found.

The investigation revealed that the well or spring serving as Lausen's water supply had as its source this subterranean stream. Thus, the excreta from typhoid patients two miles distant and on the opposite side of the mountain contaminated the town's water supply.

The 1892 cholera epidemic in Hamburg, Germany stands out as a classic example of a water-borne epidemic. It was not only one of the most devastating epidemics of its kind, but also one of the most instructive. The conditions of this naturally occurring epidemic paralleled those of a well-controlled laboratory experiment. The relation between the infected water and the disease was conclusively proven and the value of slow sand filtration was demonstrated.

In a period of a little over two months, from August 17 to October 23, 1892, nearly 17,000 cases with 8,065 deaths occurred in Hamburg, a city of 640,000 people. During the height of the epidemic, over 1,000 new cases occurred in a single day.

The epidemic principally involved Hamburg and Altona which are adjacent but separate cities. Hamburg, being an old Hanseatic city, had its own government, while Altona was in Prussia. Both cities rest upon the banks of the river Elbe and were furnished drinking water from this grossly polluted stream. At the time of the epidemic, the intakes for the water supplies of both cities were directly at the river front and the sewers of Hamburg emptied into the river at various points along the same river front. Altona was downstream and hence was drinking Elbe river water, plus Hamburg's sewage; however, its water supply was treated by the slow sand filtration process. Hamburg, on the other hand, furnished its citizens with raw unfiltered Elbe river water.

Both cities had homogeneous populations, the same site, the same climate and all other conditions were similar, the only difference being their water supplies. Relatively few cases occurred in Altona and most of these were on the boundary where people probably had access to Hamburg's raw unfiltered Elbe river water.

Germany's own great bacteriologist, Robert Koch, studied this epidemic and stated: "Cholera in Hamburg went right up to the boundary of Altona and there stopped. In one street, which for a long way forms the boundary, there was cholera on the Hamburg side, whereas the Altona side was free from it."

The year 1892 was a pandemic one for cholera. The disease followed the routes of trade, travelling from the Valley of the Ganges, through Persia to Russia and into Germany and other countries of Europe. It was even brought to the shores of the United States with several cases occurring in New York City.

The sources of Hamburg's epidemic were traced to Russian immigrants crowded in barracks on one of the wharves pending their embarkation for the United States. At the time of the outbreak there were on an average about 1,000 of these people on hand all the time.

Many of them came from districts in Russia which had been, and were then, suffering severely from cholera. All were well supplied with dirty clothing and blankets, some of which they washed while they were being detained. It is believed that among those that had arrived there must have been some mild cases of the disease, or at least some convalescents and carriers. All of the sewage and waste matters from these people were discharged directly into the river at the wharf. After the Elbe River once became seeded with the cholera vibrio the people in Hamburg who drank this infected water took the disease, and their discharges, returning to the river, added fuel to the flames. A vicious circle was thus set up, so that the infection became exceedingly concentrated and intense, and as the circle was a short one the time interval was correspondingly brief and the virulence unusually severe.

The Hamburg epidemic will ever remain as a classic and historical account of a water-borne epidemic. The facts and circumstances surrounding it were clear-cut and complete. Absolute proof of its water-borne nature was furnished by Robert Koch, who isolated the cholera organism from the polluted waters of the River Elbe.

The annals of public health record so many water-borne epidemics that time and space only permit a historical review of some of the most famous. However, it is impossible to conclude this historical review without some comments on Chicago's famous drainage canal.

The great midwestern metropolis of Chicago is located on the south-western shores of Lake Michigan. Prior to the turn of the century the city discharged its sewage via the Chicago River into Lake Michigan and also obtained its drinking water from the lake. As the city grew in size the area of the lake polluted with Chicago's sewage became greater and greater. Despite the fact that the city pushed its water intakes further and further out into the lake, the pollution increased. As a result, typhoid fever and other intestinal diseases occurred both endemically and epidemically within the city. It became obvious that something drastic had to be done.

Chicago decided to divert and exclude its vast daily river of sewage from the city's drinking water. In so doing, it performed a bold and miraculous feat of sanitary engineering. It reversed the natural flow of the Chicago River, causing it to discharge into the Mississippi

River 357 miles away, instead of into the lake at its doorstep. Early in the twentieth century Chicago built its famous drainage canal, into which it poured its sewage, taking waters from Lake Michigan to dilute it and to send it on its way.

Although the construction of the drainage canal temporarily solved Chicago's public health problem, it in turn created other problems. The State of Missouri tried to get an injunction to restrain Chicago from dumping its sewage into the Mississippi. The case was tried before the U. S. Supreme Court and the court refused to grant the injunction. Another problem created by the drainage canal arose from the enormous amounts of water that were diverted from Lake Michigan. Charges were made by the Great Lakes cities of both the United States and Canada, that the water levels of the lakes were being lowered to a point where shipping was interfered with. The courts ruled that Chicago was to build adequate sewage treatment plants and to limit and later cease diverting waters from the Great Lakes.

Thus, in order to protect its public health, Chicago built the drainage canal, altered the course of a river, built extensive sewage treatment plants and chlorinated the lake water it drank. As a result, the rates for typhoid fever and other intestinal diseases fell to almost zero.

During the Chicago World's Fair of 1933 and 1934, that city experienced an interesting and unusual water- and food-borne epidemic of amoebic dysentery. Approximately 932 cases and 52 deaths were traced to this epidemic.

The epidemic originated in two first-class Chicago hotels and was spread in part by fecally contaminated food and in part by sewage polluted water. The plumbing in these two hotels was antiquated and cross connections existed between the potable water supply and the sewers. Investigation revealed that the two involved hotels used essentially the same water supply and hence pollution occurring in one affected the supply of the other.

Carriers were responsible for the spread of the disease and examination of 1,100 employees of both hotels revealed that 165 food handlers and 141 other employees were harboring the entamoeba histolytica.

As set forth in previous chapters of this book, mankind had very early in his history recognized that cleanliness, pure water and the proper disposal of human body wastes was of paramount importance for the maintenance of good health and the prevention of disease. Unfortunately, the Biblical admonitions in this regard were not generally observed by the peoples of the world. The early sanitary engineering accomplishments of the Romans with their system of sewers and magnificent water supplies fell into disrepair and disuse after the fall of the Roman Empire. For all practical intents and purposes the concepts and practices of good sanitation all but disappeared. Thus, during the Dark and Middle Ages the sanitary conscience of the world fell asleep. People lived in a dirty, disease-ridden world amid an indescribable assortment of smells, stinks and stenches.

The sanitary conscience of the world was slow to awaken and the science of sanitary engineering and its practical application did not really come into being until approximately the middle of the nineteenth century. However, sporadic spurts of sanitary progress can be found several centuries prior to this time.

A remarkable milestone in the history of sanitation was Sir John Harington's invention of the water closet in 1596. Harington was the witty godson of Queen Elizabeth, who affectionately referred to him as her "Boye Jack." A popular member of the Royal Court, he was well educated and possessed both the Bachelor's and Master's degrees. A clever and merry young fellow, Sir John enjoyed a reputation as a scholar, wit and poet.

In the course of his literary pursuits, Harington translated a salacious Italian poem into English verse and circulated this "baudie tale" among the "Ladies of the Court." The Queen, prompted by jealous and hostile courtiers, became displeased at this and other antics of her merry godson, and banished him. The royal ruling stated: "That this merry poet, her godson must not come to court till he hath grown sober and leaveth the ladies, sportes, and frolics."

Sir John Harington was thus forced to retire to the family estate at Kelston, 3½ miles from Bath. Here, away from the glittering Elizabethan court, with time on his hands, and faced with the discomforts of rural life, he supposedly invented the water closet.

Harington had the device constructed and installed in his fine manor house at Kelston. In order to introduce his sanitary device of water-carried sewage disposal to a needful world, he wrote a book entitled, *A New Discourse of a Stale Subject, Called the Metamorphosis of Ajax*. The word "ajax" is a pun and refers to the old English term for a privy which was "a Jakes" or "a Jacks," comparable to our current slang term "a John." His book not only set forth the basic utility of his invention, but also contained instructions and diagrams on how to construct and assemble his water closet. Although the book is full of Elizabethan puns and delights in word play, its chief importance is the fact that it is a vivid social document portraying the customs and problems of the time.

Sir John delves back into Roman history and tells of the edict that the Emperor Vespasian issued against the custom of "pissing on the palace walls." He relates how the Emperor erected "diverse and sundrie places of faire polished marble" for this special purpose and charged all persons "to refrain from shedding their urine" against the walls of his royal palace and also against the walls of the temples of the gods and goddesses. He further relates how the Romans, in addition to using their engineering skills to build the Cloaca Maxima and other fine sewers and drains, insured their proper operation by appointing a set of minor deities to preside over the whole business. The god Stercutius was the god of dung, while the goddess Cloacina presided over the drains. Cloacina was euphemistically addressed as "Sweet Cloacina" and her powers were invoked for protection against the diseases that arose from the stench of the drains.

Harington continues his entertaining discourse and alludes to the "French Courtesy." This was the custom of French Royalty to receive visiting nobles and dignitaries while "setting on the stoole." This custom displayed implicit trust in the visitor, because a person cannot be more helpless or defenseless than when "caught with his breeches down."

He relates how it was the common custom for royalty and members of the nobility to be served by a "groome of the stoole," whose function it was to "pot and powder" these pampered people. Thus, they were spared the discomforts of the filthy privies of their day. He goes on to tell of the "groome of the stoole" to a French prince who wrote a "beastly treatise" on what was the "fittest thing to wype with." This treatise stated that; "white paper is too smooth, brown paper too rough, woolen cloth too stiff, linnen too hollow, satin too slippery, taffeta too thin, velvet too thick or perhaps too costly; but concluded that a goose neck be drawn between the legs."

Sir John brings out the universally deplorable conditions and methods of sewage disposal of his day. He tells of the filthy privies, the dirty dung heaps and the futile attempts of cleaning out privy vaults and how the "dung carters" carried their stinking loads out of the cities for the "gong-farmers" to spread on their fields.

He sums up two of the pertinent problems of Elizabethan times by stating that "an excellent rule to keepe a chimnie from smoking and a privie from stinking, was to make your fire in the privie and to set your stoole in the chimney."

Sir John Harington stated; "that the matter itself (the disposal of human body wastes) has been of concern in all ages." He never loses sight of the basic utility of his water closet and insists on its usefulness, "in poor cottages, stately houses, or the goodliest palaces of the realm." He further states that his invention would be, "a great benefactor to the citie of London and all other populous places." He concludes that his book tells; "How unsavorie places may be made sweete; noysome places, wholesome; filthie places, cleanly," and "that his work was published for the common benefit of builders, housekeepers and home-owners."

Unfortunately, Sir John Harington and his invention were several centuries too early for general acceptance. The concept and practice of water-carried sewage disposal was not put into general use until well into the nineteenth century.

Following the Report of the Health of Towns Commission in England in 1844, water closets were rapidly introduced. In 1847 it was required that they be connected to sewers and the use of cesspools in towns was prohibited. Although the introduction and use of water-carried sewage disposal did away with the accumulation of filth around urban dwellings, it gave rise to serious problems of pollution where their contents discharged into streams and lakes.

What is frequently referred to as the "Great Sanitary Awakening" occurred in the mid-nineteenth century. It was brought about by the growth of cities and was part of the industrial revolution. As people flocked to the cities, lack of community organization and facilities created teeming slums with indescribably horrible sanitary conditions. Pestilence and death reigned unchecked and the need for sanitary reform was great. Decent housing, safe and adequate water supplies and the effective disposal of human body wastes were urgently needed.

Edwin Chadwick (1800-1890) introduced the "sanitary idea" and focused public attention on the need for sanitary reforms. Chadwick was an English lawyer who became interested in sanitary and public health conditions while serving as the secretary of the Poor Law Commission. He became convinced that poverty and disease were almost inextricably entwined. In 1842 he wrote a volume entitled *The Sanitary Condition of the Laboring Population of Great Britain.*

His book revealed such horrifying facts as, that more than half of the children of the poor died, as compared to one-fifth of the gentry. That sections of Manchester existed where there was only one privy for 245 people. That the poor had to depend on the polluted waters from dirty drainage ditches for drinking purposes and that a glass of clean water was an unheard-of novelty.

Unfortunately, Chadwick was not a tactful man and in his burning zeal to bring about social reforms and to "clean up the cities" he made thousands of enemies. Although a number of physicians gave him excellent support and cooperation, he held a low opinion of the medical profession. He felt that most physicians were indifferent to the problems and that some actually wanted to perpetuate disease for their own financial gain. He believed that sanitary engineering along with the enactment of forceful laws and strict enforcement was the "key to health."

As a result, he incurred the wrath of many vested interests as well as the politicians and physicians. He soon became the "most abused" man in all of England and was forced to retire from public administration at the age of fifty-four with a pension of 1,000 pounds.

Despite all this opposition, his book exerted great influence on Parliament and started Commissions on Public Health that led to the building of a sewage system for London and finally culminated in the Public Health Act of 1848. This marked the beginning of modern public health in Great Britain and exerted a worldwide influence.

Dr. Southwood Smith (1788-1861), an epidemiologist and physician to the London Fever Hospital, was another of the pioneers of English public health. He had vigorously called public attention to bad environment as an important cause in the production of fevers. In 1838 he had made a report on the "Physical Causes of Sickness and Mortality." In 1841 he made a report on the "Physical aspects of Child Labor" and in 1842 a report on the "Moral Aspects of Child Labor." He also proposed and outlined an excellent program of community sanitation.

Because of Chadwick's prejudice towards doctors, the first General Board of Health formed in 1846 had no medical member. However, when the National Board of Health was formed in 1848, Southwood Smith was appointed to it as the medical advisor. He served on this Board with great distinction along with Chadwick, Lord Carlysle and Lord Shaftesbury.

In 1848 the City of London appointed Doctor John Simon as its first Medical Officer of Health. Simon was a brilliant, able and tactful administrator, and was one of the first designers of modern public health practice. He stated that, "Sanitary neglect is mistaken parsimony, that fevers and cholera are costly items to count against the cheapness of filthy residences and ditch-drawn drinking water. That widows and orphanages made it expensive to sanction unventilated work places and needlessly fatal occupations."

A great mass of data collected while he was medical officer, on overcrowding, inadequate ventilation, general filth, lack of drainage, contaminated water supplies, as well as proposals for correction, is preserved in two thick volumes of general reports. Causes of death in London were presented regularly by Simon to the City Council. The great threat to health from dumping the city sewage into the tidal Thames, as well as the medical hazards of cesspools, was pointed out by him.

Dr. John Simon served the City of London for a period of twenty-one years and in 1887 was knighted at Queen Victoria's Jubilee. He died at the age of eighty-eight and his obituary in the London Times described him as:

> The master of sanitary science, the organizer, and for years the official head of a system of public health preservation which is without equal in the world, the philosopher whose teaching has saved the lives of hundreds of thousands of our people, whose name is a household word wherever preventive medicine is studied, and whose writings form the classical literature of the subject to which much of his life has been devoted.

The works of Chadwick, Smith and Simon in England exerted a profound influence upon the development of public health and preventive medicine in the United States. The cornerstone of American public health was laid in 1850 with the publication of the "Shattuck Report."

Lemuel Shattuck (1793-1859) was a Boston bookseller, schoolmaster, city councilman, state legislator and vital statistician. Through his interest in geneology, he recognized the need for accurate vital statistics and in 1842 secured the passage of a law in Massachusetts initiating the statewide registration of vital statistics. In 1845 he published a census of the city of Boston. This census revealed a high general mortality rate and a shocking infant and maternal mortality rate. Communicable diseases were widely prevalent and conditions of general sanitation and living facilities were grossly inadequate.

Stimulated by the ideas and activities of the English sanitary reformers, Shattuck engineered the appointment of a commission to make a sanitary survey of Massachusetts. He was named chairman of the commission and was the principal author of the report.

Published in 1850, Shattuck's "Report of the Sanitary Commission of Massachusetts" prescribed the first general plan for the promotion of public health in America. Of the fifty specific recommendations in the report, thirty-six are fundamental activities of present day public health. His report recommended and led to the establishment of State Boards of Health. Lemuel Shattuck thus assumed his place in the history of preventive medicine and became known as the "father of American sanitation."

As a result of the awakening of the sanitary conscience and the work of the sanitary reformers there was a need for the discovery and development of procedures for the purification of water supplies and the proper disposal of human body wastes.

Simple procedures for purifying water are age-old. Sanskrit medical lore dating back to 2000 B.C. advises: "Keep water in copper vessels, to expose it to sunlight and filter through charcoal" and "to treat foul water by boiling and exposing to sunlight."

In 1804 the entire water supply of Paisley, Scotland, was filtered. The Chelsea Water Company, under the direction of James Simpson, installed the first sand filter about one acre in area, in London to clarify the Thames River water in 1829. This installation was so successful that by July 1852 filtration of all river water supplied to London was made compulsory by Parliament.

The development of sand filtration had progressed to the extent that by 1865 many European cities were using this system of clarification. Recognizing the value of these slow sand filters, the Water Commission of St. Louis, Missouri, in 1865 sent James P. Kirkwood to Europe to study their operation. In 1872 Kirkwood built the first successful slow sand filter plant in this country in Poughkeepsie, New York.

The Massachusetts State Board of Health established the Lawrence Experimental Station in 1887 to study and devise methods for the purification of sewage and industrial wastes. Studies were undertaken with slow sand filters for water purification. As a result of these investigations Lawrence, Massachusetts constructed a slow sand filter plant in 1889, considered to have been "the first filter plant built in America for the express purpose of reducing the death rate of the population."

In about 1800 Guyton de Morveau in France and Cruikshank in England first used chlorine to treat water, and Thomas Henry in England proposed the use of lime for water softening. Dr. Robley Dunglinson in 1834 recommended the use of chlorination for making marsh water potable. However, it was not until 1908 that G. A. Johnson initiated the use of chlorine compounds for disinfecting water and applied this process to the water supply of the Chicago stockyards. In the same year, this process was applied on a large scale to the water supply of Jersey City. Brigadier General Carl R. Darnell discovered that liquid chlorine effectively sterilizes water in 1909. Thus, the effective disinfecting of water supplies by chlorination did not come into use until the first part of the present century.

In 1861 Graham developed colloidal chemistry, gels, emulsions, and coagulation, which led to water purification with alum. Hyatt and Leeds in 1884 were the first to apply and patent the principle of coagulation with an electrolyte to remove turbidity from water on a plant basis.

Drainage systems of various types have been used from the earliest of times. However, these invariably consisted of a simple system of drains or sewers that were used to carry wastes directly to the soil or into a stream. As the cities developed and provided community water supplies, sewers and water-carried sewage disposal gradually came into general use.

Serious problems of stream pollution occurred and in London the tidal Thames became so foul that an English commission in 1854 used chlorination in the treatment of sewage. In the United States the gross pollution in eastern Massachusetts became so serious that special committees were set up to study the problem in 1881 and 1884. This led to the establishment of the Lawrence Experiment Station on the banks of the Merrimac River in 1887, under the direction of Allen Hazen. The fundamental facts developed at this Experiment Station led to methods of sewage purification by the slow oxidation of organic matter carried on by living bacteria. Upon this general principle depends the functioning of the contact bed, the sprinkling filter and the activated sludge process.

Intermittant sand filtration was used in England as far back as 1870 and Lowcock in 1892 introduced the trickling filter in the same country. W. T. Lockett is credited with the discovery and use of the activated sludge process in Manchester, England in 1912.

Progress in rural sanitation was also made, and E. A. Parks gave an excellent description of sanitary privies, water closets and latrines in his widely used *Manual of Practical Hygiene* in 1864. The fermentation of stored sewage in septic tanks was developed in 1891 by Sir Colin Scott-Moncrief who was with the British Foreign Service. In the United States, septic tanks were also developed by A. N. Talbot of Illinois in 1894. However, Donald Cameron is credited with developing the modern septic tank at Exeter, England in about 1895. His design was an outgrowth of experiments which were suggested by similar tanks, some of which were built as far back as 1852. Although Cameron was granted a patent for his design in 1896, considerable litigation ensued challenging his patent. At one time septic tanks were commonly called Cameron tanks.

The popular and widely used Imhoff tanks were invented by Karl

Imhoff, who first used them in the Essen District in Germany in 1907. This is a two-story tank with a combination of a sedimentation chamber and a digestion compartment.

Actually, water-carried sewage disposal and its effective treatment is less than a century old. The sanitary progress made during the current century in safeguarding our water supplies and effectively treating sewage has been so successful that the days of the great waterborne epidemics are a thing of the past.

Chapter 27

CHOLERA AND TYPHOID

ALTHOUGH THESE TWO devastating diseases have been described in the preceding chapter on "The Water-Borne and Fecal Discharge Diseases," their importance is so great that they merit additional historical review.

In the annals of pestilential pandemics none have been more deadly and devastating than those of Asiatic cholera. During the nineteenth century, this deadly disease made no fewer than four murderous journeys around the world, killing untold millions.

Hippocrates and other ancient medical writers described a disease called cholera. In 30 A.D. Celsus in his book, *De Medicina,* explained that the disease owes its name to the vari-colored or bile-like appearance of the watery discharge from the bowels. The term is derived from the Greek word "chole" or bile.

There is a great deal of historical doubt that the cholera referred to by the ancient medical writers was true Asiatic cholera. The term in all probability referred to a whole "clinical wastebasketful" of severe diarrheal diseases. It is sometimes assumed that all diseases are as "ancient as mankind" and that there are no "new diseases," but only diseases that achieve recognition by being differentiated from a welter and confusion of similar diseases, by better diagnosis and scientific advancement. It is of interest to note that the older medical writers did differentiate the dysenteries from what they called cholera, by the fact that cholera was far more severe and was characterized by simultaneous vomiting and purging, along with early collapse and a high fatality rate. However, the first unmistakable report of what is now known as Asiatic cholera was the description of an epidemic written in 1768 by Sonnerat in India.

Asiatic cholera has been known for centuries in India and from here it is reported to have spread to China during the seventeenth century. Cholera is and has always been present and endemic in the regions of the lower Ganges River in India. From this endemic focus, due to some unknown and mysterious reason, it broke forth during the nineteenth century to rampage around the world.

Cholera is a fearful and fantastic disease. For long periods of time, it lies slumbering and smouldering, hidden in a small geographic corner of the world. Then, suddenly, it flares and flames to life and like a raging prairie fire, breaks its bounds to encircle the globe. For the individual, death strikes suddenly like a bolt from out of the blue. A young man, strong and healthy in the morning, soons begins to feel weak and dizzy. By noon, he is dreadfully ill with intractable vomiting and continuous diarrhea. He soon collapses with sunken eyes and a cold and clammy skin. Helpless and hopeless, he soon falls into a stupor and is dead by evening. During an epidemic the dead and dying are everywhere and like the plague of old, it spares neither prince nor pauper. Villages, towns and cities become paralyzed with fear and people everywhere are panic-stricken and terror-ridden.

Cholera is spread by man from place to place and the organism enters the digestive tract through the mouth. Infested water is the common medium of transferance and is probably the chief vector responsible for the great epidemic outbursts of the disease. It may, however, be transferred from man to man directly. It can also be transferred indirectly by flies, fingers, food, and all the innumerable channels from the anus of one man to the mouth of another.

During the nineteenth century cholera followed the flag and traveled the routes of trade, encircling the globe in four separate virulent pandemics. From 1811 to 1817 cholera began its epidemic extension over India and it soon overran the entire peninsula. In 1818 British troops helped spread it to Hindustan, Eastern India and Ceylon. As it left India, the disease spread in two directions at once, going both east and west.

The first pandemic occurred from 1826 to 1837. Starting from India in 1826, it reached Poland, Siberia and Russia in 1829 to 1830. In 1830 the disease reached China and in 1831 it broke out in Germany and England as well as striking Turkey and Africa. From England the disease leaped the channel and invaded France.

In 1832 cholera reached the American shore, coming by sea and entering the continent at Quebec and New York. In 1833 emigrant ships brought the disease to New Orleans, from where it traveled up-river, spreading throughout the entire Mississippi Valley. The attack rate of this pandemic has been placed at about $2\frac{1}{2}$ percent of the world's population, while the mortality rate was said to have approached 50 percent.

The second pandemic originated in India in 1840 and afflicted the world until about 1862. British troops carried the disease into China and from there it returned to India. Invading Russia in 1848-49, it killed approximately one million people, and during the same period of time, France is said to have lost about 150,000 people.

The disease penetrated the United States in 1848 and during the next year the "Forty-Niners" on their mad rush for gold, dragged cholera across the continent. Thus, thousands of unfortunate gold-seekers found death from cholera instead of the El Dorado of their dreams.

The third pandemic extended from 1863 to 1875. However, due to improved transportation it now traveled faster and took a shorter time to spread from India to Europe. Although the disease again reached the United States in 1873, it fortunately failed to gain a real foothold and the epidemic was a limited one. Since that time only sporadic cases have occurred in our country.

The fourth and last of the great cholera pandemics rampaged around the world from 1883 to 1894. In 1883, as the disease reached Egypt from Bombay, India, the great German bacteriologist, Robert Koch, responded to a stricken world's plea for help and went to Egypt to study the disease. He soon discovered the causative organism to be the vibrio cholera which he isolated from the stools of cholera cases. Later, he went to India and at the Medical College of Calcutta, he conclusively reconfirmed his previous findings.

Hamburg's famous cholera epidemic of 1892 dramatically demonstrated the water-borne transmission of the disease and highlighted the protective value of water purification by means of sand filtration. In 1893 Koch's studies of this epidemic led him to point out the important role of the "vibrioentraeger" or cholera carrier in the transmission of the disease.

The first attempt to immunize man against cholera was made by

Ferran in Spain in 1884. However, Waldemar Mordecai Haffkine (1860-1930), a Russian-English bacteriologist, introduced the first successful anticholera vaccine in 1893. He first used an attenuated culture of vibrio cholera and later a virulent culture. In 1896 the German bacteriologist, William Kolle, developed an effective killed cholera vaccine.

Due to modern preventive medicine, worldwide pandemics of cholera are now a thing of the past. However, the disease still exists and occurs in its ancestral home in India and also parts of the Orient.

For many centuries typhoid fever was confused with other long-continued fevers such as typhus, recurrent fever and septic infections. The first full description of what was probably typhoid fever was written by Thomas Willis, an English physician, who in 1643 described an epidemic that occurred in Parliamentary troops. In 1826 Bretonneau wrote a monograph further describing the clinical characteristics of the disease, and called it "dothienenteritis" or abscess of the small intestine.

The recognition of typhoid fever as a disease, and also its name, we owe to Charles Alexandre Louis (1787-1842) a popular French professor of medicine. In 1829 after searching long and vainly for a suitable name he wrote, "I still retain the expression 'typhoid fever' as the one least open to objection." He coined the word "typhoid" from the disease named typhus by adding the Greek suffix "eidos" or like, thus meaning a typhus-like disease. The Greek word "typhus" means a cloud or haze and was used to designate a stupor or delirium due to a fever.

Louis was an eminent French clinician at the Charite in Paris. It is interesting to note that he taught almost two score American physicians, most of whom became leaders of American medicine. He is probably best known for his clinical-pathological description of typhoid fever. This was prepared in 1829 in two volumes from data based on notes collected in preceding years. He compared 138 cases of fevers with gastroenteric symptoms and morbid states classed as typhoid or typhus fever, with a controlled group several times this size. The accurate observations that he reported first established typhoid fever as a clinical entity, although he did not clearly differentiate typhoid from typhus fever.

William Wood Gerhard (1809-1872), the most distinguished American pupil of Louis, bested his teacher in the clear differentiation of the two diseases. Previously, the diverse manifestations of both diseases had been described and the afflicted treated as typhoid fever victims, without discrimination.

Gerhard was born in Philadelphia, received his undergraduate training at nearby Dickinson College (founded by Benjamin Rush and others), and in 1830 obtained his doctorate in medicine at the University of Pennsylvania. This was followed by a two-year period of postgraduate study in Paris where he sought and received instruction under Pierre Charles Alexandre Louis.

Upon his return to Philadelphia, Gerhard was resident physician at the Philadelphia Hospital. He held a staff appointment until 1868, with an overlapping appointment in the Institutes of Medicine at the University of Pennsylvania. Gerhard's studies on fevers begun under Louis in Paris were continued in America. He had the good fortune of observing and studying epidemics of typhus and typhoid occurring in Philadelphia at the same time. In 1837 he published his observations stating: "The fact that the morbid changes pathognomonic of dothienenteritis (typhoid fever), are not met with in the typhus fever, would of itself seem conclusive that the two diseases are no more identical than pneumonia and pleurisy."

Sir William Osler is credited with assigning priority to Gerhard for the typhus-typhoid differentiation, although undoubtedly others had some appreciation of the clinical and pathological characteristics of these maladies, alike in name but dissimilar in many respects.

In 1856 William Budd (1811-1880), an English general practitioner, published a classic study on the epidemiology of typhoid fever. By inductive reasoning he concluded that typhoid fever was a contagious disease spread thru the alvine discharges of typhoid fever patients.

William Budd came from a family of physicians and was born in 1811 in Devonshire, England. He received an excellent medical education, studying in London, Edinburgh and Paris. While serving as a young naval surgeon, he survived a serious bout of typhoid fever; hence, this disease commanded his interest throughout his medical career.

Budd began his remarkable epidemiological studies and investigations of typhoid fever in 1839. However, his conclusions were not stated in print until 1856 when he wrote:

> This species of fever has two fundamental characteristics. The first is, that it is an essentially contagious disorder; the second, that by far the most virulent part of the specific poison by which the contagion takes effect is contained in the diarrhoeal discharges which issue from the diseased and exanthematous bowel.

Thus twenty-five years prior to the identification and discovery of the Salmonella typhosa as the causative organism, Budd had clearly defined the epidemiology of the disease.

In 1873 he summarized his findings and published his best known treatise which was entitled, *Typhoid Fever: Its Nature, Mode of Spreading, and Prevention.* To William Budd belongs the credit for proving that, by disinfecting the alvine discharge and isolation of the sick, the pollution of drinking water could be prevented and the disease held in check. Unfortunately, Budd's views aroused no great interest and remained without impact upon official public health practice.

The causative organism of typhoid fever was first identified in 1880 by Karl Joseph Eberth (1835-1926), a pathologist from Halle, Germany. A short time later, Gaffky grew it in pure culture. Metchnikoff and Besredka in 1900 conclusively established it as the causative agent by producing the disease in anthropoid apes and inoculating them with a pure culture.

In 1896 Gruber and Durham reported the discovery of agglutinins in the blood serum of typhoid patients; this greatly enhanced the knowledge of typhoid immunity and formed the basis for the diagnostic agglutination test by Widal a few years later.

Georges Fernand Isidore Widal (1862-1929) was an Algerian-born bacteriologist and pathologist. He was graduated in medicine from the University of Paris in 1885. With bacteriological research in the forefront of medicine at that time, he gravitated to that field.

His contribution to public health is in connection with the diagnosis of typhoid fever. In 1896 he demonstrated that the blood serum of typhoid cases would agglutinate typhoid bacilli. This practical and well-known test is called the Widal test or reaction in his honor.

The development of antityphoid vaccine forms another interesting chapter in preventive medicine. In 1893 and 1894 Pfeiffer reported the result of a series of investigations on the nature of immunity in typhoid infection, and elaborated a test for the presence of protective bodies in the blood serum, which became classic under the name Pfeiffer phenomenon. In 1896 Pfeiffer and Kolle prepared a typhoid vaccine by killing typhoid bacilli as grown in culture mediums. Antityphoid vaccination was extensively applied during the following decade in the English Army under the direction of Sir A. E. Wright and Sir William B. Leishman and in the German Army under the direction of Professor Robert Koch.

In 1908 Major F. F. Russell of the Medical Corps, United States Army, began the preparation of antityphoid vaccine on a large scale at the Army Medical School Laboratory in Washington, D. C. The vaccination of troops began in 1909, during which year in an army of 57,124 there were 173 cases of typhoid infection and 16 deaths. Vaccination became compulsory in 1911 for all Army personnel under forty-five years of age; in 1913 with a mean strength of 59,608 men, there were only two cases of typhoid and no deaths.

In the past typhoid was primarily a water-borne disease; some of the great water-borne epidemics of the past have been described in the chapter on "The Water-Borne and Fecal Discharge Diseases."

Another important manner of disseminating typhoid fever and one which still constitutes an important problem is the carrier condition. In fact, chronic carriers at present are the greatest source of the disease. The amount of harm which a single carrier can cause is amazing.

The story of "Typhoid Mary" is the classic example of how typhoid fever can be spread by a chronic carrier. Mary Mallon found her place in medical history through the dubious distinction of disseminating death and disease.

Aptly nicknamed "Typhoid Mary," she was a walking epidemic, who over a long period of time excreted the deadly Salmonella typhi in her stool. A careless cook with little regard for her fellow human beings, she carried disease with her from kitchen to kitchen. She moved from one home to another as a cook for wealthy families, and everywhere that Mary went she left a trail of typhoid. Some accounts claim that she was responsible for over two hundred cases and at least three deaths in and around New York City.

The story begins in 1901 when Mary Mallon, who had been employed as a cook for a New York family for three years, developed typhoid fever at about the same time that a visitor to the family had the disease. One month later, the laundress in this home came down with typhoid.

In 1902 Mary obtained a new position as a cook and two weeks after her arrival one of the servants was taken ill. The following week a second case of typhoid developed and soon seven members of the household were sick.

In 1904 Mary went to cook for a family on Long Island. The household consisted of four family members and seven servants. Within three weeks of her arrival four of the servants became ill.

In 1906 Mary again changed positions and six of the eleven members of this new family came down with typhoid between August 27 and September 3. At this time, she first came under suspicion as a carrier. She entered another family on September 21 and on October 5 the laundress developed typhoid fever.

In 1907 Mary again changed positions and two months after her arrival in this new family, two cases of typhoid fever developed, one of which proved fatal.

During this time, George A. Soper, a Sanitary Engineer with the New York City Health Department and other staff members, traced Mary Mallon's movements from one typhoid-stricken home to another. The Health Department took Mary into custody and hospitalized her on March 19, 1907. Repeated cultures showed that she was a chronic carrier and excreted enormous numbers of typhoid bacilli in her stools.

Mary Mallon was then placed under strict surveillance by the New York Health Department. She signed a pledge to abandon her career as a cook and to be careful of her personal hygiene. She was also required to report to the Health Department every three months. However, this arrangement was relatively short-lived and lasted for only about three years. In 1910 Mary vanished and was lost from sight for five years.

In January and February of 1915 an outbreak of typhoid fever struck the Sloane Hospital for Women in New York. Twenty-five cases occurred, principally among the doctors, nurses and help. An investigation of the outbreak placed the cook under suspicion. As soon as this occurred the cook left the hospital premises and did not return or leave her address. However, she was located by the Health Department hiding under an assumed name. Her identity was soon established as the familiar and infamous Typhoid Mary Mallon.

Thereafter, health officials took no chances and Mary Mallon was confined in an institution and remained there until her death in 1938.

A subsequent study of Mary's career showed that she had infected many others beyond those already mentioned. She may have been the source of a widespread water-borne typhoid epidemic that occurred in Ithica, New York, in 1903 involving over 1,300 cases. A person by the name of Mary Mallon was known to have been employed as a cook in the vicinity of the place where the first case appeared and from which contamination of the water supply occurred.

Chapter 28

BITING BUGS
THE HISTORY OF ARTHROPOD-BORNE
DISEASE

A GREAT EXTENSION of knowledge took place during the last decades of the nineteenth century when it was demonstrated that bacteria were not the only cause of our infectious diseases. It was a great accomplishment to learn that various protozoa and other parasitic organisms were capable of infecting man and producing disease. Of fundamental importance was the demonstration of the role of insects and animals as vectors or carriers of disease. Complex patterns of parasitism and disease were revealed when it became known that these arthropod vectors not only transmitted disease from man to man and from animals to man, but also frequently served as intermediate hosts for disease-producing organisms.

Two types of disease transmission were recognized. In one, the biting arthropod acted merely as the mechanical agent in transferring the germ, as in the transmission of plague by the bite of the rat flea, or the transmission of typhus by lice. In the second type, the arthropod vector also acted as the intermediate host, as demonstrated by the role played by the mosquito in the transmission of malaria.

This knowledge closed the last gap in the germ theory of disease. Prior to this, the clinical case of a disease in man was regarded as the sole source of infection, and hence, all control measures were directed toward the case. The patient was isolated and his household and contacts were quarantined, while his clothing and the articles used by him were disinfected. To explain the lack of association between cases, it was assumed that particles of infectious material were disseminated by air currents or were carried for great distances and long periods of time by persons or inanimate objects.

The arthropod vectors of disease belong to many genera and species. They may be grouped as bugs, gnats, lice, fleas, flies, mosquitoes, ticks and mites. The discovery of the part played by them as carriers of disease has rounded out our modern concept of communicable disease transmission and control. A striking burden of global illness was, and still is, attributable to the arthropod-borne diseases. In the past, these diseases have limited the population of man, shaped history, decided battles and determined the sites of human habitation.

The concept of parasitism was so commonly accepted by the late seventeenth and early eighteenth centuries that it inspired the famous English satirist, Jonathan Swift to write:

> So, naturalists observe, a flea
> Has smaller fleas that on him prey;
> And these have smaller still to bite 'em.
> And so proceed 'ad infinitum."

The knowledge concerning arthropod-borne diseases and the existence of intermediate hosts did not come about as the result of any one single great discovery, but was the culmination of a long series of observations, theories and experiments. The Viennese physician, Joseph Jakob Plenck, recognized parasitic diseases in his classification of diseases in 1776 and this work influenced subsequent publications. In 1790 a Danish veterinarian and physician named Peter Christian Abildgaard observed that animal parasites may pass various stages of their life cycles in different animal hosts.

This phenomenon, known as metoxeny, was also demonstrated experimentally in cestodes by F. Küchenmeister in 1851. However, the first determination of the life cycle of a parasite was accomplished by Karl Theodor Ernest von Siebold in 1854. He worked out the development of Taenia Coenurus which carries sheep gid or sturdy. Siebold showed that this parasite is the larval form of Taenia multiceps which passes its adult stage in the intestine of the dog. Further general knowledge on the biology of parasitism was provided by the zoologist Rudolf Leuckart (1822-1898) whose outstanding work on human parasites helped lay the foundations for subsequent research in this field.

In 1858 the Russian naturalist Fedschenko, following Leuckart's suggestions, demonstrated the life cycle of the Guinea worm of man and showed that a small arthropod water flea transmitted the worm. Leuckart and Melnikoff in 1868 demonstrated that the dog tapeworm was transmitted by the dog louse, thereby showing that a parasite which fed on an animal could act as an intermediate host in the transmission of disease.

Unfortunately all of this work attracted little medical attention and it was not until 1879, when Patrick Manson successfully unravelled the life history of the Filaria bancrofti that medical progress began to be made. Manson is frequently called "the father of modern tropical medicine." His work provided a major impetus for the further study of human parasitology and ultimately led to the solution of the mysteries surrounding the arthropod-borne diseases.

Patrick Manson was born in 1844 near Aberdeen, Scotland, the son of a well-to-do land owner. He terminated his early education at the age of fifteen to become an apprentice in the ironworks of his mother's relatives. This heavy work soon impaired his health and his interests turned to natural history and medicine. In 1860 he entered the University of Aberdeen and obtained his medical education there.

After graduation he served as a physician at the Durham Lunatic Asylum for a short time. Manson then obtained an appointment as medical officer to the Chinese Imperial Maritime Customs. This appointment took him to the Far East where he remained until the age of forty-five, serving first at Formosa, then at Amoy and later at Hong Kong. His professional activities were divided between his official duties and the private practice of medicine and surgery. However, as an avocation he carried on a series of remarkable original investigations in parasitology.

Although Manson had received no special training in laboratory research, a microscope and a few accessory items purchased with his own personal funds, were sufficient tools with which to begin his remarkable work. As a result of his investigations, Manson introduced the concept of the transmission of infection by arthropods; this concept opened up a totally new understanding of disease.

Manson's most important medical contribution was the culmination of his search for the intermediate host for filaria, which is the cause of elephantiasis. The filaria embryos had been recognized in human blood by Lewis in 1872 and the parent worm had been discovered in 1876 by Joseph Bancroft of Brisbane. Manson observed that the incidence of filariasis in infested areas might be as high as 50 percent of the population. He found that most of those affected were in apparent good health, despite the finding of parasites in their blood. In other cases with clinical symptoms, he could not recover the parasite. This led him to speculate that the parasites might appear in the peripheral blood intermittently, diurnally or nocturnally. He therefore arranged to examine patients periodically through a twenty-four hour period and thus discovered that there was a diurnal migration of the parasite.

This information provided Manson with the clue needed for his next step in identifying a supposed vector. He reasoned that the vector must be a nocturnal bloodsucker with a geographic range corresponding to that of the filaria. This led him to investigate the common tropical mosquito, the culex fatigans. He took a culex mosquito that had not previously been fed on patients with filariasis and placed it under a mosquito net with an infected person. The next morning he retrieved the mosquito, fed it on fresh bananas for a time and then examined it. Microscopic sections revealed the filaria in the mosquito's stomach and thoracic muscles. Thus the life cycle between man and mosquito was exposed.

Manson's work included a number of other notable accomplishments which he pursued while in the Far East or after his return to London. These included a description of Sparganum mansoni, the larval stage of filaria loa, the eggs of Schistosoma mansoni, Trypanosoma gambiense, the fungus Trichophyton mansoni, and a clinical description of tinea imbricata and tropical sprue. After his return to London, Manson encouraged Ronald Ross, who was studying public health in England at that time, to investigate the mosquito as an intermediary host for malaria.

Manson provided the major impetus in the establishment of two schools of tropical medicine. In 1886 he helped found the Hong Kong Medical College and one of his first pupils was Sun Yat-sen, who later became president of the Chinese Republic. In 1898 he founded the London School of Tropical Medicine and established the Royal Society of Tropical Medicine.

Although Manson proved that filariasis was transmitted by mosquitoes, the experimental transmission of a disease of man or lower animals through an intermediary host still remained to be accomplished. Theobald Smith in 1893 furnished the final link in the chain of evidence by infecting healthy cattle with the offending parasite of Texas Cattle fever, recovered from the host tick.

Theobald Smith was born in Albany, New York in 1859, the son of an immigrant German tailor. He studied biology and mathematics at Cornell and received his M.D. from Albany Medical School. Smith was a doctor who never practiced medicine or treated human beings. At the age of twenty-five he was appointed Director of the Pathological Laboratory of the United States Bureau of Animal Industry at Washington, D. C. This appointment was due to chance and to two small pieces of histologic research he had carried out with his friend and teacher, Professor Gage of Cornell.

The Bureau of Animal Industry had been charged with the investigation of Texas Cattle fever which was causing severe losses in the livestock of the Southwest. Smith and his colleagues conducted a remarkably thorough study of this disease, using clinical and epidemiologic as well as laboratory methods. Smith was a field as well as a laboratory investigator. He worked in the corral and on the range to better pursue his epidemiologic, clinical and postmortem studies.

After years of toil and study, Smith and his colleagues demonstrated that the severe anemia of Texas Cattle fever was caused by an intercellular parasite transmitted by a tick. The critical observation was the identification of the parasite Babesia (Piroplasma) bigemina in the red blood cells of the infected cattle. The studies on Texas Cattle fever were summarized in a monograph published by the Government Printing Office for the Bureau of Animal Industry in 1893. The conclusions summarized in this monograph set a standard for epidemiologic excellence and revealed the potentialities for the investigation of other arthropod-borne diseases such as yellow fever, sleeping sickness, bubonic plague and typhus.

In 1895 Smith was invited to become the first incumbent of the endowed chair of comparative pathology at Harvard. He also became Director of the State of Massachusetts' Antitoxin and Vaccine Laboratory. Later in life Smith accepted the position of director of the Department of Animal Diseases for the Rockefeller Institute for Medical Research.

During his lifetime Theobald Smith made a number of bacteriological and scientific contributions. He demonstrated that dead virus can give an immunity against living virus and differentiated human and bovine tubercule bacilli. His work brought him international fame and he was the recipient of many honors. However, Smith's most important contribution was the development of basic concepts and epidemiologic principles through his studies on parasitism and disease.

In 1894 David Bruce brought another of the arthropod-borne diseases into focus, when he worked out the etiology of nagana, a disease of cattle and horses in Zululand. He demonstrated that it was due to a trypanosome and was transmitted by the tsetse fly.

Trypanosomes are among the most deadly of the protozoan parasites that plague mankind. Two species, trypanosome gambiense and trypanosome rhodesiense, cause the terrible scourge of sleeping sickness that hangs like a black cloud over tropical Africa. There are a great many kinds of trypanosomes inhabiting many different animals. Most trypanosomes are not specific for one host. Thus the trypanosome of sleeping sickness infects not only man, but also monkeys, dogs, rodents, domestic animals and a large number of wild game animals.

A nonpathogenic type of trypanosome was discovered by Lewis in 1870, and in 1880 Griffith Evans was the first to discover a pathogenic trypanosome. The organism that Bruce identified as the cause of nagana is named Trypanosoma brucei in his honor. It infects the large wild game animals of Central Africa which serve as the natural reservoir of the disease. Although they are immune to the effects of the organism, the trypanosome is carried from them to cattle and horses by the bite of a tsetse fly known as the Glossina Morsitans. The disease is always fatal to horses and few cattle recover from it. Thus domestic animals that are brought into the "fly belt" soon die and the development of a vast area of Africa is impossible without control of this disease.

The cause of African sleeping sickness in humans, the trypanosoma gambiense, was discovered by Dutton in 1901. Dutton and Todd found that tsetse flies were prevalent wherever sleeping sickness existed. In 1903 Bruce showed that tsetse flies may carry the disease twenty-one days after feeding upon a monkey infected with sleeping sickness. Next to the mosquito the tsetse fly is the most dangerous of the biting insects.

In 1909 the Brazilian physician Carlos Chagas described American Trypanosomiasis. The organism carrying this disease was studied by another Brazilian physician Osvaldo Cruz and is named the trypanosoma cruzi in his honor. This disease is spread by the bite of a bloodthirsty, bedbug-like insect called the Lanus Megistus.

Dengue, dandy or break-bone fever is an acute febrile infection that had been frequently reported as occurring in explosive outbreaks in various parts of the world. It had long mystified medical men as to its cause and means of spread. In 1902 and 1903 Graham working in Beirut demonstrated that it was a mosquito-borne disease. It is now classified as one of the arthropod-borne, viral hemorrhagic fevers.

Relapsing fever, febris recurrens, or spirillum fever are terms applied to a large group of acute infectious diseases which are characterized by an initial febrile period, followed by apparent recovery and then one or more relapses. The relapsing fevers are caused by various closely related spirochetes which are either tick- or louse-borne. The first known description of this condition was given in 1739 by Rutty who reported on an epidemic in Dublin. Because of the typical recurrences or relapses seen in this disease the name "relapsing fever" was proposed by Henderson in 1843. He also differentiated the disease from typhus. In 1868 Obermeir discovered the causative spirochete. In 1891 Flügge and in 1901 Mackie concluded that the body louse acted as the vector. In 1905 Dutton and Todd reported that ticks also acted as vectors.

When the secret of man's most deadly disease, the terrifying bubonic plague, was finally revealed, it was found to be an arthropod-borne disease. Plague was discovered to be primarily a disease of rats, transmitted to man by the bite of a flea.

After devastating the Medieval World for almost 400 years and nearly exterminating the human race, plague mysteriously retrogressed. After a last deadly epidemic in Marseilles, France in 1720, plague left Europe, never to return. During the next 172 years, epidemics progressively waned throughout the world, so that by the last decade of the nineteenth century the Black Death appeared to be a disease of the past.

However, plague continued to smoulder in the East where its existence had been maintained by the native rodents of Central Asia since time immemorial. At the end of the nineteenth century plague erupted in Hong Kong and Canton and then moved on to Bombay and Calcutta. From the distant reaches of the Gobi Desert and the plains of Central Asia, the rats, fleas and germs of plague came to Hong Kong in 1893. Carried by trade and travel, it took three years for the plague to go from Hong Kong to India. Spreading from Bombay to Calcutta, the plague went on to ravage India. Millions were swept away and died, before the pestilential tide finally ebbed. It is estimated that plague killed over 10 million people in India and the Orient during the twenty-five years between 1893 and 1918.

In 1894 Yersin and Kitasato, while investigating the Hong Kong epidemic independently of each other and almost simultaneously, discovered the causative organism of plague. Their searching microscopes found it lurking in the buboes and blood of patients who had died from the plague.

Alexandre Emil Jean Yersin (1863-1943), a French bacteriologist and former pupil of Pasteur's, succeeded in isolating the organism and growing it on culture plates. He proved his case and fulfilled the postulates of Koch by producing plague in rats that were inoculated with organisms from his cultures.

The brilliant Japanese bacteriologist Shibasaburo Kitasato (1856-1931) also discovered the bacillus of plague. A thorough worker, he had studied medicine under Koch in Germany. Kitasato's independent isolation of the same organism in the same year, served to prove beyond a doubt that at long last the deadly organism of plague had been discovered.

Yersin soon attempted to find a vaccine against plague. He developed his so-called Yersin's serum, obtained by immunizing horses, first with dead and then with living plague bacilli. Unfortunately his serum was only of slight therapeutic value and gave a rather feeble and transient type of prophylactic protection. In 1898 the Russian-

English bacteriologist Waldemar Mordecai Wolff Haffkine, working in India, also developed an antiplague vaccine. Known as "Haffkine's prophylaxis," this vaccine has been successfully used to protect doctors, nurses and others working in plague areas.

The organism was fittingly named the Pasteurella pestis, thereby coupling the name of the world's greatest bacteriologist with the world's deadliest pestilence. The association of rats with plague had been observed since ancient times and was so obvious that it had been accepted long before it was proved. Hence, almost simultaneously with the discovery of the organism it was demonstrated that the epizootic among rats was identical with the epidemic among men. The problem was how to link them together.

The important thing that remained to be discovered was how the infection was transmitted from rats to humans. In 1897 Masaki Ogata of the Hygienic Institute of Tokyo while working on plague in Formosa observed the plague bacillus in rat fleas. He not only demonstrated that fleas from plague-infected rats contained the pathogenic organism, but also was the first to suggest that they might transmit the infection to man.

The hypothesis that plague was primarily a disease of rats, spread by rat fleas was conceived in 1898 by the French epidemiologist P. L. Simond (1858-1947). His theory that plague was conveyed by fleas was based on observations and supported by some experimental evidence. By carefully examining plague-infected patients he was able to find the tiny puncture wound where the flea had first bitten its victim. Usually these were single punctures and Simond observed that a typical bubo always appeared in the glands draining the area of the bite. He also recovered plague bacilli from fleas which had fed on infected rats. His work attracted sufficient medical attention so that it was studied by the First Indian Plague Commission. Unfortunately the Commission erroneously concluded that Simond's hypothesis lacked proof and stated that they could find no connection between fleas and plague.

Fortunately a number of plague investigators were dissatisfied with the findings of the Commission. This dissatisfaction continued to mount as new evidence accumulated showing that rats and fleas were invariably and closely associated with human plague. Finally, Captain Glen W. Liston of the Indian Medical Service, along with others, succeeded in securing the appointment of a Second Indian Plague Commission which restudied the rat-flea theory.

In 1907, almost ten years after Simond had set forth his hypothesis, the Commission definitely announced that fleas were the vectors of plague and were responsible for transmission of the disease. They proved their case by the simple experiment of hanging cages containing rats at different heights above hopping, plague infected, fleas. The rats whose cages dangled safely above the flea's four inch jump escaped the plague, while those that hung at lower levels sickened and died.

Thus the whole story of plague was unravelled. Bubonic plague is primarily a disease of rats and small rodents, caused by a germ known as the Pasteurella pestis. When an epizootic explodes among rats, they sicken and die in large numbers.

Rats have fleas. The fleas leave the dead rats and seek warm living rats, carrying with them the deadly germs of plague. When fresh rats are not to be found, the fleas reluctantly bite men, thereby infecting them with plague. The fleas themselves are infected and like rats and men, they too sicken and die from plague. The Xenopsylla Cheopis or Oriental rat flea is the chief transmitter of plague. Through commerce this flea has attained worldwide distribution. However, other species of fleas are also capable of transmitting plague.

It was found that from a primary rat-borne case of bubonic plague in man a secondary plague pneumonia could develop as a complication. Pneumonic plague is swift, deadly and highly contagious. The sputum teems with plague bacilli and thus pneumonic plague can be spread from man to man.

In August, 1903 a blacksmith died of plague contracted from a squirrel in Contra Costa County, California. While investigating this case, Rupert Blue became impressed with the fact that ground squirrels might be infected with Pasturella pestis and thus could serve as an important reservoir of plague. However, it was not until 1908 that McCoy and Wherry discovered natural plague in ground squirrels and demonstrated its existence among wild rodents in fourteen western states. Because the disease existed primarily in wooded areas it was descriptively called "sylvatic" plague.

In 1911 McCoy of the United States Public Health Service described "a plague-like disease of rodents" occurring in Tulare County, California. In 1912 he and Chapin discovered the causative organism, which has since been named the Pasteurella tularense. In 1907 Martin, an Arizona opthalmologist, described five human cases which were contracted from skinning jack rabbits. Francis in 1919 and 1920 described "deer fly" fever in Utah and recognized it to be identical with McCoy's "plague-like disease of rodents." He named the disease "Tularemia" in honor of the California County where it first was found. Tularemia is primarily a fatal bacteremia of wild rodents, especially rabbits and hares, and secondarily an accidental infection of man. Bloodsucking insects such as ticks, lice, fleas and flies transmit the infection from animal to animal in nature.

Chapter 29

LICE, FLEAS AND DDT

ANOTHER FASCINATING CHAPTER in the history of arthropod-borne disease was revealed in 1909 when Charles Nicolle discovered that the lowly louse was responsible for the transmission of typhus. One of the oldest of pestilential diseases, typhus was discovered to be self-limiting. It was found that the disease does not pass from man to man, but is transmitted from man to louse to man.

Historically, typhus has always accompanied man in misery and misfortune. It follows in the wake of war, famine, flood and disaster. Whenever and wherever men are crowded or confined together in dirt and misery, their unkempt, unwashed bodies soon become louse infested and deadly typhus then erupts. Typhus has been called jail fever, ships' fever, camp fever, military fever, hospital fever, and famine fever, to mention just a few of the hundred or more names that the disease has been known by.

Typhus ravaged populations long before its symptoms were sorted out from the welter of pestilential fevers that afflicted the world. Perhaps the first identifiable symptoms of typhus were recorded in 1083 at the Monastery of La Cava near Salerno. However, our formal knowledge of the disease began in the Middle Ages, which was a most flourishing time for lice and typhus.

The concepts of cleanliness and the bathing customs of ancient Greece and Rome had long been forgotten and were left behind in history. Few people bothered to bathe, everybody stank and everybody itched and was lousy. At medieval funerals, the spectators frequently occupied themselves during the long ceremony by counting and commenting upon the steady parade of lice that marched away from the body of the dead.

The Spaniards called typhus "Tabardillo" or "little cloak" in a fanciful allusion to the discoloration of the skin caused by the typical purple petechial spots of the disease. The army of Ferdinand and Isabella lost 17,000 soldiers from typhus during the Seige of Granada in 1489-90. This is reliably estimated to have been six times as many as were killed by the Moors. Early in the sixteenth century, the Spanish explorers and Conquistadores carried their lice and typhus to Mexico, thereby introducing the disease to the New World.

Severe and devastating epidemics of typhus ravaged Italy in 1505 and again in 1528. The disease was described by Girolamo Cardano in 1536. He stated that most Italian physicians called it the petechial disease and frequently confused it with measles. Cardano proposed calling it "morbus pulicans" or flea-bite disease. Typhus was also clearly and accurately described in 1546 by Fracastoro in his famous *De Contagionibus.*

Known as gaol fever, typhus was the terror of the medieval English jails. Because the sick and the well, the clean and the verminous were indiscriminately locked up together, typhus frequently ravaged the near-starved inmates of these filthy jails.

No respector of persons, the jail-starved lice would commonly crawl from the lowly prisoners in the dock to the exalted judges on the bench. Thus, while the judge and jury dispensed justice, the typhus-bearing lice would sentence the court to death. In England these deadly sessions of the court mingled with typhus became known as the "Black Assizes."

One of the first and best documented of the Black Assizes occurred at Oxford in 1577. A Catholic bookbinder named Rowland Jencks was accused of treason and profaning the Protestant religion. The court found him guilty and sentenced him to have his ears cropped.

However, Jencks had his revenge for this cruel and inhuman punishment. Typhus-bearing lice crawled from his sick and verminous person to feed upon the members of the court. Shortly after his trial, the chief baron of the exchequer, the sergeant at arms, two sheriffs, one knight, five justices of the peace and most of the jury, sickened and died from typhus. The deadly lice then crawled from the court room into the town of Oxford and before the epidemic subsided, over five hundred had died. Strangely enough, the prisoner survived both his illness and punishment and lived for another thirty-three years.

This Black Assizes was followed by a number of others. One of the last occurred at the Easter session of "Old Bailey" in London in 1750. Typhus was raging in Newgate Prison and once again the prisoners brought their lice to court with them. This time the toll included the lord mayor, an alderman, two judges, an under-sheriff, the jury and many of the lesser court attaches.

In the eighteenth century James Lind practically banished typhus from the Royal Navy by improving British Naval Hygiene. During the eighteenth and nineteenth centuries a general improvement in personal cleanliness, together with the increased use of cotton clothing and the introduction of underwear reduced lousiness and thus lessened typhus. However, historical records show that innumerable typhus epidemics continued to plague the world.

The great Napoleon had reason to know typhus well. As his "Grand Army" of 500,000 marched east through the endemic typhus areas of Poland and Lithuania his sickness rates increased tremendously. After the Battle of Ostrowo in July of 1812, it is estimated that over 80,000 of his troops were stricken with typhus. During his tragic retreat from Russia, his defeated army was further decimated by disease until only a straggling remnant of his once Grand Army returned. Deadly typhus was responsible for a large share of his losses.

Typhus derives its name from the characteristic stupor that accompanies the fever. The disease was so named by the French pathologist Sauvages in 1760 and is derived from the Greek word "typhos," literally meaning smoke, haze or a cloud. Typhus and typhoid fever were hopelessly confused until 1829 when the French physician, Pierre Charles Alexandre Louis, recognized typhoid fever as a distinct disease entity. He also coined the word "typhoid" from typhus by adding the Greek suffix "eidos" or like, thus meaning a typhus-like disease. In 1836 William Wood Gerhard of Philadelphia, who had studied under Louis, thoroughly established typhus and typhoid as two distinct diseases and thus ended the confusion.

In 1909 Charles Jules Henri Nicolle exposed the lowly louse as the villian responsible for the transmission of typhus. Born in Rouen on September 21, 1866, Nicolle was educated in his native city and in Paris, where he was a pupil of Pasteur's. After receiving his medical degree in 1893, he was appointed professor of bacteriology at Rouen. Here, his outstanding work attracted the attention of the French government and in 1903 he was invited to inaugerate a government health service in Tunisia and to direct a branch of the Pasteur Institute.

Nicolle was the first to show that serum from patients convalescing from typhus, measles or undulant fever would protect susceptible individuals from these diseases. He also demonstrated that the blood of typhus fever patients is infectious. In 1909 Nicolle discovered that the louse was a carrier of typhus and served as its chief transmitting agent. He also demonstrated that the disease could be transmitted by crushing a louse and rubbing its infected remains into the excoriated skin.

In 1928 Nicolle was awarded the Nobel prize in physiology and medicine for his work on typhus. He died in Tunisia on February 28, 1936.

By the end of the nineteenth century and the beginning of the twentieth century, a whole group of typhus-like diseases came into focus. These are now known as rickettsial diseases and are caused by a family of microorganisms that are intermediate between bacteria and viruses. These diseases were gradually differentiated as to their etiology, pathology and epidemiology.

In 1898 Nathan Edwin Brill, a New York physician, encountered a number of sporadic cases of an atypical typhoid-like disease in which the Widal tests and blood cultures were negative. In 1910 he reported 255 such cases and called attention to their several common features: the disease usually occurred in immigrants from Russia or Poland, there was no infectiousness, and the most characteristic aspect of the disease was a macular or maculopapular rash beginning on the fifth or sixth day. Clinicians in other large cities of the eastern United States promptly reported cases which were referred to as "Brill's disease." In 1912, Anderson and Goldberger showed by cross-immunity tests in monkeys that Brill's disease was a form of typhus.

In 1934 Hans Zinsser advanced the hypothesis that the disease was a recrudescence of typhus and he postulated the persistence of typhus rickettsia during the latent interval somewhere in the tissues of the human subject. Further work verified Zinsser's hypothesis and Mooser in 1953 suggested the term "Brill-Zinsser's disease."

Flea-borne or murine typhus fever probably has occurred for centuries as a sporadic or endemic disease, but only since 1931 has it been clearly distinguished from classic epidemic louse-borne typhus. Sporadic cases of typhus were reported occasionally in Europe in the medical literature before Brill's disease was defined as an entity. Attention has already been called to the erroneous use of the term "Brill's disease" for cases of murine typhus.

In 1922 Hone reported isolated cases from Australia and Wheatland described a noncontagious typhus-like fever in Queensland at a time when a plague of mice afflicted that part of Australia. Maxcy suggested a nonhuman reservoir of typhus in southeastern United States and specifically mentioned mice and rats. He further suggested that fleas, mites or ticks could be the vectors.

Mooser in 1928 observed a basic difference in behavior of certain strains of typhus rickettsia in the tissues of guinea pigs. Dyer and his colleagues isolated typhus rickettsia from rat fleas in Baltimore in 1931. Mooser, Zinsser and Ruiz-Castenada found the agent in rats in Mexico City. Mooser then named the disease "murine typhus" to indicate that it is a natural infection of rats. The causative organism was named Rickettsia mooserii in recognition of Mooser's work. Reports rapidly accumulated showing a worldwide distribution of murine typhus.

Historical evidence points to the fact that Rocky Mountain spotted fever was known to the Indians and existed in Idaho and Montana long before the arrival of the white man. The disease was first described by Surgeon Major W. W. Woods in 1896. In 1899 Dr. Maxcy, an Idaho physician, published the first clinical description of the disease in a medical journal. Dr. John F. Anderson reported the existence of "spotted fever" in the Rocky Mountains in 1903.

In 1902 Wilson and Chowning made some important laboratory and field investigations and suggested that the disease was transmitted by the wood tick. In 1906 Howard Taylor Ricketts, an American pathologist, described the microorganism which is the cause of Rocky Mountain spotted fever. He demonstrated the presence of infected ticks in nature and in 1909 reported the successful transmission of spotted fever by the wood tick Dermacentor andersonii. His work defined most of the problems of the disease and its causation. The disease has now been recognized in more than three-fourths of the United States, as well as in Mexico and South America.

In 1910, during the course of some of his experiments, Ricketts died of typhus in Mexico City. In Serbia, Stanislaus Josef Mathias von Prowazek was also studying typhus and searching for its cause. He too, unfortunately contracted the disease and died from it at not quite the age of forty.

The causative organism of typhus was isolated in 1916 by the Berlin physician Henrique da Rocha-Lima. He named it Rickettsia prowazeki in honor of the two researchers who lost their lives to typhus. The studies of Wolbach, Todd and Palfrey in 1922 established beyond a doubt the relationship of Rickettsia-prowazeki and typhus fever.

Derrick in 1937 reported another typhus-like disease which he observed in Australia. Because it was a fever of unknown origin he named it "Q fever," taking the Q from the word "query" or question. In 1938 the disease was identified as endenmic in western Montana where it was known as "nine-mile fever." The causative organism was isolated and named the Rickettsia burnetti. The infection is spread to man by the bite of ticks.

Rickettsial pox, another typhus-like disease, was first observed in 1946 when it became epidemic in a New York City housing development. A clinical description of the disease was given by Greenberg in 1947. The causative agent is Rickettsia akari which is transmitted to man by a rodent mite that is ectoparasitic on mice. Control consists of the suppression of mouse infestation.

True to its historical pattern of following in the wake of war, famine and disaster, epidemic typhus erupted in Serbia during World War I, where it caused over 100,000 deaths in six months. In the years following the Russian Revolution, typhus took an estimated toll of three million lives in that country.

During World War II, the threat of typhus and other arthropod-borne diseases was once again greater than the dangers of battle. Naples, an Italian city of close to a million, was devastated by allied bombings and the retreating Germans. With the water supply destroyed, the people were living in overcrowded shelters with the most primitive of sanitary arrangements. Food and soap were scarce and as dirt and poverty increased, the lowly louse took over.

When the Allies entered Naples in October of 1943, an epidemic was already under way and winter was approaching. Typhus soon was raging and threatened to block the Allied advance, when DDT joined the fight and effectively controlled the epidemic in a few short weeks. Thus, DDT made medical history with its miraculous pesticidal powers. It not only checked typhus in Italy, but also in the war-torn areas of the Near East, Korea, Japan, North Africa and Germany.

The term DDT is a contraction of the chemical name of this compound, which is dichloro diphenyl trichloroethane. DDT was first synthesized in 1874 by the German Chemist Othmar Zeidler. However, its potent insecticidal properties were not discovered until about the beginning of World War II. The final research and development of this compound was carried out in the laboratories of the J. R. Geigy Company of Basle, Switzerland.

After the war, DDT became available for civilian use and its powerful pesticidal properties were immediately thrown into man's never-ending battle against his insect foes. The results were phenomenal. Man could at long last protect his food supply, and crop losses due to insect pests were drastically reduced. However, more important was public health's use of this powerful pesticide to combat such arthropod-borne disease as typhus, malaria and yellow fever.

Unfortunately, after a number of years it was found that some insects became resistant to DDT. However, DDT had ushered in the era of chemical pesticides and numerous new and effective compounds were rapidly developed. Lindane, Chlordane, Dieldrin, BHC, Malathion and numerous other insecticides and pesticides were able to take over whenever and wherever DDT failed.

The discovery of DDT and the other chemical pesticides can be ranked among the top scientific discoveries of the age. By making possible the chemical control of the arthropod-borne diseases, these potent pesticides have saved millions of lives.

Chapter 30

WINGED DEATH
THE STORY OF MALARIA AND
YELLOW FEVER

THE INCRIMINATION of the mosquito as a carrier of death and disease forms one of the most fascinating chapters in the history of preventive medicine. The unmasking of the lowly mosquito as the winged vehicle of infection in such deadly and devastating diseases as malaria and yellow fever represents one of mankind's greatest accomplishments. The translation of this knowledge into action has made "mosquito control" one of public health's most powerful and effective weapons. It has made possible the prevention and control of these and other tropical diseases, thereby saving millions of lives.

The story of "Winged Death" logically starts with malaria, one of the most ancient of all diseases and one which has probably killed more people than any other single disease in the world. Although the actual discovery that malaria is spread by mosquitoes is a modern one, the association between insects and disease had been suspected since the earliest of times. The signs and symptoms of malaria are so characteristic that when they are described in ancient writings they can easily be detected as such.

The earliest of medical records recognized malaria as a definite clinical entity. The Brahmin physician Susrata in about 500 B.C. gave an excellent description of malaria and definitely suspected the mosquito as a cause. We thus know that the disease was widespread from the earliest ages in the Mediterranean basin, India, and South China. The disease became common in Greece in about 400 B.C. It was so common in the Roman Empire that the Ancient Romans created a goddess of intermittent fevers named Dea Febris, who was worshipped in an effort to control the disease. In fact most medical historians believe that malaria was an important cause in the decline of the Grecian and Roman civilizations.

Hippocrates described the disease and differentiated the fever into the quotidian, tertian and quartan types. He further described how these intermittant fevers were associated with the swamplands and occurred most often during the warm summer months. In about 100 A.D., Columella in his *De Rustica,* a book on hygiene, spoke on the need of choosing a healthy location for a dwelling. He wrote, "Nor indeed must there be a marsh near the building, nor a public highway adjoining, for the former always throws up noxious and poisonous steams during the heats and breeds animals with mischievous stings which fly upon us in exceeding thick swarms . . . . whereby hidden diseases are often contracted."

The ancient idea that malaria was closely associated with mosquitoes continued to reappear throughout the pages of medical history. It was well known that the disease had a seasonal incidence, occurring during the summer and autumn and disappearing with the first frost. It was also clearly understood that the disease had a definite geographic distribution and commonly occurred in swampy, low-lying areas and adjacent to ponds and marshes. Although many workers tried to incriminate the mosquito, this grain of truth was repeatedly lost in the chaff of a vast amount of blundering folly. Unfortunately, medical thought was dominated by the miasmic theory of disease spread and malaria was believed to be due to the noxious vapors and miasma that arose from swampy low-lying areas. In fact, the disease owes its name to this erroneous concept and the term malaria is derived from the Italian words "male" (bad) and "aira" (air). It was so named by Torti in 1718 in a classical treatise upon various climatological fevers.

We know that malaria was present in Europe during the Middle Ages and that from the sixteenth to the eighteenth century it was endemic and frequently epidemic. There is some dispute as to when and by what route malaria reached the New World. Some believe that the Spaniards found it already present when they came to South America, while others believe that they carried the disease with them.

There is, however, abundant evidence that malaria did not exist in

North America prior to its discovery. The disease was introduced into the West Indies either by the Spaniards directly, or it was carried by Negro slaves brought to the New World in 1563. There is no question but that the introduction of Negro slaves into the West Indies caused the disease to flourish there.

Negro slaves were first delivered to the Jamestown Colony from Africa in 1619 and by bringing the malarial parasite with them, they became the most important source of malarial infection on the North American Continent. During the first half of the eighteenth century, the disease became highly endemic throughout a zone below Chesapeake Bay and soon all of the southern States suffered from severe epidemics of malaria. The disease then spread northward and all of New England was widely invaded by short, sharp summer epidemics. In 1800 with the opening of the West, the disease followed the settlers on their westward migrations and they were severely plagued by intermittant fevers, chills and the ague.

In 1850 the pioneer physician Daniel Drake in his great classic, *Principal Diseases of the Interior Valley of North America,* described malaria as the principal disease of North America. In his observations on the epidemiology of malaria he came close to the solution. He set forth the hypothesis that the disease might be transmitted by an insect like the mosquito; unfortunately proof for his hypothesis still lay fifty years in the future.

A curious feature in the history of malaria is that its treatment was discovered in advance of the knowledge of its cause. For many centuries the Peruvian Indians had successfully treated their fevers with the powdered bark of the quina-quina tree. Presumably the knowledge of the curative powers of this miraculous drug had been handed down to them by their forebearers, the Incas. According to legend, the Countess of Chinchon, wife of the Spanish Viceroy of Peru, was stricken with malaria while in Lima in 1630. She was saved from death by the timely arrival of an Indian who cured her with the miraculous powder of the fever bark tree. The Countess supposedly introduced the drug into Europe where it was called Chinchona in her honor.

Quinine was also called Jesuit's bark, or Cardinal's bark after the Jesuit Cardinal Lugo who successfully treated Louis XIV with it and promoted its use during the 1640's. However, the popularity of quinine in the treatment of malaria was largely due to the English physician Robert Tabor. Tabor successfully cured Charles II from an attack of tertian malaria and then was called to France to treat the Dauphin who was suffering from the ague. When the jealous physicians of the French Court asked him what the fever was, he replied, "I do not know; you gentlemen may explain the nature of the fever; but I can cure it, which you cannot." Full medical approval was given to quinine after the great Sydenham reported his successful use of it in treating an outbreak of the ague in England.

Quinine not only was a cure for malaria, but proved to be a valuable diagnostic agent. It was used as a therapeutic test and cases of chills and fever that failed to respond to its use could almost without exception be classified as nonmalarial.

However, the battle was being fought against an invisible and mysterious foe until the first great forward step was made by Charles Louis Alphonse Laveran's discovery of the causative organism in 1880. Laveran, a French army surgeon serving in Algeria, found the microscopic parasite of malaria in the blood of patients suffering from the disease. He published four treatises on the subject and received a Nobel Prize for his work in 1907. He observed the various stages through which the parasite passed and noted that with each new brood of parasites in the blood a fresh bout of fever began. However, Laveran's discovery, important as it was, did not supply the means of controlling malaria. The knowledge of the transmission of the parasite by the mosquito was needed before his discovery could grow to practical usefulness.

The mystery of malaria was solved by Ronald Ross, a young officer in the Indian Medical Service. Ross was born in 1857 in the Himalayan Mountains of India, the son of a Commander of the British forces on the Northwest frontier. He was the eldest of ten children and at the age of eight was sent to England to begin his education. In obedience to his father's wishes, he enrolled at St. Bartholomew's Hospital in London at the age of seventeen. In his "Memoirs" Ross himself wrote as follows:

> I wished to be an artist, but my father was opposed to this. I wished also to enter the Army or Navy; but my father had set his heart upon

my joining the medical profession and, finally, the Indian Medical Service, which was then well paid and possessed many good appointments; . . . But I had no predilection at all for medicine and, like most youths, felt disposed to look down upon it.

Ross graduated five years later and, in accordance with his father's wishes, took the entrance examinations for the Indian Medical Service. He failed to pass and served as a ship's surgeon while waiting for a second try. In 1881 he passed his examinations "without distinction" and upon receiving his commission as a surgeon in the Indian Medical Service he sailed for India.

His first years in India were rather idle medically and he spent a great deal of time in literary pursuits composing poetry and prose. However, Ross could not escape becoming interested in malaria and mosquitos early in his career. Malaria was an ever-present scourge and it is estimated, that at this time, over a million persons a year died of this disease in India. He expressed his feelings on the need for finding the cause of malaria in the following verse:

> In this, O Nature, yield I pray to me.
> I pace and pace, and think and think, and take
> The fever'd hands, and note down all I see,
> That some dim distant light may haply break.
>
> The painful faces ask, can we not cure?
> We answer, No, not yet; we seek the laws.
> O God, reveal thro' all this thing obscure
> The unseen, small, but million-murdering cause.

Mosquitos were everywhere and he was personally plagued by them. While stationed at Bangalore he was nearly devoured by them before he discovered that they were breeding in a tub outside the window of his bungalow. He solved the problem and got rid of them by simply upsetting the tub. Ross later wrote of this incident as follows:

When I told the Adjutant of this miracle, and pointed out that the Mess House could be rid of mosquitos in the same way, much to my surprise he was very scornful and refused to allow men to deal with them for, he said, it would be upsetting the order of nature, and as mosquitos were created for some purpose, it was our duty to bear with them! I argued in vain that the same thesis would apply to bugs and fleas, and that according to him it was our duty to go about in a verminous condition! I did not know then that this type of fool is very common indeed.

In 1889 Ross returned to London to study bacteriology and became a diplomat in public health. While in London he met Sir Patrick Manson, the great parasitologist and expert on tropical diseases. Manson in 1879 had discovered the life cycle of the Filaria bancrofti, the parasite which caused elephantiasis. He had demonstrated that part of this life cycle occurred in the body of the mosquito and that the disease was transmitted to humans through the bite of the Culex mosquito. Manson showed Ross the malaria parasite in human blood and expressed the opinion that this probably represented only a single phase of a more elaborate life cycle. He advised Ross to pursue this avenue of research and suggested that malaria like filariasis was probably spread by mosquitoes.

Ross returned to India and began his long relentless search to find the role of the mosquito in the transmission of malaria. His work was done with a dilapidated microscope in a makeshift laboratory with equipment that would be considered primitive by present-day standards. Manson continued to encourage Ross and a great deal of correspondence was exchanged between the two parasitologists during the years of 1895-97.

Ross met with success in 1897 when at Secunderabad he discovered the parasite in the stomach of an Anopheles mosquito which had been fed on a human sufferer from malaria, a patient named Husein Khan. He traced the development of the plasmodium in the mosquito, finding the zygote, or sexual forms, in the stomach and the sporoblasts, or progeny, in the salivary glands. In the summer of 1898 Ross furnished the final proof that the mosquito was the intermediary host for malaria when he infected healthy birds by the bite of mosquitoes fed on malarious birds.

Ever the poet, Ross expressed his victory in the following verses:

> This day designing God
>   Hath put into my hand
> A wondrous thing. And God
>   Be praised. At His command,
>
> I have found thy secret deeds
>   Oh million-murdering Death.

I know that this litle thing
A million men will save—
Oh death where is thy sting?
Thy victory oh grave?

Later Ross wrote of his discovery as follows: "The exact route of infection of this great disease which annually slays its millions of human beings and keeps whole continents in darkness was revealed. These minute spores enter the salivary glands of the mosquito, and pass with its poisonous saliva directly into the blood of men. Never in our dreams had we imagined so wonderful a tale as this."

Ross retired from the Indian Medical Service in 1899 and was appointed lecturer on tropical medicine at the University of Liverpool. He was awarded the Nobel Prize in medicine in 1902 and became Sir Ronald Ross in 1911 when he was knighted. In 1926 the Ross Institute of Tropical Hygiene was dedicated and named in his honor.

In 1932 death closed the career of this remarkable man who in addition to being a great parasitologist was an accomplished poet, novelist, musician and mathematician. Starting his career as a reluctant physician with no great love of medicine, Ross became one of medicine's immortals by his solution of the mystery of malaria and thus made possible the saving of millions of lives.

Another dramatic chapter in the story of Winged Death is that of yellow fever. There are many similarities between the two tropical diseases malaria and yellow fever. Both diseases are of great antiquity and each has taken a tremendous toll of human life. Both mystified medical science as to their means of spread until it was discovered that they were mosquito-borne.

The origin of yellow fever is controversial; some historians believe it to be a New World disease, while others believe that it originated in Africa. From our modern scientific knowledge we now know that the tiger mosquito (the Aedes Aegypti or Stegomyia fasciata) is a highly domesticated species which can live and multiply on board ship. In the light of this knowledge it is possible to trace the journey of yellow fever from continent to continent along the trade routes of the old sailing vessels.

While European medical writers did not mention the disease before the days of Columbus it must be remembered that old medical records are not easily interpreted and yellow fever has borne at least 152 names during its history. The disease was often confused with dengue and infectious jaundice and was probably first recognized as a separate disease entity in the sixteenth century. Although yellow fever had frequently been carried from Africa to Spain and Portugal, the European physicians frequently failed to recognize the disease and were for the most part ignorant of it.

The disease received its chief recognition in the New World and the name "yellow fever" was first employed by Griffith Hughes in his *Natural History of the Barbados,* published in 1750. In this book he gave a classic description of the arrival of this "new distemper" in the West Indies in 1715. The disease was widely prevalent in the Caribbean and all along the tropical and subtropical coastal regions of South and Central America. In all probability it was brought from West Africa to the New World by the old slave traders.

Yellow fever was one of the most dreaded diseases of the Atlantic trade routes. The legend of the Flying Dutchman which was described by Sir Walter Scott was probably founded upon the story of a ship that was condemned to haunt the seas forever because, after a murder had been committed aboard, yellow fever broke out amongst the crew and no country would allow the stricken ship to enter its harbors. The disease commonly struck ships trading with West African ports and would frequently wipe out a whole ship's company. These ships soon learned to anchor some distance offshore because they observed that those who went ashore and slept on land were most frequently afflicted. The disease was nicknamed "yellow-jack" because vessels with the disease aboard had to fly a yellow flag or "jack." To this day, vessels arriving in quarantine are required to fly a yellow flag which stands for the letter "Q" of the International Code.

One of the first authenticated records of an epidemic of yellow fever was the outbreak that occurred on the populous little island of Barbados in 1647. It struck with such terrific force that over 5,000 died within a few months. Governor Winthrop of Massachusetts called the disease the "Barbados distemper" and in order to protect his Colony he instituted the first regulations for ship's quarantine in North America. In 1648 outbreaks of yellow fever were recorded in Yucatan and on the West Indian island of St. Kitts. From 1700 on there are abundant historical records of devastating epidemics not only in the Caribbean, but also along the coastal regions of North, Central and South America, as well as Spain, Portugal and France.

One of the most dramatic records of the devastation caused by yellow fever is the account given by Dr. Benjamin Rush of the tragic epidemic which struck Philadelphia in 1793. Brilliant and well educated, Rush was the leading physician of his day and the founder of American medicine. He was not only a famous physician and medical teacher, but was also an outstanding civic, political and patriotic figure. He was a member of Congress from Pennsylvania and was one of the signers of the Declaration of Independence. During the Revolutionary War, Rush served as surgeon general of the Middle Department of the Army. At the end of the war he returned to private practice and medical teaching in Philadelphia.

Rush's greatest test as a medical leader came with Philadelphia's tragic yellow fever epidemic in 1793. At this time Philadelphia was the nation's capitol with a population of over 35,000. The summer was hot and dry and the fever first appeared in July near the docks. Rush was one of the first to recognize the disease and its epidemic potential. His suggestions for preventive and control measures were at first treated with contempt by his medical colleagues. In mid-August the epidemic reached alarming proportions and by the end of the month people panicked and fled the city. The roads leading from the city were crowded with fleeing families, leaving the city nearly deserted, while business came to a standstill.

Although Rush sent his family to Princeton for safety, he stayed on to fight the epidemic. He estimated that by mid-October, 6,000 people were ill with the fever and "only three physicians were able to do business out of their houses." One hundred or more people were dying daily and Dr. Rush worked day and night. In the light of modern medicine his treatment was atrocious and consisted of drastic purging and copious bleeding. He himself came down with the fever, but managed to survive his own vigorous treatment.

Although Rush never stated or suspected that the disease was mosquito-borne, his recommendations almost foreshadowed this truth. He noted and complained on numerous occasions about the swarms of mosquitos that plagued the city. He recommended cleaning of the streets and advocated the draining of puddles, ponds and marshes. Other popular preventive measures were the burning of gun powder in the streets and the smoking of tobacco. The latter was so popular that even women and children had cigars in their mouths. As a preventive against the "fever-producing miasmic air" many relied on vinegar and camphor sprinkled on a handkerchief and held to the nose. Others relied on garlic or cloves which they chewed all day. Whiskey was ever-popular as both a preventive and cure.

Finally when frost ended the epidemic, Philadelphia had lost 5,000 people or one-tenth of its population. The following year Rush recorded the experience in *An Account of the Bilious Remitting Yellow Fever, As It Appeared in the City of Philadelphia, in the year 1793.*

In 1800 an epidemic of yellow fever defeated the ambitious schemes of Napoleon who had dispatched an army of 30,000 men to Haiti to fortify that island and use it as a base for his plans of colonization of Louisiana and Mexico. However, yellow fever intervened causing 23,000 casualties, thereby decimating his army and changing the course of history.

One of the riddles surrounding yellow fever was the fact that an epidemic never began promptly, but that there was always a lag of at least two weeks between the appearance of the first case and the occurrence of an outbreak. The first man to suggest the correct answer to this riddle was Dr. Josiah Clark Nott or Knott, of Mobile, Alabama. In 1848 in an article published in *The New Orleans Medical and Surgical Journal* he advanced the theory that the mosquito was a carrier of yellow fever. Unfortunately his article attracted little attention and his theory was soon forgotten. Others who suggested that insects played a part as carriers of yellow fever were Dr. J. C. Crawford of Baltimore in 1807 and Dr. L. Beauperthuy in 1854.

The first man to specifically accuse the mosquito as a carrier of yellow fever was Dr. Carlos J. Finlay of Havana, Cuba, who on August 11, 1881 at a meeting of the Royal Academy in Havana read a paper entitled "The Mosquito Hypothetically Considered as the Agent of Transmission of Yellow Fever."

Carlos Finlay was born in Camagüey, Cuba in 1833 of a Scotch father and a French mother. His early education was obtained at Le Havre and Rouen and his medical education at the Jefferson Medical College of Philadelphia, from where he graduated in 1855. He returned to Cuba and entered general practice in Havana. Becoming interested in epidemiology he made a number of contributions in the fields of leprosy, beriberi, filariasis, trichinosis, relapsing fever and cholera, as well as yellow fever. After many years of study he became convinced that yellow fever was transmitted by the bite of a mosquito, then known as the "Culex fasciata." His claims were supported with a report on a series of experimental inoculations of humans with infected mosquitos.

Unfortunately, Finlay was unable to gain medical support or attention and his theory was ignored for two decades. When the Spanish-American War broke out, Carlos Finlay, then sixty-five years old, went to Washington and offered his services to the United States Army and served in the Santiago Campaign. In 1899 the provisional government of Cuba appointed him chairman of its Yellow River Commission. In this capacity he met Dr. Walter Reed and explained to him his theories on the mosquito transmission of yellow fever. Although Finlay failed to convince Reed of his theories at this time, he later greatly assisted the work of the Yellow Fever Commission and supplied them with the first mosquitos used in their experiments.

After the occupation of Havana during the course of the Spanish-American War the losses among the United States troops from yellow fever were so great that Surgeon General Sternberg appointed a commission to go to Cuba and study the cause of transmission of the disease. As chairman of this commission, Sternberg appointed one of his most able and trusted medical officers, Major Walter Reed. The other members of the commission were Dr. James Carroll, a bacteriologist; Dr. Jesse W. Lazear, a specialist on insects; and Dr. Aristide Agramonte, a pathologist.

Walter Reed, the son of a minister was born in Gloucester County, Virginia, September 13, 1851. He entered the University of Virginia at the age of sixteen and being extremely bright, graduated third in his class at the age of eighteen. He then went to New York where he entered Bellevue Hospital Medical College and received his M.D. in 1870. After an internship and some years of practice in that city he received a commission as a First Lieutenant in the Medical Corps of the United States Army in 1875.

Reed spent thirteen years in various frontier army posts until 1890 when he was sent to Baltimore. There he worked in bacteriology and pathology at Johns Hopkins Hospital under Dr. William H. Welch. In 1893 he was appointed professor of bacteriology at the Army Medical School and curator of the Army Medical Museum in Washington. Reed did some significant work on the contagiousness of erysipelas in 1892 and in 1898 headed a commission to study typhoid fever in army camps which reported on the importance of flies as carriers. Along with Dr. James Carroll he studied the Bacillus icteroides which was claimed by its discoverer, Sanarelli, to be the cause of yellow fever. Their findings on this study were negative.

When the Yellow Fever Commission went to Havana they received the hearty cooperation of William C. Gorgas and Carlos Finlay. Gorgas was the Army's chief sanitary officer in occupied Havana and had been unsuccessful in his attempts to stamp out the disease. He was familiar with Finlay's mosquito hypothesis which he rejected in the belief that the disease was spread by filth. While Reed also rejected the mosquito theory as unproven he was sufficiently impressed so that he determined to test it out.

On August 27, 1900 Dr. James Carroll allowed himself to be bitten by a mosquito which had previously fed upon four yellow fever patients. He became severely ill four days later and very nearly died. Dr. Lazear was accidently bitten and died of yellow fever on September 25, 1900. These events emphasized the importance of testing the mosquito theory thoroughly.

Major Walter Reed now established a fully controlled experimental station a mile outside of Quemados, which he named Camp Lazear. Two heavily screened wooden structures were erected in which to carry out the experiments. One of these was deliberately poorly ventilated and was outfitted with beds, bedclothes and personal effects that were soiled and saturated with the excrement and vomitus of patients who had died from yellow fever. He had two separate groups of volunteers live in this contaminated environment for a period of twenty days. They came through this test healthy and unharmed, thus proving that the disease was not spread by filth or fomites.

The other experimental building was light and well ventilated. It was divided by a screen wall into two compartments. Equipped alike, one side was used by volunteers who allowed themselves to be bitten by mosquitoes; the other by control volunteers carefully protected from mosquitoes, but living under identical conditions and breathing the same atmosphere.

Private John Kissinger was the first man to be exposed to contaminated mosquitoes and on December 8, 1900 he came down with a well-defined case of yellow fever. In addition to Kissinger, three other volunteers were bitten by mosquitoes which had previously been fed on yellow fever patients. They all developed typical cases of yellow fever, the diagnosis of which was confirmed by the physicians of the combined Commissions. At the same time the nonimmune controls who slept in the other half of the building and shared the same atmosphere suffered no ill effects. Thus the Commission conclusively proved that yellow fever was transmitted by the bite of the Stegomyia mosquito.

On October 15, 1901 the study was carried one step further when filtered serum from an experimentally infected patient was injected into three human volunteers. Two of these developed yellow fever thus proving that the organism of yellow fever was a filterable virus. This was the first time that a filterable virus had been proven to be the cause of a specific human disease.

The conquest of yellow fever is the story of many heroic men. It cost the life of Dr. Jesse W. Lazear and in Johns Hopkins Hospital there is a memorial tablet to him. It reads as follows: "With more than the courage of the soldier, he risked and lost his life to show how a fearful pestilence is communicated and how its ravages may be prevented." Of Private John Kissinger, the first volunteer to be exposed to the bite of an infected mosquito, Major Reed said, "In my opinion this exhibition of moral courage has never been surpassed in the annals of the army of the United States." Reed also acknowledged the work of Finlay with the following statement, "To Dr. Carlos J. Finlay, of Havana, must be given . . . full credit for the theory of the propagation of yellow fever by means of the mosquito. . . ."

Unfortunately, Reed did not live very long after his scientific triumph, but died suddenly of appendicitis on March 22, 1902. General Leonard Wood at a memorial service said of him: "I know of no man who has done so much for humanity as Major Reed. His dis-

covery results in the saving of more lives annually than were lost in
the Cuban war and saves the commercial interests of the world a
greater financial loss in each year than the cost of the entire Cuban
war." Today in his honor, the Army's great research hospital near
Washington, D.C. bears Walter Reed's name.

Carlos Finlay enjoyed a kindlier fate and was appointed chief sanitary officer of Cuba, a post he held for many years. He died in 1915
at the age of eighty-two and was acclaimed as an international medical hero and had a number of institutions named after him.

The practical consequences of the findings of Reed's Yellow Fever
Commission were tremendous and immediate. Dr. William Crawford
Gorgas, the Army's Chief Sanitary Officer in Havana, applied vigorous, rigid antimosquito measures to the city. His mosquito control
measures were so effective that he was able to rid the city of yellow
fever within a period of three months. In recognition for his work in
Havana Gorgas was raised to the rank of Colonel and in 1904 was
appointed chief sanitary officer for the Panama Canal Commission.

Winged Death in the form of yellow fever and malaria had made
the Panama Canal Zone "The White Man's Grave." It is doubtful
if the canal could ever have been built or used without the discoveries
of preventive medicine. The Panama Canal Zone was probably the
unhealthiest and most unsanitary place in the two Americas. A French
Company headed by De Lesseps, the successful builder of the Suez
Canal, went bankrupt in its attempt to build the canal. Its failure
was not due to a lack of engineering skill, but was because for eight
grueling years the workers who labored on the Canal died by the
thousands from yellow fever, malaria and other tropical diseases.

A new start was made on the partly completed canal when the
United States bought out the rights of the French company. President
Theodore Roosevelt provided adequate financial backing and a determined effort was made to overcome the greatest obstacle to the
construction of the canal, which was the problem of protecting the
health and lives of the workers.

Colonel Gorgas was appointed chief sanitary officer of the Canal
Zone with full authority and was elevated to the rank of General.
He started with the basic fundamentals of good sanitation by waging
a determined war on dirt and filth. The workers were provided with

clean, airy, screened-in, living quarters and were given an adequate nutritious diet. Gorgas instituted the most intensive and effective mosquito control program the world had ever seen. He drained and ditched swamps and marshes, eliminated puddles of stagnant water and applied oil and chemicals to ponds and lakes, thus eliminating all possible breeding places for mosquitos. In a short time he transformed the Canal Zone from a death-dealing area that had been aptly nicknamed "The White Man's Grave," to a safe and healthy land where men could live and work. The canal was successfully finished in ten years and its construction was truly a triumph of preventive medicine.

However, the fight against yellow fever had really just begun. The Rockefeller Foundation appointed General Gorgas to head up its Yellow Fever Commission when his work in Panama was completed. During the next thirty-five years the Foundation spent over $14 million on research and grants to various countries to stamp out yellow fever. The fever fighters met with success in the populated areas of the world, but from time to time unexplained outbreaks occurred. Researchers found that a reservoir of the disease existed in the jungles of Africa and South America. They found that monkeys and marsupials were susceptible to the disease and that several species of forest-dwelling mosquitoes served as the intermediate hosts.

Over the years a number of researchers besides Dr. Jesse Lazear lost their lives to this deadly disease. The list includes, Dr. Howard B. Cross in 1921, Dr. Adrian Stokes in 1927, Dr. Hideyo Noguchi in 1928, Dr. Paul A. Lewis in 1929, Dr. William A. Young in 1929 and Dr. Theodore B. Hayne in 1930.

Another great forward step in the fight against yellow fever occurred when Dr. Max Theiler and his associates, working under the auspices of the Rockefeller Foundation, managed to attenuate two strains of the live virus. From these attenuated strains it was possible to develop an effective yellow fever vaccine. Dr. Theiler was awarded the Nobel Prize for 1951 in recognition of this achievement.

Despite the knowledge that has been gained and the progress that has been made, malaria and yellow fever still remain as major public health problems. Millions of people in the underdeveloped countries of the world still sicken and die from malaria. Although the techniques and methods of malaria control are known, their effective application is hampered because of poor socioeconomic conditions.

While yellow fever has virtually vanished from the major cities of the world, pools of virus still lie deep in the tropical jungles of Africa and South America. In this day and age of rapid worldwide travel and exploding populations, the frontiers of the jungle are being invaded and these reservoirs of yellow fever constitute an ever-present health hazard.

Chapter 31

THE GREAT WHITE PLAGUE

T UBERCULOSIS IS A DISEASE that antedates recorded history. Archeological discoveries of prehistoric skeletons have revealed the indelible record of its ravages. Its antiquity is further attested to by the fact that spinal caries, undoubtedly due to tuberculosis, have been found in Egyptian mummies.

Early medical records reveal that tuberculosis, under a variety of names, was familiar to most ancient civilizations. The code of Hammurabi which was written before 2000 B.C. indicates a knowledge of the disease.

In the Bible (Lev. 26:16) Jehovah admonished the people of Israel: ". . . I will even appoint over you terror, consumption, and the burning ague, that shall consume the eyes, and cause sorrow of heart." In Deuteronomy 28:22 we find: "The Lord shall smite thee with a consumption, and with a fever, and with an inflammation . . ."

Undoubtedly the "consumption" referred to in the Bible included other wasting diseases as well as tuberculosis. However, it is interesting to note that the word "consumption" is used to translate the Biblical word "schachepheth," a word that is still used to designate tuberculosis in modern Hebrew.

The ancient Greeks knew tuberculosis well. To Aristotle and Hippocrates should go credit for early descriptions of the disease and for giving it the name "phthisis." This term, which is dervied from the Greek, is descriptive and literally means, "to waste away." Gradually, this term was replaced by the word "consumption," which is a translation of phthisis into English, via Latin, and comes from the word "consumere" literally meaning to consume or to wear away.

The ancient Romans also knew tuberculosis well. Celsus in his great medical text, *De Medicina* written in about 30 A.D., gave an excellent description of the disease and recognized its communicability. The great Galen (A.D. 131-200) regarded tuberculosis as incurable and contagious. He advised avoiding the disease and stated that it is dangerous to live with consumptives. His recommended treatment consisted of rest in a cool well-ventilated room, along with a nutritious diet which included a plentiful supply of fresh milk.

During the Dark Ages or Early Middle Ages little or nothing was added to our knowledge of tuberculosis. It was not until the Post-Renaissance period that progress occurred as a result of the contributions of the great clinicians of the sixteenth and seventeenth centuries.

The contagiousness of tuberculosis was first emphasized in 1546 by Girolamo Fracastoro in his great book *De Contagione*.

The great English clinician, Thomas Sydenham, who is frequently called the "English Hippocrates," described tuberculosis in the seventeenth century. He ascribed the frequency of its occurrence in London as being due to the foggy, polluted air of that city.

Franciscus Sylvius, or Franz de la Boe, the great Dutch physician and anatomist who taught at Leyden from 1648 to 1672, wrote a classic description of the disease. He was the first to describe the typical nodular lesions of tuberculosis that are found on postmortem examination and applied the Latin term "tubercle" to these lesions. The term literally means little lump or nodule, and from it grew our modern term "tuberculosis."

In Medieval England tuberculosis, and especially scrofula, was commonly called the "king's evil," because of the firm belief that the "laying on" of royal hands could cure the condition.

In the seventeenth century Richard Wiseman, who served as King Charles' "Principal Chirugion" wrote an interesting essay entitled "A Treatise of the king's evil." Although he himself treated the disease, both by hygienic methods and with surgery, Wiseman stated that his methods could not compare with the success obtained by his Sacred Majesty the King, who could cure scrofula and struma with his "royal touch."

Wiseman stated that through the "goodness of God" the kings of England, from Edward the Confessor downwards, were given by hereditary right, the "extraordinary power" and "immortal gift" of curing "the Evil" with their "royal touch."

Richard Morton in 1689 in his book *Phthisiologia* recognized the early stages of the disease and also its recurrences. He also expressed the belief that most people harbor the disease at one time or another.

However, the first great advance in our knowledge of diseases of the chest, and especially tuberculosis, began with the introduction of percussion and auscultation. The discovery of these two great diagnostic techniques by Auenbrugger and Laennec ushered in the era of clinical diagnosis and advanced the physical diagnosis of the chest as far as it could go until the discovery of the x-ray.

Percussion was discovered by the Austrian physician Leopold Auenbrugger. He noted that, when the thorax of a healthy person is struck lightly, a sound resembling that of a drum muffled with a thick woolen cloth is produced. In sick persons, such sounds vary in accordance with the nature of underlying change, its location, and its extent.

In 1761 Auenbrugger published his epochal contribution to medicine in a small ninety-five page book entitled *On Percussion of the Chest*. His work was unappreciated until forty-seven years later when Jean Nicolas Corvisart in 1808 translated his book into French.

Corvisart, who was Napoleon's personal physician and a leader of French medicine, recognized the importance of Auenbrugger's work and promoted the use of percussion. He was one of Laennec's teachers and thus provided the link between Auenbrugger and percussion, and Laennec's discovery of the stethoscope and indirect auscultation.

René Théophile Hyacinthe Laennec was born at Quimper, in Lower Brittany, France on February 17, 1781. His mother died of tuberculosis when he was five years of age. His father, an advocate, preferred literature to the law, and accepted little responsibility for the rearing of his children. Hence, early in life Théophile was sent to live with an uncle who was a professor of medicine at Nantes.

This uncle saw to it that he received a sound basic education despite the turbulent times of the French Revolution. At the age of fifteen, Théophile was apprenticed to his uncle as a military surgeon third class, and began work in the military hospitals of Nantes.

At the age of nineteen Laennec went to Paris to complete his medical education. Here a shortage of funds and poor living conditions impaired his already delicate health. He studied at the Ecole de Médicine and attended clinics at the Hôpital de la Charité under Corvisart and his assistant, Bayle. Corvisart stressed bedside instruction and trained his pupils thoroughly in autopsy examination. Laennec studied carefully and methodically and Corvisart, sensing a great medical future for his pupil, fathered his career at every opportunity.

During the last three years of his formal medical training, Laennec prepared meticulous histories on more than four hundred cases. He was honored with the first two prizes in medicine and surgery. His capacity for composition was appreciated early in his professional career, and for five years he was the chief editor of the Journal de Médicine. He assumed this responsibility immediately following graduation at the age of twenty-three. A prolific writer, he prepared numerous monographs on peritonitis, sclerosis of the liver and other diseases. Tuberculosis, in particular, attracted his attention and percussion was one of his favorite diagnostic methods.

In 1814 Laennec was appointed visiting physician to the Necker Hospital. He soon found himself extremely busy and routinely employed percussion and direct auscultation on his patients. Direct auscultation consists of listening to the sounds in the thorax by placing the physician's ear directly on the chest wall. Many patients were not accustomed to bathing and some were verminous, so many physicians were reluctant to use this diagnostic method. Layers of fat that sometimes obstructed transmission of sounds, and modesty of women patients were further deterrents.

One day in 1816, while walking along and pondering the problem of a modest, obese woman suffering from heart disease, Laennec observed a group of children playing around a pile of wooden beams. One would put his ear against the end of a beam, while another would tap the opposite end. To their childish amazement the sounds were conveyed from one end to the other. Laennec, grasping the physical principle involved, hurried back to Necker and his overweight patient.

Later, Laennec, in the introduction to his great book on auscultation wrote:

> I rolled a quire of paper into a kind of cylinder and applied one end of it to the region of the heart and the other to my ear, and was not a little surprised and pleased to find that I could thereby perceive the action of the heart in a manner much more clear and distinct than I had ever been able to by immediate application of the ear. From this moment I imagined that the circumstance might furnish means for enabling us to ascertain the character, not only of the action of the heart, but of every species of sound produced by the motion of all the thoracic viscera and consequently for the exploration of the respiration, the voice, the rhoncus (rale), and perhaps even the fluctuation of fluid extravasated in the pleura or the pericardium. With this conviction I forthwith commenced at the Hospital Necker a series of observations from which I have been able to deduce a set of new signs of diseases of the chest . . . to render the diagnosis of the diseases of the lungs, heart, and pleura.

Laennec experimented with various forms of his instrument and at first tried a compact roll of paper, then a wand with no aperture. This he found would convey heart sounds, but a cylinder with a central aperture and a funnel-shaped opening at the end proved best suited for chest examinations. He finally settled on a cylindrical instrument made of wood, about an inch and a half in diameter and a foot long, perforated longitudinally by a quarter-inch bore and hollowed out to a funnel shape at the end. He fitted this end with an insertable perforated plug that would convert the device to a simple cylinder. The instrument was divided into two portions of equal length that would screw together. This had the double advantage of being more convenient for carrying in a pocket, and when desired, of providing a shorter instrument.

At first Laennec called his instrument the baton, cylinder or pectoriloque. Later he changed it to the more euphoneous name of "stethoscope," derived from the Greek words "stethos" (chest) and "scopeo" (to view or explore).

The invention of the stethoscope was remarkable, but what Laennec did with this instrument was more remarkable. He founded a new method of diagnosis by describing, naming and identifying the sounds heard on auscultation. He gave us many masterly descriptions of diseases of the chest and especially of tuberculosis. In 1819 he published his findings in his famous book *A Treatise on the Diseases of the Chest and On Mediate Auscultation.*

From biographical sketches we get a picture of Laennec as a somewhat austere, proud and sensitive person, racked with tuberculosis, who made one of the most important contributions to physical diagnosis in the history of medicine. He rose to the pinnacle of French clinical medicine and became one of the most famous consultants of his time. All the while he himself was a victim of tuberculosis and battled diligently against his disease.

Laennec was well aware of his own disease and his impending death. He gave a heroic personal account of his own fatal illness and noted among other things the sounds generated from his own precordial region. On August 13, 1826, dread tuberculosis, which had claimed the life of his mother and so many of his patients, took his life at the early age of forty-five.

In the latter part of the nineteenth century the infectious nature of tuberculosis was established by the work of the French physician Jean Antoine Villemin. The existence of a microorganism or germ that was the specific cause of tuberculosis had long been suspected. Villemin demonstrated that phthisis was a specific disease and that it is caused by an inoculable agent or germ.

In 1865 he published a paper entitled "On the Cause and Nature of Tuberculosis and Its Inoculation from Man to Rabbit." In this paper he gave an account of his experiments whereby he had produced tuberculosis in rabbits and guinea pigs by injecting them with sputum or other material from a known tuberculous person.

In his book *Etudes sur la Tuberculose* written in 1868, Villemin noted that "healthy young men from country districts often became consumptive within a year or two after their arrival in army posts." He further noted that, "the dwelling together of persons in close, badly ventilated houses is followed by tuberculization of many of them." He concluded from his observations and studies that the disease is caused by a specific agent, which multiplies and transmits itself under certain conditions.

For the prevention of tuberculosis, Villemin recommended the improvement of housing and working conditions, the maintenance of a high standard of health and the disinfection of things and places which may have been contaminated by consumptives.

However, Villemin did not succeed in isolating the tubercle bacillus and it remained for the great Robert Koch to accomplish this in

1882. With his infinite care and patience, Koch devised a way of culturing the tubercle bacillus and of staining slides in such a manner that the organism stood revealed under the microscope.

When he was unable to get results with the methylene blue dye he had used successfully in earlier work with bacteria, Koch introduced alkali into the dye with the addition of potash and finally treated his specimens with a solution which stained the background brown and left the tubercle bacilli "beautifully blue."

Koch did more than "see" the invisible agent which is the specific cause of tuberculosis. He demonstrated that the bacillus was always present in tuberculous disease. He proved that a number of diseases, such as scrofula, miliary tuberculosis and tuberculosis in cattle, which were thought by many physicians at that time to be separate and distinct, were of tuberculous origin.

Koch publically announced his discovery of the tubercle bacillus on March 24, 1882. At a meeting of the Berlin Physiological Society he announced: "I have succeeded in discovering the real cause of tuberculosis. It is the tubercle bacillus, a true parasite."

The audience that listened to Koch's paper greeted it with a "profound and utter silence." Paul Ehrlich, who was later to become famous as the discoverer of salvarsan, was present at this meeting and later wrote: "That evening remains graven in my memory as the most majestic scientific event in which I have ever participated."

In his paper Koch gave suggestions as to preventive measures that could be taken to control the disease. He stated that:

Tuberculosis has so far been habitually considered to be a manifestation of social misery, and it has been hoped that an improvement in the latter would reduce the disease. Measures specifically directed against tuberculosis are not known to preventive medicine. But, in the future the fight against this terrible plague of mankind will deal no longer with an undetermined something, but with a tangible parasite, whose living conditions are for the most part known and can be investigated further.

He further stated:

. . . The sources from which the infectious material flows must be closed as far as this is humanly possible. One of these sources, and certainly the most essential one, is the sputum of consumptives, whose disposal and change into a harmless condition has thus far not been accomplished.

Koch's work was immediately regarded as a great scientific landmark and produced a tremendous impact on both the lay public and the medical world. Overnight, Koch's name became a household word and he was publicly acclaimed as the "father of the bacillus."

Koch had discovered the true cause of the "Great White Plague" and had pointed the way towards its extermination. The heretofore unseen killer was now visible and formed a tangible target for preventive medicine to aim at. With the aid of the microscope it was now possible for physicians to single out the afflicted and to isolate them.

Following his discovery of the tubercle bacillus Koch continued his research, hopefully seeking to find a preventive vaccine or a specific remedy. In 1890 he announced to the Tenth International Congress of Medicine in Berlin that he had discovered such a protective and remedial agent. His announcement was greeted enthusiastically by the medical world and hopes ran high for the great results that could be expected from the use of "Koch's lymph."

However, Koch marred his own scientific record considerably, by refusing to reveal the nature of this substance. In addition to being secretive he was prematurely enthusiastic. Ensuing experience showed that the employment of the vaccine was useless and even dangerous. Koch was soon condemned for his unethical behavior in attempting to keep the composition of his substance secret and for his lack of scientific judgment in recommending it as a preventative and remedy.

Koch's conduct has been defended on the grounds that he felt that the preparation and use of his material required much skill and that therapeutic accidents would occur if the method was used too soon by untrained practitioners. Other historians state that the policy of secrecy was dictated by the German Ministry of Health, which wished to retain a monopoly on the manufacture of the vaccine.

Koch later disclosed that his substance was a glycerin extract of the tubercle bacillus, a substance that is now known as "tuberculin." Although Koch's tuberculin proved valueless in the prevention and treatment of tuberculosis, it eventually was found to be a valuable diagnostic agent and is widely used in the performance of the "tuberculin test."

A great advance and fundamental contribution to the diagnosis of tuberculosis was made by Roentgen's discovery of the x-rays in 1895. Within a year after their discovery, Roentgen's new rays were being used as a diagnostic tool by medical men around the world. It was soon discovered that these wonderful new rays could penetrate the chest wall and reveal hithertofore unseen pulmonary disease. Over the next fifty years the newly born science of radiology rapidly expanded and further discoveries such as the fluoroscope and stereoscopic x-rays led to our modern methods for the early and accurate diagnosis of tuberculosis. Finally, the development of photo-fluorographic x-ray machines capable of taking rapid and relatively inexpensive miniature chest films made possible our modern mass x-ray case-finding procedures.

In 1882, the same year that Koch announced his discovery of the tubercle bacillus, artificial pneumothorax was introduced as a form of treatment. In that year, Carlo Forlanini (1847-1918), an Italian physician of Pavia, published a paper on this subject. Having observed that the presence of pleural fluid and pneumothorax favorably influenced the course of phthisis, Forlanini began his research with the intrapleural injection of nitrogen. Despite his successful clinical use of artificial pneumothorax and his favorable results, Forlanini's work at first met with indifference. It was not until 1912 that artificial pneumothorax was finally given official recognition and approval at the meeting of the International Congress of Tuberculosis in Rome.

From that period on pneumothorax became an effective and widespread method of treatment. After World War I much progress was made in the surgical treatment of tuberculosis and all forms of collapse therapy became popular, including thoracoplasty and phrenic crush. The great surgical advances of World War II, which included improved methods of anesthesia and the effective use of blood, made possible the surgical resection of diseased lung tissue, and this procedure has largely supplanted collapse therapy.

Among the earliest of weapons against tuberculosis were rest, good food, fresh air, sunshine and a salubrious climate. The "climatic treatment" of tuberculosis became especially popular and was much in vogue during the late eighteenth and early nineteenth centuries. Large numbers of tubercular patients travelled long distances to seek out and avail themselves of the supposedly healing properties of the sea, mountain or desert air.

In Europe the seashore and the mountains were especially favored and an extended sojourn at a marine or alpine resort was a favorite remedy. In the United States, the desert air of the southwest was considered especially beneficial. Arizona and New Mexico became so renowned for their health-restoring climates that they became veritable "meccas" for hopeful tuberculars. It was jokingly said that "Albuquerque had two businesses, the Santa Fe Railroad and tuberculosis."

Sanatoria for the treatment of tuberculosis were introduced during the nineteenth century. A German botanical student named Herman Brehmer was advised by his physicians to seek a better climate because of his tuberculosis. He went to the Himalaya Mountains where he combined botanical research along with search for a cure. Returning home cured, he studied medicine, and in 1854 published a thesis entitled *Tuberculosis Is Curable*. In that same year he built a house in Goerbersdorf in the middle of a pine forest for the open air treatment of tuberculosis. This was the forerunner and model for all of the future sanatoria that were to become such a potent force in the treatment of tuberculosis.

The father of the sanatorium movement in the United States was Dr. Edward Livingston Trudeau. Trudeau became involved in the fight against tuberculosis because of an unfortunate incident that changed the course of his life. Born of well-to-do parents in New York City in 1848, Trudeau spent most of his early years in France. Returning to the United States, he planned to enter the Naval Academy at Newport, Rhode Island. However, the death of his older brother from tuberculosis caused him to change his mind and to embark upon a medical career.

After the completion of his medical studies and at the start of his marriage and career, tragedy struck again. At the age of twenty-four Trudeau was stricken with tuberculosis. Having made an especial study of tuberculosis he was well aware of the serious and hopeless nature of his disease. He decided to go to the Adirondack Mountains where he hoped to regain his health or at least relieve his suffering.

Frail and fevered, he travelled by rail, boat and horse-drawn carriage to the Adirondacks. Here, as he later stated, he could "lead an open-air life in the great forest, alone with nature." Much to his own and everyone else's surprise, Trudeau did not succumb to his disease. Instead his health steadily improved.

From his own experience, Trudeau was convinced that a life of proper rest in the open air of a mountain climate had an arresting effect on tuberculosis. He also believed that the curative effects of the Adirondack Mountain climate should be made available to other victims of tuberculosis. Recognizing the difficulty of obtaining suitable accommodations for patients of moderate means, Trudeau established his cottage sanatorium at Saranac Lake in 1884.

From a single "little red" cottage that housed two factory girls from New York City during its first year, Trudeau's sanatorium developed into a world famous institution. As the victims of tuberculosis flocked to Saranac, the Trudeau Sanatorium became a nation-wide model for the care and treatment of tuberculosis. Twenty-five years later more than four hundred such sanatoria were to be found throughout the United States.

Koch's discovery of the tubercle bacillus brought about the universal acceptance of the fact that tuberculosis is an infectious bacterial disease that is commonly communicated from the sick to the well. The implications for community action were soon recognized and men's minds turned toward organizing congresses and societies for the prevention of tuberculosis.

In 1887 Robert W. Philip, an Edinburgh physician, organized the Victorian Dispensary for Consumptives. His program included home visiting, health education and an occupational farm colony for patients. This pioneer endeavor was followed in 1898 by the organization of the National Association for the Prevention of Consumptives in Great Britain. Similar organizations developed independently in France, Germany, Denmark and other European countries.

The United States was also influenced by these developments and in 1889 Herman Biggs, J. Mitchell Prudden and H. P. Loomis of the New York Health Department prepared a report on tuberculosis. In this report they emphasized the preventability of tuberculosis, recommended Health Department surveillance of the disease, and advocated public education concerning the dangers, manner of spread and means of preventing tuberculosis.

The first organization for the prevention of tuberculosis in the United States was founded in Pennsylvania in 1892. Lawrence F. Flick, a Philadelphia physician, who himself was a victim of tuberculosis, organized the Pennsylvania Society for the Prevention of Tuberculosis. Not only was this pioneer association the first tuberculosis society in the United States, but it also was the first to combine lay and professional membership and to concentrate its activities against a single disease. Flick and the Pennsylvania Society set a pattern for the voluntary health movement. Their example was followed elsewhere and by 1904 twenty-three state and local tuberculosis associations had been formed.

The year of 1904 marks a turning point in the battle against tuberculosis in the United States. In that year the idea of a nationwide organization was adopted and the organization that was later named the National Tuberculosis Association was formed. Dr. Edward L. Trudeau, the famed founder of the sanatorium movement in the United States, was elected its first president.

The rallying cry of the new association was "Tuberculosis is communicable, preventable, and curable." Like all crusades, the need for an emblem was recognized and in 1906 a red double-barred cross was adopted as the official insignia of the National Tuberculosis Association. An excellent method of financing was found, when in 1907, Jacob Riis, a Danish born journalist and reformer called attention to the idea of selling special stamps or seals. This device had been hit upon by Einor Holboell, a postal clerk in Denmark and was rapidly adopted in this country. As a result the annual sale of Christmas Seals to fight tuberculosis became a fund-raising device without parallel that assured the financial success of the Tuberculosis Association.

There was a rapid increase in the number of state and local organizations and the antituberculosis movement became both popular and powerful. The tempo of the fight against the Great White Plague now increased tremendously. Public health programs, both official and voluntary, expanded rapidly. Tuberculosis reporting became mandatory and official health department programs for tuberculosis control were initiated and expanded. Specially trained public health nurses were employed to conduct case investigations and follow-up programs for source and contact finding. The isolation or hospitalization of open active cases became compulsory.

At the same time, the powerful crusades of the voluntary tuberculosis associations were at work. They carried on intensive mass educational programs stressing the communicability of tuberculosis and methods of prevention, emphasizing the importance of early diagnosis and adequate treatment. They frequently joined forces with official health agencies and sponsored mass case finding programs.

Treatment progressed from the climatic concept of the health resort era to the founding of special sanatoria that emphasized rest and the open air life. These sanatoria gradually evolved into modern tuberculosis hospitals which stressed bed-rest and utilized all forms of collapse therapy. Thus, within a period of less than one hundred years, we went from a shack on a mountain top or in a forest, to modern hospitals.

The rapid industrial growth of the late eighteenth and early nineteenth centuries bettered socioeconomic conditions. As a result working and living conditions improved and the general level of community sanitation and personal hygiene was raised. There was better housing, better food, better education and better medical care. Working hours were shortened and people enjoyed more rest, sunshine and fresh air.

The failure of Koch's tuberculin did not prevent other investigators from searching for an effective antituberculosis vaccine. In 1908 at the Pasteur Institute at Lille, France, Dr. Albert Calmette, a physician-bacteriologist, and his capable veterinarian colleague, Dr. Camille Guerin, began work on a vaccine which they hoped would parallel Jenner's achievement against smallpox.

The basic concept of their research centered on the idea of producing a live attenuated vaccine. They started with a virulent culture of tubercle bacilli taken from a diseased cow's udder and modified it by repeated passages through culture media until it had lost its virulence. Thirteen years and 230 generations later the culture, nurtured on potatoes impregnated with beef bile and glycerine, yielded the desired result. They had succeeded in producing a strain of live attenuated bacilli, incapable of producing disease, but possessing sufficient protective power so that it could be successfully used as a vaccine. They named their attenuated bacillus after themselves, calling it the Baccillus Calmette Guerin, or BCG.

On July 1, 1921 the first of a series of three immunizing doses of BCG was administered in oral form to an infant in Paris. In the following year the vaccine was given by Dr. Weill Halle to more than 600 infants at the Paris Charity Hospital. No ill effects were evidenced, and the use of BCG began to spread rapidly. Intradermal injection of the vaccine was tried, and gradually replaced the oral method in most areas. As its use continued to grow, large numbers of persons, mainly children, were inoculated in Eastern Europe, Spain, Latin America, West Africa and Indochina.

Reports on the results obtained from the use of the vaccine were excellent and it seemed as though BCG vaccination would prove to be a highly effective means of preventing tuberculosis. Then in 1930 the unbelievable happened. Of 249 infants given the vaccine in Lubeck, Germany, 73 died. As the result of an investigation it was concluded that the lethal dose was caused not by the BCG strain but by an alien, virulent strain of bacilli which, through a human error, had accidently been substituted for the vaccine in the laboratory. In judicial proceedings arising out of the incident, a doctor at the laboratory in Lubeck was sentence to two years' imprisonment, and Calmette and his Institute were exonerated.

This unfortunate incident caused many bacteriologists to believe that the vaccine strain had reverted and become virulent. As a result the general acceptance of BCG vaccination was slowed down. In the United States, BCG failed to gain recognition and was not used except on a very limited scale. However, elsewhere, particularly in the Scandinavian countries, any tool holding out the hope of increasing immunity to tuberculosis was considered worthwhile. BCG vaccination of infants became compulsory in many countries of northern and eastern Europe and its use gradually spread over most of the world.

As the drama of scientific advancement unfolded and accelerated, decade by decade, during the last half of the nineteenth century and the first four decades of the twentieth century, results were reflected in a marked decline of the tuberculosis death rate. In mid-nineteenth century, when our knowledge of tuberculosis first began to increase, the death rate approximated 400 to 500 deaths per 100,000 population. At the turning of the century, it had fallen in the United States to about 200. In 1910 it decreased to 153.8 and in 1920 it had fallen to 113.1. It continued to decline as our knowledge and efforts increased, and in 1930 it fell to 71.1 and by 1940 it had fallen to 45.9 deaths per 100,000 population.

This then was the story of tuberculosis until 1943. Although tremendous progress had been made, a really effective cure for tuberculosis had not yet been found. Treatment was still uncertain, lengthy and costly. Morbidity and infection rates had not fallen as rapidly as the death rate, and preventive procedures were cumbersome and expensive. Despite the optimistic talk of public health leaders that the complete control of tuberculosis was possible, the fact remained that the Great White Plague was still widespread, highly infectious and drastically deadly.

In 1943 a major breakthrough in the fight against tuberculosis occurred. In that year Selman A. Waksman's discovery of streptomycin ushered in the era of "chemical control." Dr. Waksman, chairman of the microbiology department of the New Jersey Agricultural Station at Rutgers University, had been studying soil microbes in their relation to agriculture for over a quarter of a century. On August 20, 1943 he and his research group isolated two cultures of an organism later called streptomyces griseus from the swab of a chicken's throat. From these cultures came the new antibiotic streptomycin, the isolation of which was announced in January 1944.

Two months later Schatz and Waksman reported that streptomycin possessed decided tuberculocidal and tuberculostatic properties. This report attracted the attention of Drs. William F. Feldman and H. Corwin Hinshaw of the Mayo Clinic who were searching for an antituberculosis drug. They contacted Dr. Waksman and the result was that the first clinical trials for the treatment of tuberculosis with streptomycin were carried out at the Mayo Clinic during the winter of 1944-45. Within two years after its discovery, streptomycin was established as an effective antituberculosis drug and it became available for general use in 1947. Dr. Waksman was awarded the Nobel prize in 1952 in honor of his achievement.

Thus at last, the final chapter in the long battle against tuberculosis was ready to be written. The successful chemotherapy of tuberculosis was now an accomplished fact. Streptomycin, by breaching the chemical defenses of the tubercle bacillus, had opened up a new world of therapy.

Unfortunately, this first great antituberculosis drug soon showed flaws in its character. Germs resistant to streptomycin tended to develop in patients who received treatment with this antibiotic over a period of time.

In 1948 a second drug was introduced into the treatment of tuberculosis: para-aminosalicylic acid—PAS, as it has come to be known. This drug is relatively ineffective against the tubercle bacillus when used alone, but it has the remarkable property of preventing the tubercle bacillus from becoming resistant to streptomycin when the two drugs are prescribed together. Streptomycin and PAS, therefore, make an extremely powerful team, and since the early part of 1949 the two drugs have been used together.

In 1952 the third member of the present chemotherapeutic family was discovered: isoniazid. Like PAS, isoniazid is a simple chemical compound which can be easily manufactured. It is administered by mouth, it is cheap, relatively nontoxic and is as effective as streptomycin.

Ironically enough, isoniazid had first been synthesized in 1912, but unfortunately lay dormant for nearly 40 years. Its antituberculosis activity was studied in 1951 by three large pharmaceutical companies, each independently of the others (Bayer, Hoffman-LaRoche and Squibb).

Chemoprophylaxis made its appearance in 1958, after clinical trials had established the prophylactic value of isoniazid. The chemical control of tuberculosis was now a reality with the advent of these powerful new drugs that could be used both therapeutically and prophylactically.

Within a short period of approximately thirteen years (1947-1960) the antituberculosis drugs came into widespread general use. As a result, the mortality rate for tuberculosis dramatically decreased and by 1963 had fallen to 5.1 deaths per 100,000 population.

Undoubtedly many things contributed to this dramatic decline. BCG vaccination certainly had an effect. By 1961 it was estimated that BCG had been administered to over 130 million people.

Most of the countries involved in these projects have shown sharp declines in their TB case rates. But any attempt to draw a clear cause-and-effect relation between the immunization program and subsequent case rates runs into difficulty. During the Fifties, postwar recovery in many parts of the world produced marked upturns in nutrition, housing, and general health. Tuberculosis case rates dropped dramatically in many countries, including the United States, where BCG had not been used to any extent. This was also the period when spectacular gains were being made by treatment with the new anti-TB drugs.

How much the general decline of tuberculosis has been due to BCG vaccination and how much to other factors remains a matter of guesswork. It can be expected that with the extended use of the new antituberculosis drugs, BCG vaccinations will become of secondary importance.

Modern chemotherapy and chemoprophylaxis has not only radically reduced the tuberculosis death rate, but has also completely revolutionized care and treatment. One of the most significant developments of specific therapy has been that it has divorced the patient from the hospital. It has reduced the time spent in hospitals from years to months and has changed tuberculosis from an inpatient disease to an ambulatory outpatient disease. Tuberculosis hospital beds are now standing empty and sanatoria are closing or being converted to other uses.

The chemical control of tuberculosis has brought us into the era of "The Closing of the Sanatoria." Mankind's ancient enemy, the Great White Plague, has almost been conquered and it is now possible to speak realistically of the eradication of tuberculosis. We have but to make better use of the tools we now have to completely control and even eradicate tuberculosis.

Chapter 32

GONORRHEA
CRIPPLER OF MEN, WRECKER OF WOMEN AND BLINDER OF BABIES

THE ORIGIN OF GONORRHEA is lost in the dim and distant past. The disease is as ancient as the history of mankind itself. The antiquity of gonorrhea led Philippe Ricord, the great venereologist of the early nineteenth century, to say: "God created venereal disease along with the first human beings on earth."

The earliest records go back about five thousand years and are a part of the history of Chinese medicine. The ancient Chinese Emperor, Tsin-Chi-Hoang, was an imperious, self-centered autocrat and wanted all civilization to begin with his reign. He therefore ordered all manuscripts and writings destroyed and thus became known as the "Burner of Books." Being a personal coward, he spared all medical writings because he feared that if he became ill his physicians would have no references in which to find a cure for him. Thus were spared the medical manuscripts of Hoang-Ty, which go back to approximately the year 2637 B.C. The third chapter of this work is devoted to venereal diseases and gives an excellent description of a disease which undoubtedly was gonorrhea. The inflammation and discharges from the sex organs are described and it is stated that the disease is contracted "from women who live with too many men."

An authentic and respectable antiquity is given to gonorrhea in the Bible. The Bible is the classic of ancient records on illnesses of sexual origin and contains many references to gonorrhea. It shows that the Biblical Jews knew their venereology and that gonorrhea was no mysterious malady to them. They knew it was sexual in transmission and resulted from intercourse with an infected female. They knew gonorrhea was a distinct entity, and had effective though stern laws and measures to control its spread. This knowledge was thousands of years in advance of that of all other contemporary people and much of this knowledge was later rediscovered and verified by medical men.

That gonorrhea existed and was known to the ancient Egyptians can be shown from the Papyrus of Ebers which describes a sexual disease which undoubtedly was gonorrhea and recommended remedies to relieve it.

The beginnings of sexual hygiene originated in ancient Egypt, and as Egyptian history is intermingled with the history of the ancient Jews, there is little doubt but that this civilization exerted a tremendous influence upon Moses and thus upon the Jewish hygienic laws and indirectly upon our present day hygiene. Circumcision was practiced by the ancient Egyptians as well as by the Biblical Jews. It is argued that this was really of more importance as a hygienic practice and was only made a religious rite in order to secure its continued practice. Be that as it may, it is a well-known medical fact today that all venereal diseases and especially gonorrhea are less severe, less damaging and less liable to complications in the circumcised male than in the uncircumcised.

The ancient Greeks unquestionably knew of gonorrhea, and regarded the "whitish-yellow catarrh of the genitals" as a terror. Hippocrates, "the father of medicine," who lived from 460 to 370 B.C., dissertates upon it at some length. He stated that when one with this "catarrh of the genitals urinates, he feels a biting and burning." He also recognized gonorrhea in the female, for he stated: "The woman's uterus becomes ulcerated from it and she has fever and great distress." In his writings mention is made of joint affections occurring during the course of gonorrhea. This is probably the first mention and recognition of gonorrheal arthritis.

Herodotus, a contemporary of Hippocrates, writes: "The Scythians made an eruption into Palestine and pillaged the temple of Venus Urania. The angry goddess sent upon them and their posterity the women's disease, which is characterized by a running from the penis. Those attacked by it are looked upon as accursed."

Gonorrhea is alluded to in the writings of Plato (429-347 B.C.), Aristotle (384-322 B.C.), Epicurus (342-270 B.C.), and Seneca (5 B.C.

to 65 A.D.), who were all well aware of the disease. Seneca relates how Epicurus, who suffered from chronic gonorrhea for many years, spent fourteen days in a bath suffering with an attack of urinary retention, and failing to get relief, ended his agony with suicide.

It is interesting to note that in ancient Rome, with all its licentiousness and immorality, gonorrhea was labeled a "shameful disease." Celsus (63 B.C. to 35 A.D.) attributed gonorrhea to a loss of semen and cautioned patients with the disease against too much walking and exertion. Mussa, a physician of ancient Rome, gained fame because of his many prescriptions against gonorrhea. The story is that he was a Greek slave who was liberated by Augustus for curing him of a disease "acquired through the misfortunes of love." Shortly after Mussa, Ezio Valens became famous for his writings on the "diseases of love." It was reputed, but unsubstantiated, that Cleopatra, queen of Egypt, was a patient of his.

Galen (131 A.D.), the greatest Greek physician after Hippocrates, mistakenly believed gonorrhea to be an involuntary flow or loss of semen. He is generally credited with naming the disease gonorrhea, which literally means "flow of seed"; however, some historians credit Hippocrates with naming the disease. Galen is credited with having cured the Emperor Marcus Aurelius of an attack of gonorrhea. Galen's reputation for wisdom was so great that his ideas held sway for many centuries and the idea that gonorrhea was due to an involuntary flow of semen persisted until the Middle Ages.

While gonorrhea and descriptions of the disease and methods of treatment are included in the writings of many famous medical men, little of value was contributed until about the eleventh century.

Constantinus Africanus (1015-1087 A.D.) suggested that coitus was the cause of gonorrhea, and used urethral injections of human milk and barley water as a treatment. Frederico Scotto, who treated Emperor Frederick II of Naples, stated: "The man who has intercourse with a woman who has a discharge will himself acquire a discharge from his penis."

Moses Maimonides (1155-1204), a Hebrew philosopher and physician, states that the cause of gonorrhea is lasciviousness and licentiousness. He also describes the discharges of gonorrhea and correctly concludes that they are different from a flow of semen.

By the year 1200, it was generally accepted throughout Europe that gonorrhea was a distinct and separate infection, caused by sexual contact with an infected female. Over fourteen hundred drugs, most of them of little value, were used as a treatment of the condition.

By the thirteenth century surgical writers specifically wrote of a disease called the "chaude pisse," or "the burning," and differentiated it from the general term gonorrhea which, until that time, had included all forms of disease accompanied by a discharge from the sexual organs. The term "chaude pisse" became the vulgar French term for gonorrhea. So prevalent was "chaude pisse," or gonorrhea, that various laws were passed in an attempt to curb licentiousness and regulate prostitution.

Falck writes of such regulations made in 1375 and 1390 at Southwark as follows: "Such wenches as had the burning were to be separated from the rest, and forbid to lie with any man, while she had it." Another regulation concerning a brothel in Avignon in 1347 reads:

> The Queen commands that the superintendent and a surgeon appointed by the authorities examine every Saturday all the whores in the house of prostitution. And if one is found who has contracted a disease from coitus, she shall be separated from the rest and live apart, in order that she may not distribute her favors, and may thus be prevented from conveying disease to the youth.

Lacroix relates that the prostitutes of Paris in the Middle Ages were housed in quarters known as Clapiers, and that from this is derived the commonly used term "clap" which, even today, is the accepted vulgar name for gonorrhea.

From this time on and up until the end of the fifteenth century gonorrhea was a clearly defined and well understood disease. At the end of the fifteenth century a great epidemic of the disease we now know as syphilis swept through Europe. Soon the two diseases, gonorrhea and syphilis, were hopelessly confounded and confused.

This sudden severe widespread epidemic of syphilis totally eclipsed gonorrhea, and as a result much of the previous knowledge of the disease was lost sight of. The fact that both diseases were transmitted and acquired through sexual intercourse soon led to a confusion of the two diseases.

Paracelsus falsely believed gonorrhea to be an initial stage of syphilis and the famous Paré supported his false belief. Sydenham also believed this error and interpreted gonorrhea as a symptom or stage of syphilis. In the face of all the weight of these medical authorities, the two diseases were hopelessly confused until the eighteenth century.

However, there were dissenters to this "unicist doctrine" of venereal disease; Cockburn in 1715 published the statement "that gonorrhea was not usually followed by syphilis." Other medical writers also expressed the idea that gonorrhea and syphilis were two separate diseases.

The rediscovery of gonorrhea as a separate disease entity was well on its way when one of the greatest mistakes in medical history set it back another hundred years.

The great John Hunter undertook to solve this problem once and for all. So on a Friday in May 1767 he inoculated himself with matter taken from a gonorrheal patient. Unfortunately, this patient was suffering from both gonorrhea and syphilis and he contracted both diseases. This unfortunate error led Hunter to proclaim that the two diseases were identical and because of his preeminence in the medical world, this was generally accepted.

There were a few, however, who dared to doubt Hunter. Benjamin Bell of Edinburgh (1793) maintained that gonorrhea and syphilis were separate diseases. He even proved it by inoculation of two of his students who volunteered their services. However, it remained for Philippe Ricord in 1838 to finally establish the separate identity of the two diseases and to convince the medical profession of this duality.

Ricord was an extremely able, witty, and brilliant man. He was surgeon at the Midi or Venereal Hospital in Paris for nearly thirty years and was one of the most celebrated and popular clinicians in Paris. He was an excellent teacher and his lectures were always full of wit and humor. A favorite saying to his students was: "Gentlemen, venereal diseases are disorders to be studied without being contracted." Soon after Ricord entered the Midi Hospital in 1831, his logical mind began at once to unravel the existing chaos. He repeated Hunter's and Bell's inoculation experiments. It is said that Ricord inoculated 2,500 patients with gonorrheal discharges from every possible source and failed to produce syphilis in a single instance. He thus established forever the fact that gonorrhea is a disease entirely distinct from syphilis. He made numerous other contributions to the medical knowledge concerning both syphilis and gonorrhea; he lacked only the bacteriological evidence to have the story of gonorrhea complete.

There elapsed now a period of approximately forty years before any further definite advance was made. The discovery of the gonococcus as the causative germ of gonorrhea, by Albert Neisser in 1879, cleared up the last remaining mysteries concerning this disease, and brings us into the modern era of its history.

The cause of gonorrhea remained unknown until 1879. In that year Albert Ludwig Siegmund Neisser of Breslau, Germany, found and identified the villainous germ of gonorrhea under his searching microscope. He was the first to drag this hidden culprit from obscurity and present it to the scientific world. For a long time it had not been a secret that something microscopic was the cause of gonorrhea. Ever since the discovery of the microscope and the germ causation of diseases, many scientists had searched unsuccessfully for this elusive germ.

But Albert Neisser, a young doctor of twenty-two, was undiscouraged by this competition. With stolid persistence and unswerving zeal, he searched diligently, examining the pussy, repulsive secretions of unknown numbers of sufferers from gonorrhea under his microscope. Every moment that he could spare from his patients he was at his microscope, burning gallons of midnight oil and examining mountains of glass slides smeared with gonorrheal secretions.

The Goddess of Fame smiled upon Neisser and rewarded his intelligence and diligence only two years after his search had begun. Under the high-powered magnification of his microscope, in a watery solution of the analine dye, methyl violet, Neisser found the evil germ of gonorrhea. He did not name it the gonococcus at the time, but referred to it as a micrococcus. It was not until 1882 that he finally christened it the gonococcus. Thus, at twenty-four Albert Neisser became world famous and later in life was affectionately called "the father of the gonococcus" by his medical students.

Among the most ruthless of the ravages produced by the gonococcus is the needless blinding of babies and adults. Gonorrheal ophthalmia is the commonest and most serious form of ophthalmia neonatorum or "babies' sore eyes," and has been long a blight on innocent lives and has made tens of thousands needlessly blind for life.

Ophthalmia due to gonorrheal infection most certainly is as old as gonorrhea itself, which we know to be as ancient as the history of mankind. While accurate descriptions of gonorrhea as a genital disease exist in our earliest medical records, little or no mention is made of either gonorrheal ophthalmia or any other type of ophthalmia neonatorum. However, Aetius, who wrote about the year 500, mentions ophthalmia neonatorum in his system of medicine. It took a long time to find out that gonorrhea was a cause of ophthalmia neonatorum, and even when this fact was ascertained, it was long denied the recognition it deserved. During the eighteenth century, physicians reported the possibility that the mucus of the birth canal or more frequently a maternal vaginal discharge produced an inflammation of the eyes, frequently followed by blindness. Desessartz believed that infection of the eyes of newborn babies could be prevented by rubbing the saliva or spittle of a healthy person into the babies' eyes. It had already been the custom in many countries for unknown centuries to drop oil into the eyes of newborn babies.

In the year 1750 S. T. Quellmatz hit upon the truth; he discovered the cause to be in the vaginal discharge of the mother at the birth of the child. Unfortunately for humanity, this discovery was neglected and not accepted.

However, the truth and the keen observation of men of medicine again made themselves heard, and in 1807 Dr. Benjamin Gibson of England wrote his observations that the child's eyes were infected from the mother's gonorrheal condition. Dr. Gibson's thinking and observations were so clear and sound that they might have been written today instead of in 1807. For he says: (1) remove the disease, if possible, in the mother during pregnancy; (2) if that cannot be done, remove artifically as much of the discharge as possible from the vagina at the time of delivery; (3) at all events, pay particular attention to the eyes of the child, washing them immediately after delivery.

Two other medical men with an experimental turn of mind carried out experiments which proved that "babies' sore eyes," or ophthalmia neonatorum, was commonly caused by gonorrhea. Vetch in 1820 took pus from a baby's eye and inoculated the canal of the penis in a male patient and produced gonorrhea. Pauli of Landau in 1854 took pus from a baby's eye and introduced it into the vagina of a prostitute and produced gonorrhea in her.

Yet the truth that blindness in babies frequently came from the infection of the mother was slow in being accepted. The ignorant idea prevailed in those days that the disease represented the chastening dispensation of providence, and as such was to be meekly borne. The doctors and the public of that day ascribed all kinds of causes to account for the disease, such as exposing the child's eyes to light too soon after birth, to cold, to heat, to the condition of the bowels, or to getting into the child's eyes some of the material used in cleansing the baby.

It was not until 1879 that Albert Neisser of Breslau, Germany, the discoverer of the gonococcus, announced and proved to the world that the germs of gonorrhea were frequently to be found in the pussy secretions from "babies' sore eyes." Thus it was proven conclusively, at long last, that the gonococcus, which does so much damage to men and women, was also a blinder of babies.

Following shortly on the heels of this discovery came one of the greatest triumphs of preventive medicine. In the years 1880, 1881, and 1882 Dr. Karl Sigmund Franz Crede, professor of obstetrics and gynecology at the University of Leipsig, Germany, and director of the Leipsig Lying-In Hospital, systemized and published a method of preventing this dread disease and thus conferred upon succeeding generations an everlasting benefit. The method was unbelievably simple and sure, and made this once most dreaded, blinding disease one of the most preventable of all preventable diseases.

The method described in his own words follows: "The eyelids were gently separated by an assistant, and by means of a glass rod a single drop of the solution (2 percent silver nitrate) was placed in each eye. For twenty-four hours after the application, the eyes were cooled by means of a linen fold, soaked in salicylic acid (2:100) laid over them." Later it was found that a 1 percent solution of silver nitrate dropped into the eyes of newborn babies was as effective as the 2 percent solution and it was unnecessary to cool the eyes after the application by means of the linen fold soaked in salicylic acid, thus making the method simpler still.

In Crede's hospital in the year of 1874 there were 323 births with 45 cases of gonorrheal ophthalmia, or 13.6 percent; and in 1882 in 260 births, where the method was used, but one case developed, or only 0.5 percent. In clinics where Crede's method was tried, it was found that the rate of gonorrheal ophthalmia dropped from one out of every ten newly born babies contracting the disease to one case in one thousand births. Thus Crede became immortal as the "saver of sight" for countless thousands of newborn babies.

However, the battle against the blinding ravages of the gonococcus was not yet won. Despite the fact that the cause of the disease was clearly proven and that a simple, harmless and absolute preventive had been scientifically demonstrated, the needless blinding of babies continued.

Ignorance, carelessness and prudery on the part of doctors, mid-wives and the public held back the universal use of Crede's method. Mothers and fathers objected to the drops being instilled in their babies' eyes, feeling that the use of the preventive branded them with the stigma of having gonorrhea. Many doctors, while using the method on their charity and hospital cases, were reluctant to use it for their private patients, fearing to offend them because they felt the use of the preventive drops of silver nitrate implied their patients might have gonorrhea. Unfortunately for the doctors and their patients, and still more so for the poor helpless babies, many of the private patients did have gonorrhea and their babies' eyes became infected.

Small wonder then that the needless blinding of babies continued and constituted a serious indictment of criminal carelessness and ignorance of the doctors, midwives and parents of that day and age. However, the dramatic results that were repeatedly demonstrated in preventing ophthalmia neonatorum wherever Crede's method was used were not to be ignored. Clear-thinking doctors, medical leaders, and commissions for the blind cried out for the universal use of Crede's method and agitated for legislation making its use compulsory.

Legislation for the control of ophthalmia started in the United

States in New York State in 1890, ten years after Crede's great discovery. The legislation consisted of the required reporting of cases to the health officer or to a legally qualified physician. Dr. Lucien Howe of Buffalo, New York was one of the leaders in the fight for this legislation; the law became known as the Howe Law and was copied by many other states. As a result of the appointment of a special committee by the American Medical Association in 1906 and the organization in 1908 of the New York State Committee for the Prevention of Blindness (which later became the National Society for the Prevention of Blindness), public opinion was aroused to support and pass mandatory laws requiring the use of a prophylactic in the eyes of the newborn. Thus ophthalmia neonatorum, the dread blinder of babies, was conquered.

The history of the treatment of gonorrhea from antiquity to modern times is an interesting story. The search for a cure progresses from the magic of medicine men and the incantations and prayers of priests to the painstaking research of modern medical science. Strange, fantastic and varied were the treatments used through the ages. Among the more peculiar and outrageous methods recorded is that of the Arabian physician Avicenna. He recommended the introduction of a live flea into the urethra as a method of cure.

Philippe Ricord, who in the early half of the nineteenth century became immortal through his decisive experiments which once and for all proved gonorrhea and syphilis to be two distinct diseases, had little to offer in the way of treatment. That he frequently failed to cure his patients is shown by his oft quoted statement that "a gonorrhea begins and God alone knows when it will end." Thousands upon thousands of pills, potions, and poisons were tried and used, most of them worthless and some being more injurious than the disease. So hopeless were the methods of treatment, that it was commonly said that the patient with gonorrhea was treated "externally, internally and eternally."

Then came the modern medical miracle of the wonder drug penicillin. It was only natural that this new peerless disease fighter would be tried on cases of gonorrhea. In this country in May of 1943 Herrell, Cook, and Thompson of the Mayo Clinic reported using penicillin to treat three cases of "sulfa resistant" gonorrhea.

They administered the drug intravenously and produced a cure within forty-eight hours. Mahoney, Van Slyke, and associates in the United States Marine Hospital, Staten Island, New York soon reported the first large series of cases of gonorrhea treated by intramuscular injections of penicillin. The results of penicillin treatment exceeded the wildest hopes and expectations of doctors and public health men, by at long last producing a safe, sure, "one-day cure for the clap."

Gonorrhea being a disease as ancient as mankind, it is to be expected that prophylaxis against it should be among our earlier medical records. In the Ebers Papyrus which was probably written about 1500 B.C., we find the ancient Egyptians stating that the female genitalia could be protected against the entry of disease by injecting a douche which contained garlic and the horns of a cow as ingredients. Evidently, the precaution was not always successful because the Papyrus informs us that should this prophylactic fail and inflammation ensue, the nature of the douche should be changed to one of bile of the cow, cassia, and oil.

Moses in the fifteenth chapter of Leviticus advocates prophylaxis against gonorrhea as follows: ". . . And he that touchest the flesh of him that hath the issue shall wash his clothes and bathe himself in water." He also forbade intercourse with menstruating women and with "unclean" women or women who had a discharge.

No further historical references to prophylaxis is found until the thirteenth century, when Guillaume de Salicet attributed the onset of gonorrhea to filth retained under the prepuce after connection with an unclean woman and advised washing with water after every suspicious cohabitation. Prophylaxis was still more strongly advocated by his pupil Lanfranc, who recommended washing the parts in urine or with equal parts of vinegar and water. Thus he was the first advocate of chemical prophylaxis.

John of Gaddesden, professor at Oxford in the thirteenth century, adhered to Lanfranc's principles of prophylaxis and suggested washings with acidulated water or with urine if no water were available.

The facts concerning the invention and introduction of the condom or protective sheath are shrouded in obscurity and confusion. History indicates that this invention was introduced late in the seventeenth century or early in the eighteenth century. It was described by Turner in 1717 and its invention attributed to a Dr. Conton, an Englishman who made a protective sheath from the sheep's cecum for covering the penis. People, instead of showing their gratitude, supposedly so ridiculed him that he changed his name to Condom or Condum, which explains the name. Other historians ascribe the invention to a Frenchman, Monsieur de Condom, who was a friend of de la Rochefoucald. Other authorities seriously question the existence of either a Dr. Conton or a Monsieur de Condom and think it probable that the name is derived from the Latin "condere" or "condus," meaning to hide or to protect. Regardless of who invented this beneficent device which has prevented so much dreaded affliction and so many unwanted human beings, he should be numbered among the great inventors and benefactors of the human race and a fitting monument should be erected to his memory.

Chapter 33

DIPHTHERIA—KILLER OF CHILDREN

ONE OF THE great victories of preventive medicine has been the conquest of diphtheria. Once considered to be the "scourge of the nursery" and one of the most dreaded of the "killers of children" this disease is now, almost, of historical importance only. Due to the discovery of the causative organism along with the development of an effective antitoxin for treatment, diphtheria mortality has practically fallen to zero. The further development of a lasting prophylactic, coupled with widespread public health programs of community immunization, has reduced the disease to the vanishing point.

Diphtheria was probably known to the Ancient Hebrews and it is mentioned by another name in the Babylonian Talmud (A.D. 352-427). Aretaeus the Cappadocian, a Greek physician living in Rome in about the second or third century A.D. clearly described the disease under the name of "ulcera Syriaca." Aetius in the sixth century described epidemic diphtheria and mentioned paralysis of the palate as a sequela.

Records and writings of the disease are scant or absent during the Dark Ages and Early Medieval times. This was probably because the disease was lost from sight in the welter and confusion of the numerous epidemic and contagious diseases that ravaged the world at that time.

During the sixteenth century Guido Guidi described the disease in Spain, where it was known at "garotillo," and suggested the use of a cannula in tracheotomy. Guiloume de Bailou (1538-1616), a French physician who is remembered as one of the first great epidemiologists, described an epidemic of diphtheria in Paris in 1576. He was perhaps the first to note and comment upon the characteristic membrane and also recommended tracheotomy. In America Samuel Bard of New York published a classic description of diphtheria in 1771 entitled *Angina Suffocativa*. Little more was added to our knowledge until 1826, when Pierre Bretonneau wrote a classic monograph on the disease.

In 1818 diphtheria broke out in Tours, France, and Pierre Bretonneau, the hospital's chief physician, began his now famous studies of this disease. He was the first to describe clearly the typical clinical picture of diphtheria and to differentiate it from scarlatinal angina and spasmodic croup. Until this time these diseases were frequently and hopelessly confused. In 1821 Bretonneau read a paper before the Academy of Medicine in Paris and proposed the name of "diphtheritis" for the disease. The name is descriptive of the characteristic membrane and is derived from the Greek word "diphtheria" meaning skin, leather or a membrane. The name was later changed to "diphtheria" by his pupil Trousseau. Bretonneau advocated tracheotomy and successfully performed the operation in 1825. In 1826 he published his classic monograph which established the disease as a distinct clinical entity.

Theodor Albrecht Edwin Klebs (1834-1913) was the first to see the diphtheria bacillus and associate it with the disease. He was a native of Koenigsberg, Germany, and a contemporary of Pasteur and Koch. Klebs was well trained and studied medicine in Koenigsberg with Rathke, Helmholtz and others, and in 1855 proceeded to Wurzburg, where Kolliker and Virchow were teaching. After practicing for a short time in Koenigsberg, Klebs was appointed privat-docent in general pathology and assistant in the Physiological Institute under Wittich. In 1861, he became assistant to Virchow in Berlin; there he published his studies on paraffin embedding and designed solid media for bacterial culture. Early in 1866 he was appointed professor of pathology in Bern. In the Franco-Prussian War (1870-1871) Klebs pursued one of the first comprehensive studies of the pathology and bacteriology of war wounds.

Klebs was an advocate of the bacterial theory of infection and did much to convert the pathologists to this view. He saw and recognized the typhoid bacillus and the diphtheria bacillus before Eberth and Loeffler, whose names are associated with these bacteria. He was first to filter bacteria and to experiment with the filtrates, as well as the first to devise a method of killing off competing germs in an impure culture by successive transfers of fresh media. He investigated many other pathological conditions.

Edwin Klebs was of a restless temperament and successively served as professor of pathology at Wurzburg, Prague and Zurich. It was in 1883, shortly after accepting the post in Zurich, that he described his isolation of the specific bacillus of diphtheria from the membranes of patients suffering from laryngeal croup.

In his later years, Klebs' mercurial temperament brought him to America where he served as professor of pathology at Rush Medical College in Chicago. However, in 1900 he returned to Germany and spent his remaining years there and in Switzerland. He died in Bern, Switzerland in 1913 at the age of seventy-nine.

Although the Corynebacterium diphtheriae was shown to be the pathogenic microorganism by Klebs, it was Loeffler who in 1884 satisfied Koch's postulates for the organism and differentiated the human type from the bovine and avian. Loeffler was also able to show how the disease was spread by healthy carriers.

Freiderick August John Loeffler (1852-1915) was a famous German bacteriologist who served as Koch's assistant from 1879 to 1884. As the son of a prominent medical officer in the German Army, he received the best medical education obtainable and studied under such luminaries as Virchow, Traube and Koch.

Loeffler was a thorough worker with the result that he published little, but what he did publish has stood the test of time. His main contributions were his work with the Corynebacterium diphtheriae, the cause of glanders, swine erysipelas, and the introduction to bacteriology of several techniques, notably, his alkaline methylene blue stain and meat juice peptone gelatin medium.

Loeffler ended his career with distinction by serving as the director of The Institute For Infectious Diseases, "Robert Koch" in Berlin.

The diphtheria organism is frequently referred to as the Klebs-Loeffler bacillus to commemorate the work of these two men.

The next link in the chain of discoveries leading to the conquest of diphtheria was forged by another famous German bacteriologist, Emil Adolf Von Behring (1854-1917). Commencing his career as a Prussian Army surgeon, Von Behring achieved world fame as the discoverer of diphtheria antitoxin and the founder of serum therapy.

Von Behring was born at Hansdorf in West Prussia on March 15, 1854 and studied in Berlin. After receiving his medical qualification in 1880, he entered the Army Medical Corps and became a lecturer at the Army Medical College in Berlin in 1888. The following year, in 1889, at the age of thirty-five he became an assistant at Koch's Institute For Infectious Diseases in Berlin where he performed his most famous work.

Von Behring was familiar with the fact that in 1888, Pierre Roux and Alexandre Yersin at the Pasteur Institute had shown that the diphtheria bacillus produces a toxin or poisonous substance. He believed that if these toxins could be neutralized in the bodies of infected persons, much of the damage done by the germs could be avoided. In 1890 he found that by injecting dead or weakened diphtheria germs (toxins) into guinea pigs in a series of increasingly strong doses, he was able to produce in them a degree of immunity to the disease. He demonstrated that this was due to the appearance in the animal's blood serum of a chemical that neutralized the diphtheria toxin. Von Behring introduced the term "antitoxin" to describe this chemical.

The same results were achieved with tetanus germs. A surplus of the tetanus antitoxin was produced in the blood of experimental animals. Von Behring and a co-worker, Shibasaburo Kitasato, injected some of the serum that contained the tetanus antitoxin into other animals and found that it produced in them a strong immunity against tetanus.

On December 11, 1890 Von Behring published his important and classic paper on diphtheria antitoxin and serum therapy. However, it was not until the following year that the first human case of diphtheria was treated with antitoxin.

On Christmas night in 1891, Von Behring was called upon to supply his antitoxin for a child desperately ill with diphtheria. The injection was given by Dr. Geissler at Von Bergman's Clinic in Brick Street, Berlin. The child miraculously recovered and diphtheria antitoxin was immediately recognized as a specific treatment for the disease and received worldwide acclaim.

The large scale production of diphtheria antitoxin was soon undertaken and it was placed upon the market in 1892. William Hallock Park (1863-1939) and his assistant Alfred L. Beebe introduced diphtheria antitoxin to America; they were the first to produce it in the bacteriological laboratories of the New York City Health Department. Hallock and Beebe also carried out a series of investigations that definitely established the concept and role of the carrier in the spread of the disease.

The impact of diphtheria antitoxin upon medical practice was sensational and Von Behring found himself famous. In 1894 he accepted the chair of hygiene in Halle, but a year later transferred to a similar position in Marburg. He received many distinctions and several monetary prizes. In 1901 he was awarded the first Nobel Prize in physiology and medicine. His award read as follows: "For his work on serum therapy, especially its application against diphtheria, by which he has opened a new road in the domain of medical science and thereby placed in the hands of the physician a victorious weapon against illness and death."

Although the use of a toxin-antitoxin mixture for active immunization was first suggested by the American, Theobald Smith, it was first administered by Von Behring in 1912. The antitoxin part provides immediate passive immunity, while the toxin part stimulates the body to produce its own antitoxins, thus developing active and long-lasting immunity.

In 1913 Bela Schick (1877-1967) a Hungarian-American pediatrician and bacteriologist, introduced the skin test for susceptibility to diphtheria that bears his name. The use of this test was of great importance in the carrying on of diphtheria control programs in the early twentieth century.

Von Behring's discoveries led other scientists to seek antitoxins for a number of other diseases. He himself became financially interested in the manufacture of antitoxin by the Farbwerke Hoescht, which built and equipped an admirable laboratory for him. Von Behring died at Marburg from pneumonia at the age of sixty-three on March 31, 1917.

Widespread active immunization against diphtheria received great impetus and moved forward rapidly after the development of anatoxin or toxoid. Gaston Ramon, a French physician, demonstrated

Chapter 34

POLIO PREVENTION

HISTORICAL EVIDENCE has been discovered indicating that poliomyelitis has existed from the earliest of times. Skeletons from the Neolithic Era in Europe and an Egyptian mummy from 3700 B.C. have been found showing the ravages of what in all probability was polio. An Egyptian bas-relief, dating from about 1500 B.C., records the atrophy of an extremity in stone. In art, during the Renaissance, the paralysis resulting from poliomyelitis is depicted in "The Procession of Cripples" by Bosch.

In spite of its apparent antiquity the first recognizable description of the disease was given in 1784 by the English physician, Michael Underwood, in his textbook, *A Treatise on the Diseases of Children*. However, he did not recognize its communicable or epidemic nature, but believed it to be a scrofulous paralytic complex.

In 1840 the German orthopedist, Jakob von Heine (1800-1879), was the first to establish the disease as a clinical entity and gave it the name "infantile spinal paralysis." The epidemic nature of polio was first noted in 1887 when outbreaks occurred in Norway and Sweden. The Swedish physician, Oskar Karl Medin (1847-1927), was the first to carefully study an epidemic of polio and describe its epidemic occurrence. The disease then became known as Heine-Medins' disease.

Later, after the pathology of the disease became established, Adolf Kussmaul of Germany named it poliomyelitis acuta anterior. Poliomyelitis is a descriptive term composed of the Greek words "polio" or gray (which refers to the gray matter of the cord) and "myelos" or marrow, plus the suffix "itis" meaning inflammation.

As the nineteenth century waned and the twentieth century was born, numerous accounts of paralytic epidemics of polio began to appear in the medical literature and the concept of its infectiousness became generally accepted. As the disease became more prevalent, epidemic poliomyelitis became a phenomenon of the twentieth century, and occurred in virtually all countries of the North and South Temperate Zones.

As a result of a new wave of polio epidemics in Scandinavia from 1903 to 1906, Wickman, a pupil of Medin, published a classic monograph on the disease in 1908. He reviewed the principles of its epidemiology and described abortive cases and healthy carriers.

An important forward step in the research on poliomyelitis was made by Karl Landsteiner (1863-1943). This Austrian-American scientist, who is chiefly famed for his research on blood types and the RH factor, reported in 1909 two successful intraperitoneal inoculations of monkeys with the spinal cord from two fatal polio cases. Experimental transmission of the disease to monkeys was independently done and reported by Landsteiner and Popper, Flexner and Lewis, Leiner and von Wiesner, and Römer. These experiments proved the infectious nature of the disease, and passage of the infectious material through a Berkefeld filter demonstrated the virus etiology.

Following the successful reproduction of the disease in monkeys, and the identification of the infectious agent as a virus, it was possible for Kling and his associates to demonstrate its presence in the stools and nasopharyngeal secretions of persons sick with the disease and some of those in contact with them. This work was confirmed and extended by Flexner and his co-workers. The experimental disease in the rhesus monkey was fully described, and this provided a means of identifying the virus of poliomyelitis and differentiating it from other viruses. Monkeys paralyzed following inoculation were found to be solidly immune to a second paralytic attack induced by the same virus material. Furthermore, it was found that this immunity was indicated by the presence of neutralizing antibodies in the serum of the convalescent animal.

Meantime another fact about polio had been discovered. Tests which had been developed showed that the blood of some polio victims contained polio antibodies. On this assumption, various researchers began experimenting with vaccines, and it was found that vaccination did, in fact, give some protection to rhesus monkeys.

In 1935 two men in different parts of the country felt ready to undertake experiments of humans. Dr. John A. Kolmer of Temple University's school of medicine used live but highly diluted polio virus secured from the ground-up spinal cords of monkeys and mixed with a chemical derivative from castor oil. Dr. Maurice Brodie of the New York City Health Department tried to inactivate his monkey-cord fluid with Formalin. By the end of the year some 17,000 children had been inoculated. There was no provision for following the results closely. But after a time disquieting reports began to be heard by the U.S. Public Health Service. Investigation showed that twelve of the children receiving the vaccines had soon come down with polio, and six of them died. Both vaccines were judged unsafe and were dropped.

This then was the state of affairs until 1938 when the formation of the National Foundation for Infantile Paralysis focused the spotlight of public attention upon polio and gave tremendous impetus to polio research.

Polio has undoubtedly aroused greater public interest, fear, and attention in the United States than any other disease known to mankind. Although general public interest in polio had its beginning during the epidemic of 1916, it was not crystallized into action until President Franklin Delano Roosevelt founded a great voluntary health agency specifically dedicated to fight this disease.

Franklin D. Roosevelt was severely stricken with polio in 1921, but courageously learned to live so successfully with his handicap, that he was able to be elected to the nation's highest office and to ably fulfill the arduous duties of that office.

With the formation of the National Foundation for Infantile Paralysis in 1938 and the financial support that came from its annual March of Dimes campaign, the American people became actively engaged in the fight against polio. From that time on professional educational programs were financed and there was an organized exchange of scientific information regarding the disease. Most important of all, hundreds of research projects were funded and scientific interest in the disease reached an all-time high. With its millions of dollars the National Foundation was able to marshal the world of medicine into an all-out effort to conquer the disease.

The next significant advance in polio research came in 1939 when

Dr. Charles Armstrong of the U.S. Public Health Service succeeded in infecting cotton rats and subsequently white mice with polio. Previously, only the chimpanzee had joined the rhesus monkey as a susceptible laboratory animal, but it was even more expensive to get and troublesome to feed and keep in good health. Now in the cheap, prolific white mice, researchers had an extremely valuable new tool.

These discoveries laid the foundation for modern investigators to determine that there are hundreds of different strains of poliomyelitis virus. This great variety made the development of a protective vaccine appear impossible. If polio vaccine had to contain all these different strains, protection against the dread disease would remain a speculative vision.

Determining to find out how many distinct immunologic types there were, the National Foundation mounted a huge investigation enlisting virus laboratories at four universities. By 1951, after the expenditure of $1,370,000 and 30,000 monkeys, 100 strains from all over the world had been tested and the problem solved. There were three families. One was the "Brunhilde" family, so called after a chimpanzee at the Johns Hopkins Poliomyelitis Laboratory in which the first strain of that kind had been isolated by Drs. Howard Howe and David Bodian; one was known as "Lansing" after the strain first adapted to mice by Dr. Armstrong; the other was "Leon" after a small boy who had died of polio in Los Angeles and from whose body the first strain of the kind was identified by Dr. J. F. Kessel. Later, they were simply named Types I, II and III.

One of the great stumbling blocks hampering the search for a safe, effective polio vaccine was the fact that the polio viruses grew best only upon the living tissues of man and monkeys. The virus seemed to be strictly a neurotropic organism that could be grown only in the nerve tissues of humans and certain animals. In essence, this meant that there was no satisfactory or practical method of growing polio virus for the development of a safe or effective vaccine.

The great breakthrough that broke this bottleneck of research, and that undoubtedly was the most important discovery in the history of polio research, occurred in 1949. In that year Dr. John F. Enders and his associates, Drs. Thomas H. Weller and Frederick C.

Robbins, found that they could grow polio viruses on nonneural tissue in test tubes. Working under a research grant from the National Foundation at the Harvard School of Public Health they solved the problem of how to grow polio virus. They developed a method of keeping living tissue alive after its surgical removal from healthy animals. Their work won them the Nobel Prize for medicine in 1954.

The work of Enders and his associates advanced polio research to a point where the preparation of a safe and effective vaccine was both feasible and possible. The problems remaining were primarily those of approach, methods, and techniques. The answers to these problems were soon forthcoming from Dr. Jonas E. Salk, a research grantee of the National Foundation for Infantile Paralysis. Salk organized and analyzed the existing and accumulated knowledge on polio, and by incorporating his own findings and ideas, developed the now famous "Salk Polio Vaccine."

Jonas Edward Salk was born in New York City on October 28, 1914. He obtained his medical degree from New York University College of Medicine in 1939 and served his internship at Mt. Sinai Hospital in the same city. In 1942 he went to the University of Michigan's School of Public Health as a research fellow. He became a research associate in 1944, and in 1946 was advanced to the position of assistant professor of epidemiology. While at Michigan he worked with his teacher, Dr. Thomas Francis, Jr., in the virology laboratories on the development of influenza vaccines. This training and experience equipped him for his future work in the development of a polio vaccine.

In 1947 Salk transferred to the University of Pittsburgh, where he became an associate professor of bacteriology and later professor of preventive medicine, as well as the head of the Virus Research Laboratory.

At Pittsburgh he soon became deeply involved in polio research since this university was one of the four involved in the polio virus typing program. In 1951 he received a large grant from the National Foundation and concentrated upon polio immunization studies. After approximately two years of intensive work, Salk reported his preliminary results in the *Journal of the American Medical Association* (March 28, 1953) and *Pediatrics* (Nov. 1953). In these two papers, the Pittsburgh scientist recounted his experiences in the preparation of several types of polio vaccines and the results obtained with their use in almost 700 children and adults. Salk had enough faith and confidence in his vaccine to include his own three small sons among those he inoculated. Blood samples from groups of these individuals showed that the vaccine stimulated the production of antibodies capable of neutralizing all three polio virus types. None of the persons vaccinated had suffered serious toxic reactions or side effects.

After careful study and review by an Advisory Committee, composed of leading scientists appointed by the National Foundation, the vaccine was adjudged to be safe and effective. The questions that remained to be answered were, "How effective is the vaccine under natural conditions of exposure?" and "How lasting is the immunity it conferred?"

The announcement of the development of the Salk polio vaccine created great excitement and was attended by greater publicity than the development of any other vaccine in the world. With all prior vaccines and immunizing agents, such as smallpox and diphtheria, it had taken many long years to test their effectiveness and to gain general public acceptance. In order to obviate this time lag and to stop the ravages of the disease as soon as possible, the National Foundation for Infantile Paralysis conducted their now famous Polio Vaccine Field Trials of 1954.

The purpose of the project was to evaluate the vaccine's effectiveness in preventing paralytic poliomyelitis under natural conditions of exposure and to determine the duration of the immunity.

In the late spring and early summer of 1954, 1,830,000 second grade school children between the ages of six and eight volunteered to participate in the greatest clinical-trial program ever undertaken. Of these, approximately 440,000 received three injections of the polio vaccine. Some of the others received injections of a placebo resembling the vaccine in appearance, but having no medical properties. The remaining children served simply as observed controls. The trials covered 217 selected areas in 44 states of the United States. To pay for the vaccine, medical equipment, records and other costs, the National Foundation allocated $7,500,000 in March of Dimes funds.

One of the nation's leading authorities on epidemics, Dr. Thomas Francis, Jr., chairman of the department of epidemiology at the University of Michigan School of Public Health, was in charge of evaluating the trial program. This gargantuan task required the classification, tabulation, and analysis of 144 million items of information. More than 300,000 persons, including physicians, public health officials, nurses, schoolteachers and National Foundation volunteers helped to carry it out. Pharmaceutical manufacturers cooperated in producing the vaccine that was used.

The Polio Vaccine Field Trials were an extraordinary medical undertaking and conclusively proved the effectiveness of the vaccine. Following the Field Trials, millions of doses of Salk vaccine were administered in the United States during the years from 1955 to 1960. The effectiveness of the vaccine was attested to by the fact that the disease declined by over 90 percent during this period of time.

Preceeding and paralleling Salk's work on a killed virus vaccine a number of other polio researchers were busily experimenting with and developing oral, live poliovirus vaccines.

The most famous of these polio-researchers, each of whom succeeded in developing an oral live attenuated poliovirus vaccine, were Dr. Albert Sabin, Dr. Hilary Koprowsky and Dr. Herald Cox.

Dr. Hilary Koprowsky, who was formerly associated with Lederle Laboratories and later became Director of the Wistar Institute in Philadelphia, began his work on oral polio vaccine in 1955. At that time, while working with the World Health Organization on a rabies experiment in Kenya, Africa, he simultaneously was testing and evaluating live attenuated strains of poliovirus in chimpanzees. In order to protect the caretakers of the "chimp" colony against accidental polio infection he vaccinated them with attenuated poliovirus. This experiment was so successful that it led him and his associates to undertake large scale clinical trials. By 1958 they had successfully administered oral polio vaccine to approximately 250,000 natives in various parts of Africa. While this work was going on in Africa they were testing the efficiency of each vaccine preparation back in the United States by feeding the virus to small groups of infants and adults.

Dr. Herald Cox, a famed virologist who was associated with Lederle

Laboratories, also succeeded in developing an effective live oral polio-virus vaccine by 1959.

However, the pioneer researcher and the man to whom the lion's share of the credit must go for successfully developing an oral polio-virus vaccine is Dr. Albert Bruce Sabin of the University of Cincinnati.

Albert Sabin was born in Russia on August 26, 1906, and emigrated with his family to the United States in 1921. The family settled in Patterson, New Jersey, and Sabin worked his way through New York University, receiving his medical degree in 1931. He interned at Bellevue Hospital and became associated with the Rockefeller Insti-tute, where he remained from 1934 to 1939. He then accepted a teaching and research appointment with the University of Cincinnati's School of Medicine and the Children's Hospital Research Foundation. It was there that he carried on his now famous work.

For twenty-four years Sabin worked to develop an oral live-virus vaccine against poliomyelitis. His problem was to get a polio virus that would not attack the central nervous system but give immunity to the host. From breeding millions of polio viruses, he developed mutant strains that caused no paralysis even when injected into the brains of monkeys, and in 1956 when he felt he had found the best possible vaccine, he offered it to qualified scientists.

The prior development of Salk's killed virus vaccine in 1953 and its testing in the 1954 Polio Vaccine Field Trials preceeded Sabin's development of his oral, live, polio vaccine. Because of these events Sabin's vaccine was not accepted for testing and use in the United States at this time. Fears also existed in the United States that an attenuated live vaccine might be hazardous because the attenuated strains might possibly revert to their original wild state and become disease-producing.

However, Sabin's vaccine was readily accepted for testing and wide spread use in other countries of the world. The oral vaccine was widely tested and used in the Soviet Union and its satellite nations, as well as South Africa, Japan and Great Britain. The most extensive testing and use of the vaccine was in the Soviet Union where Dr. Sabin estimated that by the end of 1960 over 77 million people had taken his vaccine.

In an article in the July, 1960 issue of the *Archives of Internal*

Medicine, Dr. Sabin made the following recommendations regarding the use of his oral vaccine in the United States.

> Once the safety of oral poliovirus vaccine is accepted I can see no indication for the use of both types of vaccine. In order to rob the naturally occurring paralytogenic polioviruses of the soil on which they grow, it would be necessary, in a country like the U.S.A., to feed the oral vaccine within a relatively short period of time during the winter and spring months to most pre-school and school-age children, regardless of the number of doses of Salk vaccine they might have had. The relative cheapness of the oral vaccine and the ease of its administration should permit community-wide programs that would make the vaccine available to all without reference to ability to pay. This would provide a means of protecting not only the individual but also the community.
>
> The laboratory and field experiences with the oral poliovirus vaccine strains that I selected are now available for decisive judgment, and two American pharmaceutical companies expect to have the required number of successive lots of vaccine produced under the safeguards specified by the National Institutes of Health by autumn of 1960. The question now remains whether the health authorities and physicians of the United States are ready to take the necessary steps for an attempted elimination of poliomyelitis from the country before the summer of 1961 or whether the country will continue to pay the high current price for only partial prevention of the paralytic disease.

Shortly after this, Sabin's oral vaccine was licensed by the government, and the pharmaceutical companies produced it in sufficient quantities for widespread use. By 1962 nationwide "Sabin on Sunday" programs swept the nation and millions of doses of the oral vaccine were given. These mass immunization programs were sponsored by health departments and medical societies, and people responded by the millions to receive the oral vaccine on the designated Sundays.

Thus, between the Salk and the Sabin vaccines, polio, the once dread crippler, has become another of the vanishing diseases.

Chapter 35

THE DEFICIENCY DISEASES

THE CONCEPT that diseases could be caused by the absence of "something" was a revolutionary one and took a long time to gain general acceptance. This was a radical departure from the prevalent idea that all diseases were due to "something" and were caused by positive agents such as poisons or bacteria. It was easy enough for mankind to understand how someone could become ill from a toxic substance in his food, but to accept the idea that illness could be caused by the absence of an invisible substance in his food was contrary to common sense and experience.

The discovery of prehistoric skeletal remains showing conclusive evidence of scurvy and rickets established the fact that the deficiency diseases have existed since time immemorial. Since the days of antiquity mankind has associated disease with his food supply. The Bible contains numerous references to diet and disease. Physicians of Biblical times recognized night blindness (vitamin A deficiency) and treated it with goat's liver. The ancient Greeks placed great emphasis upon diet and health. Hippocrates advocated diet therapy and recognized that all foods might not be suitable for all peoples.

It is interesting to note that long before the discovery of vitamins, a number of the deficiency diseases had been accurately described and empiric cures for some of them had been found. Such classic deficiency diseases as scurvy, beriberi, rickets and pellagra had all been recognized and their occurrence was frequently associated with the food supply. However, it was generally believed that they were due to some debilitating substance in the food. Our food was formerly thought of in terms of sufficiency only, with little or no regard as to the essential nutrients.

Not until the late nineteenth century and the early years of the twentieth century did science begin to make inroads on the deficiency diseases. The first experiments hinting at the concept of avitaminosis were carried out by the Russian, N. Lunin in Basel in 1881. He attempted to rear young rats on a synthetic diet but found that they all died even though they were given all the calories they required. Another fundamental finding occurred when Christian Eijkman in 1893 discovered that a diet of overmilled rice caused beriberi and he was able to produce the disease experimentally in fowls. In 1911 Casimer Funk's studies led him to believe that certain chemical substances existing in minute amounts in food were amines necessary to life. Hence, he called them "vital-amines" and later shortened the term to "vitamins."

The prevention and conquest of the deficiency diseases, which has saved millions of lives, was the work of a great many men of science. Chief among these were a trio of brilliant scientists whose work illustrates three of the basic approaches to the founding of nutritional science and the solution of the mysteries surrounding the deficiency diseases. These men were: Elmer Verner McCollum, a pathfinder in the discovery of the family of vitamins; Joseph Goldberger, who found the cure and preventive for pellagra; and Robert R. Williams, who synthesized a substance capable of eradicating beriberi.

Elmer Verner McCollum was born in 1879 near Fort Scott, Kansas. His biography records that he himself was a victim of infantile scurvy and was saved from death when his pioneer mother decided to follow folklore medicine and fed the ailing infant on apple scrapings, raw vegetables and wild strawberry juice.

McCollum grew up to work his way through the University of Kansas, achieve his Ph.D. degree at Yale and, in 1907, win a post as an instructor at the College of Agriculture at the University of Wisconsin.

McCollum, thus, was launched upon a lifelong career of nutritional research. A skilled biochemist, he conducted innumerable animal feeding experiments, using both large and small animals. He varied the combinations of food substances but maintained the same chemical composition. On some combinations the animals thrived and on others they failed. However, the "why" of the missing dietary factor remained elusive. Then, in 1912 he found the answer and made one of the greatest advances ever made in nutritional science.

McCollum discovered and extracted a new essential nutrient which he called "fat-soluble A." He thus established the fact that previously unrecognized chemical compounds, now known as vitamins, are absolutely essential to life. He further discovered that the daily requirements of these substances necessary to maintain health are extremely small.

McCollum's discovery launched an intensified campaign in the war on deficiency diseases. Hundreds of investigators took up the search for other members of the vitamin family of nutrients. In 1922, McCollum himself added vitamin D to the growing list and by 1948 all 13 of the vitamins needed for human nutrition had been isolated.

In 1914, two years after McCollum had discovered vitamin A, Dr. Joseph Goldberger (1874-1929), a career officer of the United States Public Health Service, was given the assignment of investigating pellagra, which was found to be prevalent in the southern United States.

Goldberger's research utilized the epidemiologic approach, for it was believed at this time, that pellagra was probably a communicable disease. His remarkable research established the fact that pellagra was a dietary deficiency disease. He experimentally produced the disease in human subjects by faulty diets. Along with G. A. Wheeler, R. D. Lillie and L. M. Rogers he discovered the pellagra preventive factor, which was later identified as nicotinic acid.

A third type of approach toward solving the dietary deficiency disease problem was initiated by the work of Robert R. Williams. This involved the synthesis or chemical manufacture of the essential nutrients or vitamins. Through synthesis these essential nutrients or vitamins could be manufactured cheaply and in large quantities and thus be made available to all.

Robert Runnel Williams was born in India in 1886, the son of missionary parents. Thus, early in life he witnessed poverty, starvation and the disastrous effects of deficient diets. After graduating with a degree in chemistry from the University of Chicago he started his professional career with the Philippine Bureau of Science in Manila. Here he followed up the studies of Eijkman and others in seeking the causative factor of beriberi.

After his return to the United States, Williams changed positions a number of times and his researches were periodically interrupted. However, he doggedly continued his research, frequently using his own funds. He finally received a grant from the Carnegie Foundation and was able to work at Columbia. He succeeded in chemically identifying vitamin B-1 in 1935, and in 1936 accomplished its synthesis.

The further story of the conquest of the deficiency diseases is best told by individually outlining the history of each disease.

Scurvy

This disease has been known since the earliest of times and from the Bible we learn that Job was probably one of its victims. In the thirteenth century the disease ravaged the Crusaders at the siege of Damietta. During the "Age of Sail," scurvy became the scourge of the sea. Long voyages with inadequate diets of hardtack and salt-pork and a lack of fresh fruits and vegetables killed thousands of sailors. As related in an earlier chapter, the Scotch naval surgeon, James Lind, in the eighteenth century conquered scurvy by demonstrating that lime juice and other citrus fruits not only cured the disease but prevented it. His work resulted in having a daily ration of lime juice introduced into the daily diet of all British sailors. Thus scurvy was banished from the Royal Navy and British sailors were nicknamed "limeys." The real significance of Lind's discovery, however, escaped attention. His citrus juices were thought of as medicinal drugs rather than as the sources of an essential food substance, and physicians failed to see that the disease was caused by the absence of some nutrient that was contained in the fruit.

Scurvy was produced in laboratory animals by Holst and Frölich, whose studies were published in 1907.

In 1928 the Hungarian biochemist Albert Szent-Györgyi isolated from the suprarenal glands of oxen and from various plant sources a crystalline compound which he named "hexuronic acid." The wide distribution of this compound in animal tissues and in growing plants was soon appreciated, but it was not until 1932 that Szent-Györgyi determined by appropriate feeding experiments that he had been dealing with the specific antiscorbutic factor, vitamin C.

Simultaneously and independently, King and Waugh isolated a

highly active antiscorbutic compound from lemon juice and showed that it was identical with "hexuronic acid." By common agreement the latter term was abandoned in favor of "ascorbic acid."

In 1937 Szent-Györgyi was awarded the Nobel Prize for his work.

Rickets

Like many of the other deficiency diseases, rickets is age-old, and prehistoric bones showing rickets-induced deformities have been found. Generally speaking, however, the disease is of more recent origin; it first manifested itself in Europe during the late sixteenth century. Its appearance coincided with the peasants' flight from the land to the cities. This population movement—particularly in England, a country never noted for an abundance of sunlight—together with poverty, impoverished diets and bad housing produced the disease.

The name "rickets" is of uncertain and controversial origin, various authorities stating that it is derived from the Latin term "rachis," the spine; the old English word "wrikken," to twist; or the Anglo-Saxon word "hrycg," meaning back or ridge. The term first turned up in the London bills of mortality for 1634.

The disease was first observed in England and was for a time called the "English disease." One of the earliest, if not the first description of rickets is that of Daniel Whistler (1619-1684). After taking his degree in arts at Merton College, Oxford, Whistler proceeded to Leyden, where he received his medical degree in 1645. For his doctoral thesis he published an account of rickets. This thesis, written upon his graduation at the age of twenty-five, was his only contribution to medical science. Unfortunately, it attracted little attention and rickets did not find its place in pediatric text books until Glisson's work five years later.

Francis Glisson (1597-1677) was born in Dorsetshire, England and was educated at Gonville and Caius College in Cambridge where he received his M.D. in 1634. He became a member of the Royal College of Physicians and was made Regius Professor of physics at Cambridge, a chair he held until his death.

Glisson is famed for his anatomical study of the liver and his classic description of rickets. His book, *De Rachitide,* appeared in 1650 and contains a striking account of the disease. The illustrated frontispiece of this remarkable book graphically portrays a number of children afflicted with some of the various deformities of the disease.

Over the years various writers noted that rickets commonly occurred in cold, cloudy climates and was associated with poverty, a lack of fresh air and sunshine and an insufficient diet. Little further progress was made until 1885, when the German pathologist, Pommer, established its pathology.

To the English physiologist, Sir Edward Mellanby, belongs the credit of the discovery of the specific antirachitic factor or vitamin. His reports, published in 1918 and 1919, contain the first accounts of the undoubted production of true rickets in an experimental animal—in this case the dog—and of its cure by dietary means.

On diets consisting chiefly of cereal and small quantities of whole or skim milk, diets which are now recognized as deficient in vitamin D and also in calcium, there developed in Mellanby's puppies soft bones, bowed legs and other typical deformities seen in rachitic children. More definite proof of the presence of true rickets was obtained from roentgenograms and from chemical analysis of the dogs' bones, which were found to have a decidedly low calcium content. When a few cubic centimeters of cod liver oil was added to the diet, rickets failed to appear. Here was positive proof that rickets was caused by a definite deficiency in the diet and that the cure lay in the addition of certain specific foods.

Since the fats that were most potent in the prevention of rickets, cod liver oil and butter fat were also rich sources of the already known vitamin A, Mellanby drew the conclusion that the antirachitic factor was probably identical with fat-soluble A. But because of certain conflicting experimental results of their own, American investigators were not willing to accept this interpretation, and in 1922 McCollum and his co-workers at Johns Hopkins University published definite proof of the existence of two separate and distinct fat-soluble vitamins. Taking advantage of the fact, already established by Hopkins in England, that vitamin A is readily oxidized, McCollum and his associates passed a stream of oxygen through cod liver oil which was held at the temperature of boiling water for from twelve to fourteen hours. At the end of this time they found that the oil still retained its antirachitic potency when fed to rats but had lost its power to cure xerophthalmia; in other words, it still contained the antirachitic factor but had lost its vitamin A. This antirachitic factor McCollum named vitamin D.

For a number of years there had existed a more or less vague opinion that the incidence of rickets was in some way connected with sunshine, fresh air and other hygienic factors in the child's environment. That ultraviolet radiation constituted a specific cure for rickets, however, was first definitely established by Huldschinsky, a German physician working in Berlin during and directly after World War I.

For some time scientists were puzzled to reconcile these two discoveries, that of a specific antirachitic factor in the food and that of the antirachitic action of ultraviolet rays. But the riddle was solved independently and almost simultaneously by Hess of New York and by Steenbock of Wisconsin, who announced in 1924 that antirachitic potency could be developed in a number of different biologic materials by exposure to the rays of an ultraviolet light.

Further investigation developed the fact that the substance in the food or other material which was activated by ultraviolet radiation was not a fat but a substance associated with fats, an obscure sterol called ergosterol. Later work has shown that ergosterol has a wide distribution in plant and animal tissues, although it is usually found in minute quantities only, considerably less than 1 percent. It is found in larger amounts in ergot, from which it gets its name, and in yeast.

Prior to the discovery of the true cause of rickets in the 1920's, rickets was a public health problem of the first magnitude. In the northern and temperate zones of the world it afflicted as many as 90 percent of the infants and children of the larger cities.

Public health educational and nutritional programs over the past thirty to forty years have established the inclusion of cod liver oil or vitamin D preparations in all infant formulas. This together with the irradiation of milk and other foods has practically eliminated rickets. It is now a rarity to see the malformed, square-headed, pot-bellied children, with knock-knees, bowlegs or pigeon breast that were so frequently seen in the past.

Beriberi

This dietary deficiency disease was the scourge of the Orient and afflicted the rice eaters of the Far East for many centuries. Although it is an ancient disease it gained ground in more recent times, attacking those who subsisted almost exclusively on overmilled rice. Polishing preserved the rice and while preventing spoilage, it unfortunately removed the hulls and destroyed the vitamins.

The earliest descriptions of beriberi are found in the ancient Chinese medical manuscript of the Yellow Emperor written in 2697 B.C. The disease is also referred to in the early Japanese writings of Ashike in 807. However, beriberi was first accurately described and studied in the seventeenth cntury, particularly in Indonesia. A Dutch physician named Jacobus Bontius, who served with the East India Company in Java, gave an excellent description of the disease in his book, *De Medicina Indorum*, which was published in 1642, eleven years after his death.

He described it as, "a certain type of paralysis which the natives called beriberi." He stated that the name means sheep, because those afflicted with the disease walk with their legs raised up like sheep. However, other medical historians state that the term beriberi is a Singhalese word meaning "cannot" and that the disease was so named because those afflicted become so weak they "cannot" do anything.

Beriberi was again described in 1716 by Nicholas Tulp, another Dutch physician, who also served in the Indies. In the ensuing years descriptions and outbreaks of the disease were reported in the Philippines, Japan, East Africa and other parts of the rice-eating world.

During the years of 1878 to 1883 beriberi afflicted approximately 20 percent of the sailors in the Japanese Navy. Kanehiro Takaki, a high ranking medical officer was assigned to study the problem. In 1884 he came to the conclusion that the disease was most likely due to a faulty diet, since climate seemed to be without influence and the sanitary conditions on Japanese ships was as good as those in European navies which were not troubled with the disease. He, therefore, ordered that the sailor's traditional rice diet be enlarged to a mixed diet including vegetables.

Thus, Takaki freed the Japanese Navy of beriberi by simply changing the diet. He was successful, although he knew nothing of avitaminosis and simply acted on an empiric basis.

In the 1890's research conducted in the Netherlands East Indies by the Dutch biologist, Christiaan Eijkman, gave us our first insight as to the true nature of beriberi. He showed that beriberi occurred when people ate rice which was polished, but that the disease could be prevented if the rice with its bran was used. He showed definitely that beriberi, or a disease showing similar symptoms of nerve disturbance, could be produced or cured at will in hens by changing the diet of unpolished rice to milled rice, or the reverse. In 1906 he wrote: "There is present in rice polishings a substance of a different nature from proteins, fats, or salts which is essential to health and the lack of which causes nutritional polyneuritis."

Eijkman received the Nobel Prize in 1929 in recognition of his work.

Several years after Eijkman's initial work, Gerrit Grijns, an associate, announced that beriberi was cured by a substance that was lacking in the diet.

The recognition of beriberi as a deficiency disease was slow in gaining acceptance. Between 1910 and 1933 Robert Runnel Williams proved that a deficiency of vitamin B was the cause of beriberi. In 1926 Barend Jansen, a Dutch physiologist, isolated vitamin B-1 from natural sources. In 1936 Williams and Windaus synthesized vitamin B-1 or thiamine.

Pellagra

It is of interest to note that the earliest records of pellagra associated this disease with food. In 1600 Bornino described a disease answering to the description of pellagra as occurring among certain American Indian tribes which he related to their diet of maize. Since that time the consumption of maize or American corn has been consistently linked with this disease. To the extent to which maize was introduced into Europe from the New World, and its consumption increased, pellagra spread. Hence, numerous descriptions of the disease began to appear during the eighteenth and nineteenth centuries.

The first authentic history of the disease begins with its description in 1735 by Don Gaspar Casal. Casal, who was the physician to King Philip of Spain, recorded in his observations that a malady which he called "mal de la rosa" was prevalent among the peasants in the province of Austuria.

The disease was subsequently described in 1771, as occurring in northern Italy, by Francisco Frapolli, who first called it pellagra. This term refers to the cutaneous manifestations of the disease and literally means "rough skin," coming from the Italian "pelle" (skin) and "agara" (rough).

Although maize was specifically related to the disease, it was assumed that this cereal played its role by imparting a noxious agent to the dietary, a toxic substance, produced possibly by a chemical change in the process of "spoiling." As early as 1776, Venice passed legislative measures to prohibit the sale or exchange of ill smelling, ill tasting, or discolored corn. Opposed to the view that corn causes an intoxication was the hypothesis that pellagra was an infectious, communicable disease due to a parasite.

It was not until 1863 that the disease was first clearly described in the United States. The high mortality in certain of the Southern prison camps during the Civil War has been ascribed to this disease. The fact that the European form of the disease was identical with the American was not recognized until 1900. American physicians had focused their attention mainly to the skin symptoms and because they felt that these lesions resembled syphilis, they believed the disease to be infectious. In 1908 it was estimated that in the Southern United States about 100,000 cases of pellagra occurred annually.

That diet plays the predominant role in the production or prevention of pellagra was first clearly established through the investigations of Goldberger and his associates. By 1914 the incidence of pellagra in the South had mounted to such alarming proportions that Surgeon General Rupert Blue of the United States Public Health Service called for an investigation. He assigned his chief epidemic sleuth, Joseph Goldberger, to unravel "one of the knottiest and most urgent problems facing the Service at the present time."

Goldberger began his investigations by reading all the available literature on pellagra, but found it of little value. He then made a seven-state study tour of the areas where pellagra was most prevalent. At the Georgia State Sanitarium for the Insane, he found his first clue: there were several hundred cases of pellagra among the patients but not a single case among the doctors, nurses or other attendants. Following this lead, Goldberger visited other asylums and orphanages and found the same situation in each place. To Goldberger this was proof that the disease was not infectious and led him to study other factors, especially the diet.

He found that for pellagra sufferers meals were a monotonous succession of grits, corn mush, molasses, syrup, sowbelly and gravy— a diet heavy in carbohydrates but almost entirely devoid of high-quality protein foods. Goldberger soon put his dietary theory to test. Obtaining government funds he greatly enlarged the diets at several orphanages. By adding milk, meat and eggs to the diet, he effected a series of almost miraculous cures on the pellagrous orphans.

Goldberger and his associate, G. A. Wheeler, now embarked upon a new experiment to further test his dietary findings. Securing official approval, they set up a special "diet camp" at a prison farm near Jackson, Mississippi. Using healthy, pellagra-free, convict volunteers, they placed them on a special diet of fried mush, sow belly, grits and gravy. In a relatively short period of time they induced pellagra in the convict volunteers by means of this faulty diet.

However, even after the publication of his findings there were those who still held to the infectious theory of the disease. To disprove the infectious theory once and for all, Goldberger decided to conduct another experiment. Securing a group of sixteen volunteers, including himself and his wife, he tried to have them contract pellagra by infection, in every possible way.

He used a variety of tests, one being the injection of blood from a known pellagra sufferer into the systems of the volunteers. A second test involved applying secretions from a pellagra victim's nose and throat to the same areas of the human guinea pigs. A third was a particularly revolting measure; it required the swallowing of a small dough ball compounded of flour together with urine, feces and lesion scales from a person with the disease.

In April, May and June of 1916, Goldberger conducted six series of these tests. After the last one he wrote: "We had our final 'filth party'—Wheeler, Sydenstricker (another assistant) and I—this noon.

If anyone can get pellagra that way, we three should certainly have it good and hard. It's the last time. Never again." None of the "fifteen men and a housewife," as they were identified in the published report, contracted pellagra. The experiment served its purpose by putting an end to the infectious theory of the disease.

The final phase of Goldberger's work on pellagra was to try and find the "pellagra-preventive" factor in food. He did find that yeast contained the essential food factors that could prevent and cure pellagra. Goldberger died from cancer in 1929 and did not live to identify or find the specific vitamin involved.

It remained for Conrad Arnold Elvehjem, an American biochemist, in 1937 to isolate and find that nicotinic acid was the essential factor in food to prevent and cure pellagra.

Pellagra has now become one of the vanishing diseases and is a rarity.

Xeropthalmia

This eye disease consists of a dry and thickened condition of the conjunctiva and is due to a deficiency of vitamin A. The term is composed of the Greek word "Xeros" or dry and the Greek "opthalmos" or eye. The disease was known to the Greco-Roman physicians and Celsus in about A.D. 30 stated that the Greeks used this term. The disease was described in the middle of the eighteenth century under the name of "lippitudo sicca."

The true cause of the disease remained unknown until McCollum and Simmonds in 1917 demonstrated that it is due to a vitamin A deficiency. The chemistry, isolation and synthesis of vitamin A and its relation to carotene were elucidated by Karrer, Heilbron and Holmes and Corbett, between 1930 and 1937.

Vitamin K

This vitamin is associated with the coagulation of the blood and hence it was called vitamin K from the German spelling of coagulation which is "Koagulation." In 1924 Stefan Ansbacher, a German-American chemist, reported the synthesis of a vitamin K compound. In about 1939, Dam, Doisey and McKee all reported the synthesis and isolation of vitamin K.

Vitamin E

A deficiency of this vitamin results in problems of human reproduction such as sterility and habitual abortion. It has frequently been
called the anti-sterility vitamin. Herbert McLean Evans, a California
physician, in collaboration with K. S. Bishop discovered vitamin E in
wheat germ. Evans succeeded in isolating this vitamin in 1935.

In conclusion, it may be stated that the discovery and description
of the various deficiency diseases and the essential vitamins necessary
for their cure and prevention has been one of the great victories of
preventive medicine in the twentieth century. The science of nutrition and its practical and widespread application, especially through
the enrichment and fortification of various foods, has almost entirely
eliminated the frank vitamin deficiency diseases in most countries
where economic conditions are fairly good.

Chapter 36

RECENT PROGRESS AND PROMISE FOR THE FUTURE

GREAT PROGRESS in the diagnosis and treatment of syphilis, as well as the prevention of congenital syphilis and the prevention of the serious late effects of the disease, was made during the twentieth century. First, was the discovery in 1905 of the causative organism, the Spirocheta or Treponema pallida, by the German bacteriologists Fritz Richard Schaudinn and Paul Erich Hoffman. This was followed one year later by the announcement of a diagnostic test for syphilis. In 1906 August Paul von Wasserman, another German bacteriologist, and a former assistant to Robert Koch, discovered the serological test that has since born his name.

At about this time the brilliant German physician, Paul Ehrlich, who had also been a pupil of Robert Koch's, ushered in the era of chemotherapy. His researches led to the discovery in 1907 of the first effective antisyphilitic drug. Ehrlich called this drug "salvarsan" because he felt that it offered mankind salvation from this disease. It was also called "606" because it was the 606th drug tried in his extensive research. Later, in 1912, he discovered a less toxic drug called "909" or neosalvarsan. This advance in treatment was followed by the introduction of bismuth as an antisyphilitic by the French physician, Constantin Levaditi.

For a generation these drugs remained as the most potent and effective ones known in the treatment of syphilis. The discovery of penicillin in 1928 by the English physician, Sir Alexander Fleming, and the demonstration during World War II by Dr. John F. Mahoney of the United States Public Health Service that penicillin could cure syphilis, ushered in a new era in the control of this disease.

Thus, at long last, the weapons were on hand for the control of syphilis. The organism was identified, an easy, accurate test for diag-

[381]

nosis and case finding was available, and effective treatment was a reality. Along with these advances, public programs of education and mass blood testing were inaugurated. Laws requiring premarital and prenatal blood testing were passed and free treatment clinics were established. As a result, in the United States, congenital syphilis has almost been eliminated and the late complications of syphilis such as tabes dorsalis and syphilitic paresis have, by and large, been prevented. However, syphilis is still with us and every effort must be continued if its ultimate control is to be achieved.

The twentieth century's greatest pandemic was the "Spanish influenza" of 1918-19. This terrible pandemic swept over the entire world from the jungles to the polar regions. It is said to have snuffed out upwards of twenty million lives, either directly or indirectly as a result of secondary bacterial pneumonia.

The 1918-19 pandemic of influenza began in late 1917 and the early months of 1918, when, what is commonly referred to as the "first wave," passed over the European Continent in a series of relatively mild localized epidemics. This relatively mild first wave also occurred in the United States, with early spring outbreaks being reported from Camp Kearney, California; Camp Funston and Fort Riley, Kansas; as well as other army camps and among the civilian population.

In the late summer of 1918, Spanish influenza burst its chrysalis and created such unprecedented havoc and carnage that it has gone down in medical history as one of our greatest human catastrophes. During August 1918 epidemics of influenza were reported in Greece, Sweden, Switzerland, Spain, the West Indies, and late in the month it appeared almost simultaneously in Camp Shelby, Mississippi, and Boston, Massachusetts. In September it appeared in rapid succession in other Army camps and in the civilian population along the Atlantic seaboard and the Gulf of Mexico and spread rapidly westward over the country. By October the epidemic had involved the entire United States, except isolated places and some mountain areas. As a rule, epidemics affected rural areas later than cities in the same sections. In some areas there was a recrudescence of the epidemic in January and February 1919, which was most marked in cities where the autumn epidemic was less severe. Thus, the influenza epidemic of 1918-19 in the United States was characterized by a relatively mild phase in the spring of 1918, an explosive outbreak with high mortality in the fall, and a third phase or recrudescence early in 1919.

In the United States the population disruptions, troop concentrations, and the mobilization of men in overcrowded Army camps because of World War I added fuel to the flames of the pandemic and it spread like wildfire. The French claimed that the American Expeditionary Forces brought the flu, or as they called it "la grippe," with them when they came to France. Great Britain was also stricken and the English made a like claim. Regardless of its route of spread, the deadly "flu bug" struck with insane fury and claimed more lives in a matter of weeks than the combined armies of the world had accomplished in four years of fighting. Attrition in the United States was ten times that suffered by the American expeditionary forces in battle. It still remains a terrifying mystery as to how the flu traveled such great distances in so short a space of time. Coast Guard patrols, for example, discovered remote Eskimo villages in inaccessible Alaskan areas where the entire population was wiped out. By the end of 1918 and in early 1919 the Spanish influenza subsided and disappeared, and where it went nobody knew.

Outbreaks of epidemics believed to have been influenza have been recorded since ancient times. In 412 B.C. Hippocrates recorded an epidemic resembling influenza which nearly annihilated an Athenian Army. Allusions to, and descriptions of flu-like epidemics seem to have been recorded approximately every hundred or more years. In the fifteenth century the mysterious and deadly English Sweat (described elsewhere in this book) killed hundreds of thousands. Most medical historians believe this to have been influenza.

The disease has been described under a variety of names such as the sweating sickness, the jolly rant, and la grippe. During the seventeenth century when the disease was epidemic, the Italians named it influenza, believing it to be due to the unfavorable "influence" of the stars or planets. In the same century the disease was supposedly brought to the New World from Valencia, Spain and hence was called the Spanish influenza. However, some historians believe the term to be more recent and that because of the neutrality of Spain in World War I, we had most information about the early 1918 epidemic from that country. As a result, in the United States the disease was popularly called "Spanish influenza."

In the nineteenth century two pandemics of influenza occurred, one in 1847-1848 and the other in 1889. Both had a relatively low mortality rate, especially in the United States. Some physicians at that time called the disease the "Chinese distemper," and believed it to have originated from clouds of dust carried by the winds from the parched banks of the Yellow River. Others pointed an accusing finger at the heavens, believing it to be due to "cosmic dust" emanating from volcanic eruptions. Wherever it came from, the disease had a relatively low mortality rate and then vanished for a time. It lay dormant until its furious and deadly onslaught in 1918.

Following the disastrous 1918 pandemic it was generally accepted that the disease was caused by a filtrable virus. However, research techniques were not sufficiently developed at that time to identify the suspected virus.

The first successful isolation of the influenza virus took place during an epidemic in England in 1933. In that year the elusive virus was found at the National Institute for Medical Research at Hampstead in suburban London. Dr. Wilson Smith, together with Doctors W. W. C. Topley, Patrick P. Laidlow and Christopher H. Andrews, were able to grow the virus in ferrets. The virus which was obtained from the throat washings of human influenza patients produced the typical disease in these rodents. This agent is now designated as influenza virus A.

These findings were confirmed in 1934 by Dr. Thomas Francis Jr., who also found that a number of mutant strains of the virus existed. The influenza virus soon became known as "the virus that changes," because of its ability to mutate and produce new strains. In 1940 Francis and Magill independently reported the isolation of a new virus, which was designated as Type B.

Since then numerous new strains of flu virus have been discovered, such as Asian A and B. This mutation of the virus has made it difficult to produce a truly effective flu vaccine. In fact, almost all of the vaccines, from a protective point of view, are one epidemic behind. However, it should be remembered that the mortality associated with influenza is principally due to secondary bacterial infection, and that today due to penicillin and the other antibiotics we are much better equipped to combat bacterial infection than we were in 1918.

During recent years methods of active immunization against measles have been developed and that greatly underrated, almost universal disease of childhood can now be prevented.

Historically, there are on record widespread epidemics of measles in "virgin" populations accompanied by high mortality rates. This was dramatically brought to attention in 1847 by Peter Ludwig Panum's classic study of the disastrous measles epidemic that occurred in the Faroe Islands.

Although the death rate for measles in the United States is relatively low, its after-effects in deafness and mental crippling are serious. It is still a major threat to many parts of the world. In Africa and South America the death rate among children may be as high as 25 percent.

In 1954 Drs. John F. Enders and Thomas Peebles of Boston succeeded in cultivating in their laboratory a strain of measles virus from an eleven-year-old boy named David Edmonston. In order to produce an attenuated virus, the original Edmonston strain was first grown in human kidney tissue cultures for twenty-four generations, then in human amnion tissue cultures for another twenty-eight, and it was then adapted to and propagated in chicken embryo tissue. The vaccine was first tested and found to be effective in 1958. It was licensed in 1963, and large scale measles immunization campaigns were carried on in the United States during 1967 and 1968. Measles can thus be added to the long list of vanishing diseases.

A relatively recent discovery in the field of prevention is the fact that the controlled fluoridation of drinking water is a proven method of reducing cavities in the teeth of children. It has now been demonstrated that this is the most effective and least costly preventive dental health measure now available.

The relationship between dental caries and fluorides has been known for many years. In 1892 Dr. J. Crichton-Browne observed in the British medical journal, *Lancet,* that there might be a relationship between dental decay and the fluoride content of teeth. He further suggested that the high rate of dental decay in London might be due to a lack of fluorides in the diet.

The first serious investigation into fluorides was carried on in the

United States by Dr. Frederick S. McKay of Colorado Springs. McKay noticed that a number of his patients had teeth with mottled enamel. He also noticed that these teeth were surprisingly free from cavities. In questioning his patients, he learned that all of those with mottled teeth were born in Colorado Springs or had moved there as young children. Mottled enamel was not present in anyone who had moved into Colorado Springs in their teens or later. He also noted that these people had a significantly larger number of cavities. In February of 1916 McKay together with G. V. Black published an article in *Dental Cosmos* entitled, "Mottled Teeth—An endemic developmental imperfection of the teeth, heretofore unknown in the literature of dentistry."

Dr. McKay continued his studies over the years and in 1931 he investigated mottled enamel in Bauxite, Arkansas. In that year he sent samples of water from Bauxite to two industrial chemists in Pennsylvania, H. V. Churchill and A. W. Petrie. They discovered that the water from Bauxite contained some 13.7 parts of fluoride per million parts of water. Bauxite abandoned its deep wells and started using water from the Saline River, which had no fluorides. As a result the children's teeth no longer became mottled, but their number of cavities increased.

At about this point the United States Public Health Service became interested, and Dr. H. Trendley Dean and his associates began a series of investigations in 1938. They found a direct relationship between the fluoride content of drinking water and the amount of tooth decay in the children who drank the water. Late in 1938 they made detailed measurements in Galesburg and Quincy, Illinois. Galesburg used deep well water with 1.8 parts of fluoride per million parts of water. Quincy got its water from the Mississippi River, with only .1 part fluoride per million parts of water. Quincy children between twelve and fourteen had three times as much tooth decay as Galesburg children.

In 1941 and 1942 Dr. Dean, in association with Drs. Francis A. Arnold and E. Elvove, published studies of tooth decay in 7,257 selected children of the same age group in twenty-one cities of four states, checked against the fluoride content of their drinking water. They found that children drinking water that contained one part fluoride per million parts of water had approximately 60 percent fewer decayed teeth than those drinking water without any fluorides. They also found that mottled enamel only occurred where the drinking water contained more than 1.5 parts of fluoride per million parts of water.

These studies ultimately led to the conclusion that it might be possible to reduce the cavities in the teeth of children by the controlled fluoridation of water supplies.

The first test of controlled fluoridation started on May 2, 1945 in the Hudson River city of Newburgh, New York. A feeder machine was turned on at the city's filtration plant and the water delivered from that time on contained 1.2 parts of fluoride per million parts of water. A ten-year study was started in which the children of Newburgh were compared with children of the same age in the neighboring city of Kingston, where the water remained fluoride-free.

This carefully controlled, scientific study and many other subsequent ones thoroughly established fluoridation as a cheap, safe and effective method of preventing dental decay. Despite this overwhelming scientific evidence, fluoridation has encountered a great deal of irrational opposition which undoubtedly will diminish and disappear.

The twentieth century has seen much research and progress aimed at the prevention and treatment of birth defects. A vast diffuse and puzzling area, birth defects until recently were considered to be hopeless and without solution. However, a number of "breakthroughs" have occurred and the promise for the future is bright.

One of the first breakthroughs was the discovery of the Rh factor in 1940 by two American physicians, Karl Landsteiner and Alexander S. Wiener. The term Rh stands for Rhesus, because this agglutination factor was first found in the red blood cells of the Rhesus monkey. It has been determined that the Rh factor is present in the blood of about 85 percent of people. Those who have it are Rh positive and those who don't are Rh negative.

If a mother is Rh negative and a father Rh positive and the child inherits the father's blood type, the child may be stillborn or be born severely anemic or jaundiced and die from erythroblastosis. This rarely occurs in a first pregnancy, but the danger rises in subsequent pregnancies.

In the United States Rh disease each year has menaced an estimated 40,000 babies with death or damage before or soon after birth. A vaccine is now available to any woman whose Rh type might be of danger to her unborn child. An injection of the new vaccine, given to an Rh negative mother within seventy-two hours after the birth, stillbirth or miscarriage of each Rh positive baby, prevents an adverse reaction in the mother's blood which can endanger offspring.

For women already sensitized by previous births, the Rh vaccine is ineffective. But new techniques of giving blood transfusions to unborn babies can save many Rh infants who might otherwise be stillborn. Exchange transfusions immediately after birth will prevent the death of babies who are born alive, but who are jaundiced and anemic due to erythroblastosis or Rh disease.

Physicians can now prevent this major cause of birth defects, but they must first know the woman's Rh blood type and her baby's. Rh testing has now become a routine part of good prenatal care.

In recent decades, certain virus infections—often so mild that an expectant mother is not aware that she is ill—have been identified as major sources of damage to unborn babies. An example is the rubella or German measles virus, which was recognized as a cause of birth defects in 1941, and isolated in 1961. Now a new vaccine is available and birth defects due to German measles should be greatly reduced or eliminated.

Another significant new breakthrough in the field of preventive medicine has been the discovery of the disease known as phenylketonuria. Commonly abbreviated to PKU, this condition is a congenital inherited metabolic disorder associated with mental retardation. It holds a unique position in the field of mental deficiency because it is easily detected, and when diagnosed early, the associated mental retardation can be prevented or favorably modified by special dietary management.

Its discovery dates back to the early 1930's to a Norwegian family with two mentally retarded children. Seeking help for her children, the mother made the usual rounds of going from doctor to doctor. She had noted that her children had a peculiar "musty" odor about them which she mentioned to the doctors and sought relief for. She finally came to a Norwegian physician and biochemist named Asbjörn

Fölling. Dr. Fölling discovered that the urine of the two children reacted with ferric chloride to give an unusual green color. He found out that this was due to the presence of phenylpyruvic acid, which he was able to crystalize in pure form from their urine.

Because these urinary findings were associated with mental retardation a urine-test survey was conducted on several hundred patients in two nearby institutions for the mentally retarded. The survey uncovered eight additional patients with the same disorder, including two more pairs of siblings.

In 1934 Dr. Fölling published his findings in the Norwegian and German medical literature with the title, "Excretion of Phenylpyruvic Acid in the Urine, a Metabolic Anomaly in Connection with Imbecility." He postulated that the abnormality was an inherited error in the metabolism of phenylalanine, and called it "Imbecillitas Phenylpyruvica."

As information concerning this newly discovered disease spread, patients in institutions for the mentally retarded in many countries were surveyed and tested. This brought about a clearer knowledge of the incidence, the type of inheritance, and the clinical picture of the disease. Because phenylpyruvic acid, the substance which is excreted in the urine, is a phenyl ketone, the British researcher L. S. Penrose suggested that the disease be named phenylketonuria. This name became generally accepted and was soon abbreviated to PKU.

It was soon discovered that PKU is found, on the average, in 1 percent of institutionalized mental defectives. From these figures it was estimated that PKU occurred in one out of every 20,000 to 40,000 live births. Recent studies, screening newborns, indicate that the incidence may be closer to one in every 10,000 births.

Because PKU frequently involved more than one child in a family, it was recognized from the beginning as a familial disorder and was soon shown to be a Mendelian recessive trait. It was found that because the mother is essentially normal, even as a carrier, the baby is protected before birth. When the newborn PKU baby begins to take milk, phenylalanine is absorbed because the baby's normal metabolic pathways are blocked. It is believed that a continual high level of phenylalinine or its related metabolites is responsible for the mental retardation.

Dietary treatment for PKU was described by Bickel, Gerard, and Hickman in the *Lancet* in 1953. In 1955, Woolf, Griffith and Moncrief published an article in the British Medical Journal entitled, "Treatment of Phenylketonuria with a Diet Low in Phenylalanine."

Since these findings, the progress in the early detection, diagnosis, and treatment of PKU has been rapid. Most pediatricians and physicians now routinely check all newborns for PKU and in some states, laws have been passed making PKU testing compulsory. Thus, at long last it is possible to prevent at least one form of mental retardation.

Cancer, that age-old terrible disease, whose dread name is still whispered in horror, is today being examined in every aspect. The mounting tempo of worldwide cancer research gives us every promise for the future that effective procedures for the prevention of cancer will be found.

Perhaps our earliest knowledge as to the cause and prevention of any type of cancer came from England. In 1775 the famous English physician, Percival Pott, published his classic description of scrotal cancer in chimney sweeps. He pointed out that this type of skin cancer was an occupational disease due to the soot and continuous irritation of the skin that resulted from the "sweeps" working in the narrow confines of "sooty" chimneys. He advocated cleanliness and protective clothing as preventive measures.

Since that time our knowledge of occupational skin cancers has increased tremendously, until today, numerous industrial carcinogens, such as tar, pitch and oils are known. These cancers can be prevented by avoiding skin irritation and contact with these carcinogenic substances.

Cancer of the lung has recently been shown to be related to heavy cigarette smoking and the breathing of air polluted with auto exhaust fumes and industrial toxins. Lung cancer is far greater in smokers than in nonsmokers, and higher in urban industrial areas than in rural regions. The preventive moral is clear: "To prevent lung cancer, live in the country and don't smoke."

In cancer, early detection and prompt surgical or radiological treatment, can and does prevent death. One of the great advances in early detection has been the development and wide spread use of the cytologic test or "Pap" smear. This test was developed in 1943 by George Nicholas Papanicolaou, a New York physician, at Cornell Medical College.

These and other already known preventive procedures, together with those yet to be discovered, will ultimately enable us to control and prevent cancer.

This *History of Preventive Medicine* has portrayed mankind's never-ending struggle for health up through the ages. However, if we allow ourselves the luxury of looking forward we will realize that this portrayal of the past is only a beginning and that preventive medicine presents an almost unlimited promise for the future.

With the complete conquest of contagion virtually achieved, we now literally stand upon the mountain tops and look into the promised land. In our modern world of rapid scientific advancement, preventive medicine will leap from one great victory to another. As scientific research continues to unlock the secrets of nature, we will learn the cause and prevention of birth defects, cancer and the rest of our chronic, crippling and degenerative diseases.

On this new horizon of preventive medicine looms the possibility of lengthening man's life span from the biblical "three score years and ten" to a century or more. It further presents the possibility of the fulfillment of the Utopian dream, that we may all some day live at peace and prosperity in a disease-free world.

BIBLIOGRAPHY

ACKERKNECHT, E. H.: *A Short History of Medicine*. New York, Ronald, 1955.

ACKERKNECHT, E. H.: Naval surgery from 1500 to 1800. *Ciba Symp, 4* (Nos. 9-10) : 1394-1404, Dec. 1942-Jan. 1943.

ACKERKNECHT, E. H.: *History and Geography of the Most Important Diseases*. New York, Hafner, 1965.

ASHBURN, P. M.: *The Ranks of Death*. New York, Coward, 1947.

AULT, WARREN O.: *Europe In Modern Times*. Boston, Heath, 1946.

BAILEY, H., and BISHOP, W. J.: *Notable Names in Medicine and Surgery*. Springfield, Thomas, 1959.

BARON, A. L.: *Man Against Germs*. New York, Dutton, 1957.

BERCOVICI, KONRAD: *The Crusaders*. New York, Cosmopolitan, 1929.

BETTMAN, OTTO L.: *A Pictorial History of Medicine*. Springfield, Thomas, 1956.

BOLDOAN AND BOLDOAN: *Public Health and Hygiene*. Philadelphia, Saunders, 1949.

CARCOPINO, JEROME: *Daily Life in Ancient Rome*. Lorimer, E. O. (Tr) New Haven, Yale, 1940.

CASTIGLIONE, A.: *A History of Medicine*. New York, Knopf, 1947.

CASTIGLIONE, ARTURO: The medical school of Vienna. *Ciba Symp, 9*: Nov. 3-4, June-July, 1947.

CHAMBERS, J. S.: *The Conquest of Cholera, America's Greatest Scourge*. New York, Macmillan, 1938.

CHAMBERS, J. S.: *Biographical Dictionary*. New York, St. Martins, 1961.

CHAPIN, CHARLES V.: *The Sources and Modes of Infection*, 2nd ed. New York, Wiley, 1912.

CLENDENING, LOGAN: *Behind the Doctor*. New York, Knopf, 1933.

CLENDENING, LOGAN: *Source Book of Medical History*. New York, Dover, 1942.

COMEGYS, CORNELIUS G.: *Reonouard's History of Medicine*. Philadelphia, Lindsay and Blakiston, 1867.

DEFOE, DANIEL: *A Journal of the Plague Year*. Philadelphia, Morse, 1903.

DEKRIEF, PAUL: *Microbe Hunters*. New York, Harcourt, 1926.

DOBELL, CLIFFORD, F. R. S.: *Anton Van Leeuwenhoek and His 'Little Animals,'* New York, Harcourt, 1932.

Dock, Lavinia L., and Stewart, Isabel M.: *A Short History of Nursing.* New York, Putnam, 1932.

Donno, Elizabeth Story: *Sir John Harington's, A New Discourse of a Stale Subject, called the Metamorphosis of Ajax.* New York, Columbia, 1962.

Drew, Major General V. R. M.: Smallpox. *J Roy Army Medical Corps,* Jan. 1962.

Dubos, Rene: *Pasteur and Modern Science.* Garden City, Doubleday, 1960.

Dubos, R.: *Louis Pasteur.* Boston, Little, 1950.

Eberson, Frederick: *Microbes Militant.* New York, Ronald, 1948.

Epidemiology, Historical and Experimental. Bulletin. Baltimore, Johns Hopkins, 1932.

Fisk, Dorothy: *Doctor Jenner of Berkeley.* London, Heinemann, 1959.

Franklin, B.: *Some Account of the Success of Inoculation for the Smallpox in England and America.* London, Strahan, 1759.

Galdston, Iago: *Progress in Medicine.* New York, Knopf, 1940.

Garrison, F. H.: *An Introduction to the History of Medicine,* 4th ed. Philadelphia, Saunders, 1929.

Greenwood, Major: *Epidemic and Crowd Diseases.* London, William & Newgate, 1935.

Haggard, Howard W.: *Mystery, Magic and Medicine.* Garden City, Doubleday, 1933.

Haggard, Howard W.: *The Doctor in History.* New Haven, Yale, 1934.

Haggard, Howard W.: *The Lame, the Halt and the Blind.* New York, Harper, 1932.

Hanlon, John J.: *Principles of Public Health Administration.* St. Louis, Mosby, 1950.

Heiser, Victor: *An American Doctor's Odyssey.* New York, Norton, 1936.

Hobson, W.: *World Health and History.* Bristol, John Wright, 1963.

Hoehling, A. A.: *The Great Epidemic.* Boston, Little, 1961.

Holmes, S. J.: *Louis Pasteur.* New York, Dover, 1961.

Holy Bible—King James Version.

Hull, Thomas G.: *Diseases Transmitted From Animals to Man,* 3rd ed. Springfield, Thomas, 1947.

Jenner, Edward: *An Inquiry Into the Causes and Effects of the Variolae Vaccinae.* London, 1798.

Johnstone, Harold Whetstone: *Private Life of the Romans.* Chicago, Scott, 1903.

Kelly, Emerson C.: *Encyclopedia of Medical Sources.* Baltimore, Williams & Wilkins, 1948.

LeFanu, W. R.: *A Bio-Bibliography of Edward Jenner.* Philadelphia, Lippincott, 1951.

Leff, S., and Leff, Vera: *From Witchcraft to World Health.* New York, Macmillan, 1958.

Major, Ralph H.: *Classic Descriptions of Disease,* 3rd ed. Springfield, Thomas, 1959.

Major, Ralph H.: *A History of Medicine.* Springfield, Thomas, 1954, 2 vols.

Mathison, Richard: *The Shocking History of Drugs.* New York, Ballantine, 1958.

Megroz, R. L.: *Ronald Ross, Discoverer and Creator.* London, Allen & Unwin, 1931.

Mellanby, E.: Jenner and his impact on medical science. *Brit Med.:* 921-926, 1949.

Mettler, Cecilia C.: *History of Medicine.* New York, McGraw, 1947.

Munro, Dana Carleton: *The Kingdom of the Crusaders.* New York, Appleton, 1935.

New Century Cyclopedia of Names. New York, Appleton, 1954.

Newman, Sir George: *The Rise of Preventive Medicine.* London, Oxford, 1932.

Newsholme, Sir Arthur: *Evolution of Preventive Medicine.* Baltimore, Williams & Wilkins, 1927.

Nohl, Johannes: *The Black Death.* New York, Ballantine, 1960.

Pringle, Patrick: *The Romance of Medical Science.* New York, Roy Pub, 1953.

Ramazzini, B.: *De Morbis Artificum.* Wright, W. C. (Tr.) Chicago, U. of Chicago, 1940.

Rapport, Samuel, and Wright, Helen: *Great Adventures in Medicine.* New York, Dial, 1952.

Reynolds, Reginald: *Cleanliness and Godliness.* Garden City, Doubleday, 1946.

Riesman, David: *The Story of Medicine in the Middle Ages.* New York, Harper, 1936.

Robinson, Victor: *The Story of Medicine.* New York, Tudor, 1931.

Robinson, Victor: *Pathfinders in Medicine.* New York, Medical Life, 1929.

Roddis, L. H.: Edward Jenner and the discovery of smallpox vaccination. *Mil Surg, 65*:645, Nov.; 844 December, 1929; 66.6 January, 1930.

Roddis, Louis H.: *James Lind, Founder of Nautical Medicine.* London, Heineman, 1951.

Rosen, George: *A History of Public Health.* New York, M.D. Pub., 1958.

Rosenau, Milton J.: *Preventive Medicine and Hygiene,* 6th ed. New York, Appleton-Century, 1935.

Ross, R.: *Memoirs, With a Full Account of the Great Malaria Problem and Its Solution.* London, Murray, 1923.

Rush, Benjamin: *An Account of the Yellow Fever as It Appeared in Philadelphia in 1797.* Philadelphia, Dobson, 1798.

Schmidt, J. E.: *Medical Discoveries.* Springfield, Thomas, 1959.

Schneck, Jerome M.: *A History of Psychiatry.* Springfield, Thomas, 1960.

Sedgwick's Principles of Sanitary Science and Public Health. New York, Macmillan, 1935.

Seignobos, Charles: *The Rise of European Civilization.* New York, Knopf, 1938.

Shattuck, L.: *Report of the Sanitary Commission of Massachusetts— 1850.* Cambridge, Harvard, 1948.

Sigerist, Henry E.: *The Great Doctors.* New York, Norton, 1933.

Sigerist, Henry E.: *Landmarks in the History of Hygiene.* London, Oxford, 1956.

Slaughter, Frank G., M.D.: *Immortal Magyar. Semmelweiss, Conqueror of Childbed Fever.* New York, Abelard, 1950.

Smillie, Wilson G.: *Public Health, Its Promise for the Future.* New York, Macmillan, 1955.

Smith, Geddes: *Plague on Us.* Commonwealth Fund, Cambridge, Harvard, 1943.

Snow, John: *On Cholera.* Commonwealth Fund, Cambridge, Harvard, 1936.

Stearn, E. W., and A. E.: *The Effect of Smallpox in the Destiny of the Amerindian.* Boston, Humphries, 1945.

Taylor, B.: *Edward Jenner, Conqueror of Smallpox.* London, MacMillan, 1950.

Tobey, James A.: *Riders of the Plagues.* New York, Scribner, 1930.

Turner, E. S.: *The Astonishing History of the Medical Profession.* New York, Ballantine, 1961.

Underwood, E. A.: Edward Jenner, the man and his work. *Brit Med J. 1*:881-884, 1949.

Wain, Harry: *The Story Behind the Word.* Springfield, Thomas, 1958.

Wain, Harry: *The Unconquered Plague.* New York, Int. Univ., 1947.

WAKSMAN, SELMAN A.: *The Conquest of Tuberculosis.* Berkeley U. of Calif., 1964.

WALKER, KENNETH: *The Story of Medicine.* London, Arrow Bks, 1959.

WILKINSON, P. B.: *Variations on a theme by Sydenham: Smallpox.* Bristol, John Wright, 1959.

WILLIAMS, GREER: *Virus Hunters.* New York, Knopf, 1959.

WINSLOW, SMILLIE, DOULL, and GORDON: *The History of American Epidemiology.* St. Louis, Mosby, 1952.

WOODHAM-SMITH, CECIL: *Florence Nightingale.* New York, McGraw, 1951.

ZINSSER, HANS: *Rats, Lice and History.* Boston, Little, 1935.

NAME INDEX

Abildgaard, Peter Christian, 291
Aetius, 347, 353
Agramonte, Dr. Aristide, 318
Almenar, Juan, 89
Alphanus, 42
Anderson, Dr. John F., 304, 305
André, Nicolas, 139, 140
Andrews, Christopher H., 384
Ansbacher, Stefan, 379
Antoninus, 28
Appert, Nicolas, 206, 207
Aretaeus, 353
Aristotle, 98, 113, 238, 324, 342
Armstrong, Dr. Charles, 362
Arnold, Dr. Francis A., 386
Asclepius, 12, 13, 17
Ashike, 375
Auenbrugger, Leopold Joseph von,
    150, 151, 326
Auerbach, Leopold, 245
Averroes, 173
Avicenna, 33, 83, 84, 87

Bacon, Roger, 115
Bacon, Sir Francis, 103, 105
Baillou, Guillaume de, 110, 353
Baker, Dr. George, 207
Ballard, E., 252
Bancroft, Joseph, 293
Bang, 260, 261
Bard, Samuel, 353
Bartholin, Thomas, 111
Bateman, Thomas, 167
Bayle, 327
Beauperthuy, Dr. L., 317
Beebe, Alfred L., 357
Behring, Emil Adolph von, 355, 356,
    357
Bell, Benjamin, 345
Bell, Oswald, 252
Bentham, Jeremy, 207
Besredka, 286

Bethencourt, Jacques de, 92
Bickel, 390
Biggs, Herman, 334
Bishop, K. S., 380
Black, G. V., 386
Blaine, Sir Gilbert, 204
Blue, Rupert, 299, 377
Boccaccio, Giovanni, 56, 57, 58
Bodian, Dr. David, 362
Boerhaave, Hermann, 110, 146, 147,
    169
Bontius, Jacobus, 375
Borden, Gail, 257
Bornino, 376
Boyle, Robert, 113, 146
Boylston, Zabdiel, 184, 185
Brehmer, Herman, 333
Bretonneau, Pierre, 284, 354
Brill, Nathan Edwin, 304, 305
Brodie, Dr. Maurice, 361
Bruce, David, 260, 261, 295
Budd, William, 285, 286
Burnett, 259
Burton, John, 221

Cadogan, Dr. William, 139
Cagliostro, Count, 164, 165
Caius, John, 72, 85
Calmette, Dr. Albert, 336, 337
Cameron, Donald, 279
Cardano, Girolamo, 302
Carroll, Dr. James, 182, 318, 319
Cartier, Jacques, 199
Casal, Don Gaspar, 376
Castillo, Bernal Diaz del, 181
Castro, Jacob de, 174
Celsus, Aurelius Cornelius, 18, 21, 32,
    238, 281, 324, 343, 379
Chadwick, Edwin, 275, 276, 277
Chagas, Carlos, 296
Chamberland, 237
Chapin, 300

[397]

Chauliac, Guy de, 58, 59, 80
Chinchon, Countess of, 113, 310
Chowning, 305
Churchill, H. V., 386
Cline, Henry, 192
Cockburn, 345
Cohn, Ferdinand, 245
Cohnheim, Julius, 245
Coit, Dr. Henry L., 257
Collins, Robert, 222
Colombo, Realdo, 105
Columella, 96, 309
Comby, J., 255
Constantinus Africanus, 42, 168, 343
Conton, Dr. (Monsieur de Condom), 352
Cook, 350
Cook, Capt. James, 203, 204
Coram, Thomas, 138
Corbett, 379
Corvisart, Jean-Nicolas, 151, 326, 327
Couch, Dr. James F., 251
Cox, Dr. Herald, 365
Crawford, Dr. J. C., 317
Crazy Sally, *see* Mapp, Sarah
Crede, Dr. Karl Sigmund Franz, 348, 349, 350
Crichton-Browne, Dr. J., 385
Cross, Howard B., 322
Cruikshank, 278
Cruz, Osvaldo, 296
Cullen, 70, 141

Dam, 379
Darnell, Brig. Gen. Carl R., 278
Davaine, 235, 244
Dean, Dr. H. Trendley, 386
Defoe, Daniel, 63, 126, 127
De Lesseps, 321
Democritus, 238
De Paul, St. Vincent, 130, 214
Derrick, 306
Descartes, Rene, 112, 115
Digby, Kenelm, 170
Dimsdale, Thomas, **178, 179**
Dio, Casius, 28
Doisey, 379
Drake, Daniel, 251, 310

Dumas, Jean-Baptiste, 228
Dunant, Jean Henri, 218, 219
Dunglinson, Dr. Robley, 278
Durham, 286
Durer, Albrecht, 89
Dutton, 296
Dyer, 305

Eberth, Karl Joseph, 286, 354
Edmonston, David, 385
Ehrlich, Paul, 248, 330, 381
Eichhorn, Dr., 261
Eijkman, Christiaan, 369, 370, **376**
Elvehjem, Conrad Arnold, 379
Elvove, Dr. E., 386
Empedocles, 13, 14
Enders, Dr. John F., 362, 385
Epicurus, 343
Eustachius, Bartholommeo, 80
Evans, Alice C., 261
Evans, Griffith, 295
Evans, Herbert McLean, 380

Faber, Johannes, 115
Falck, 344
Fallopius, Gabrielle, 80, 149
Fedschenko, 291
Feldman, Dr. William F., 338
Finlay, Dr. Carlos J., 317, 318, 319, 320, 321
Fleming, Sir Alexander, 381
Flexner, 360
Flick, Lawrence F., 335
Fliedner, Pastor Theodore, 213
Flugge, 256, 296
Fölling, Asbjörn, 388, 389
Forlanini, Carlo, 332
Fracastoro, Girolamo, 93, 94, 95, 96, 98, 169, 173, 302, 325
Francis, Dr. Thomas Jr., 363, 365, 384
Frank, Johann Peter, 208, 209, 210, 211, 212
Franklin, Benjamin, 158, 185, 204
Frapolli, Francesco, 377
Froben (Frobenius) Johann, 84
Frolich, 371
Frontinus, Sextus Julius, 24

Fuchs, Leonard, 162
Funk, Casimer, 369

Gaffky, 247, 286
Gage, Professor, 294
Galen, Claudius, 18, 19, 20, 29, 32, 42, 43, 47, 55, 72, 79, 80, 83, 84, 85, 98, 104, 146, 325, 343
Galileo, 76, 103, 104, 115
Gariopontus, 42
Geissler, Dr., 356
Gerard, 390
Gerhard, William Wood, 285, 303
Gibson, Dr. Benjamin, 347
Gilbert, Dr. William, 102
Glauber, Johann Rudolf, 113, 114
Glisson, Dr. Francis, 110, 372
Goldberger, Joseph, 304, 369, 370, 377, 378, 379
Gordon, Dr. Alexander, 221
Gorgas, William C., 319, 321, 322
Graaf, Regnier de, 112, 118
Grafton, 70
Graham, James, 165, 278
Graunt, Capt. John, 121, 122, 123, 125
Greenberg, 306
Gregory, Bishop of Tours, 168
Griffith, 390
Grijns, Gerrit, 376
Gruber, 286
Guerin, Dr. Camille, 336, 337
Guidi, Guido, 353

Haffkine, Waldemar Mordecai, 284, 298
Hakluyt, Richard, 199
Hales, Reverend Doctor Stephen, 155, 156
Halle, Dr. Weill, 337
Haller, Albrecht von, 147
Halley, Edmund, 124
Hallock, 357
Haly Abbas, 43
Harington, Sir John, 23, 47, 272, 273, 274
Hart, Ernest, 252

Harvey, William, 80, 104, 105, 106, 107, 111, 112, 119, 146, 156
Hayne, Dr. Theodore B., 322
Hazen, Allen, 279
Heilbron, 379
Heine, Jakob von, 359
Helmholtz, 354
Henderson, 296
Henle, Jacob, 243
Henry, Thomas, 278
Herodotus, 167
Herrell, 350
Hess, 259, 374
Hickman, 390
Hinshaw, H. Corwin, 338
Hippocrates, 14, 15, 16, 29, 32, 42, 47, 49, 62, 67, 72, 82, 83, 85, 87, 98, 108, 146, 166, 167, 281, 309, 324, 342, 343, 368, 383
Hoang-Ty, 341
Hodges, Dr. Nathaniel, 127
Hoffman, Paul Erich, 381
Holboell, Einor, 335
Holmes, 379
Holmes, Oliver Wendell, 222, 223, 226
Holst, 371
Holt, Emmet L., 262
Hone, 305
Hooke, Robert, 120
Howard, John, 143, 144, 145
Howe, Dr. Howard, 362
Howe, Lucien, 350
Hughes, Griffith, 315
Huldschinsky, 374
Hunter, John, 151, 152, 153, 154, 188, 345
Hutten, *see* Von Hutten
Huygens, Christian, 124
Hyatt, 278
Hygeia, 13

Imhoff, Karl, 279, 280
Isla, Rodrigo Ruiz Diaz de, 88

Jacobi, Abraham, 253, 254, 255
Jacobs, E. G., 252
Jansen, Barend, 376

Janssen, Hans, 115
Janssen, Zacharius, 115
Jenks, Rowland, 302
Jenner, Edward, 142, 153, 171, 172,
    186, 187, 189, 190, 191, 192,
    193, 194, 195, 336
Jesty, Benjamin, 193
John of Gaddesden, 169, 351
Johnson, G. A., 278

Karrer, 379
Kennedy, Peter, 174
Kessel, Dr. J. F., 362
King, 371
Kircher, Athanasius, 119, 120
Kirkwood, James P., 278
Kissinger, Private John, 320
Kitasato, Shibasaburo, 247, 297, 356
Klebs, Theodor Albrecht Edwin, 354,
    355
Klencke, 258
Kling, 360
Knott, Dr. Josiah Clark, 317
Koch, Robert, 160, 235, 243, 244, 245,
    246, 247, 248, 249, 258, 269, 270,
    283, 287, 297, 329, 330, 331, 332,
    334, 336, 354, 381
Kolle, William, 284, 287
Kollicker, 354
Kolmer, Dr. John A., 361
Koprowsky, Dr. Hilary, 365
Krause, 244
Kuchenmeister, F., 291
Kussmaul, Adolf, 359

Lacroix, 344
Laennec, Rene Theophile Hyacinthe,
    326, 327, 328, 329
Laidlow, Patrick P., 384
Landsteiner, Karl, 360, 387
Laveran, Charles Louis Alphonse, 311
Lavoisier, Antoine Laurent, 157, 158,
    159
Lazear, Dr. Jesse W., 318, 319, 320,
    322
Leeds, 278

Leeuwenhoek, Anthony van, 112, 116,
    117, 118, 146, 205
Leiner, 360
Leishman, Sir William B., 287
Leoniceno, Nicola, 87
Lettsom, John Coakley, 141, 142
Leuckart, Rudolph, 291, 292
Levaditi, Constantin, 381
Lewis, 360
Lewis, Dr. Paul A., 322
Lille, R. D., 370
Linacre, Thomas, 85
Lind, Dr. James, 196, 199, 200, 201,
    202, 203, 204, 303, 371
Linnaeus (Carl von Linne), 159, 160,
    161
Lister, Joseph, 234, 235, 241
Liston, Capt. Glenn W., 298
Locke, 132
Lockett, W. T., 279
Loeffler, Frederick August John, 247,
    354, 355
Loomis, H. P., 334
Lowcock, 279
Louis, Pierre Charles Alexander, 284,
    285, 303
Ludlow, Daniel, 189
Lunin, N., 369
Mackie, 296
Magill, 384
Mahoney, Dr. John F., 351, 381
Maimonides, Moses, 343
Maitland, Dr., 176, 177
Mallon, Mary, *see* Typhoid Mary
Malpighi, Marcello, 119
Manson, Patrick Sir, 292, 293, 294,
    313
Mapp, Sarah Wallin (Crazy Sally),
    162, 163
Marius, 168
Marston, Jeffrey Allen, 259
Mather, Cotten, 182, 184, 185
Maxcy, 305
McCollum, Elmer Verner, 369, 370,
    373, 374, 379
McCoy, 299, 300
McKay, Dr. Frederick S., 386
McKee, 379
Mead, Dr. Richard, 138, 148, 176, 177

Medin, Oskar Karl, 359, 360
Meister, Joseph, 239, 240
Mellanby, Sir Edward, 373
Melnikoff, 292
Metchnikoff, 286
Meyenberg, John B., 257
Moncrief, 390
Monrad, 256
Montagu, Lady Mary Wortley, 175,
    176, 177, 185
Mooser, 305
Morgagni, Giovanni Battista, 135,
    148, 149, 150
Morton, Richard, 326
Morveau, Guyton de, 278
Moses, 6, 7, 8, 9, 10, 342, 351
Munro, Alexander, 147
Mussa, 343

Napoleon, 303
Neisser, Albert Ludwig Siegmund,
    346, 348
Newton, 132
Nicolle, Charles Jules Henri, 301, 303,
    304
Nightingale, Florence, 215, 216, 217,
    218, 219
Noguchi, Dr. Hideyo, 322
Obermeir, 296
Ogata, Masaki, 298
Osler, Sir William, 285

Panacea, 13
Panum, Peter, 385
Papanicolaou, George Nicholas, 391
Paracelsus, 67, 68, 83, 84, 85, 94, 96,
    344
Pare, 80, 81, 82, 169, 221, 345
Park, William H., 262, 357
Parks, E. A., 279
Pasteur, Louis, 160, 226, 227, 228,
    229, 230, 231, 232, 233, 234, 235,
    236, 237, 239, 240, 241, 242, 243,
    252, 253, 256, 297, 303, 354
Pauli, 348
Peebles, Thomas, 385
Penrose, L. S., 389

Petrarch, 56, 57
Petrie, A. W., 386
Petty, Sir (Dr.) William, 123, 124,
    125
Pfeiffer, 287
Philip, Robert W., 334
Plato, 342
Plenck, Joseph Jakob, 291
Pollender, 235
Pommer, 373
Popper, 360
Pott, Percivall, 152, 390
Priestley, Reverend Joseph, 155, 156,
    157, 158
Pringle, Dr. John, 203, 204
Procopius, 55, 168
Prowazek, Stanislaus Josef Mathias
    Von, 306
Prudden, J. Mitchell, 334
Pylarini, Giacomo, 174

Quellmatz, S. T., 347

Radcliffe, Dr. John, 148
Ramazzini, Bernardini, 133, 134, 135
Ramon, Gaston, 357
Rathke, 354
Reed, Dr. Walter, 318, 319, 320, 321
Rhazes, 33, 167, 168
Ricketts, Howard Taylor, 305, 306
Ricord, Philippe, 341, 345, 350
Riis, Jacob, 335
Robbins, Dr. Frederick C., 363
Rocha-Lima, Henrique da, 306
Roentgen, 332
Rogers, L. M., 370
Rokitansky, Carl von, 223, 225
Romer, 360
Roosevelt, President Franklin Delano,
    361
Rosenau, Milton J., 186, 262
Ross, Ronald, 293, 311, 312, 313, 314
Rossignol, 236
Rotch, Dr. Thomas M., 257
Rousseau, Jean Jacques, 132, 139
Roux, Emille, 237
Roux, Pierre, 237, 239, 356

Royer, 235
Ruiz, Castenada, 305
Rush, Dr. Benjamin, 147, 316, 317
Russell, Major F. F., 287

Sabin, Dr. Albert Bruce, 365, 366, 367
Saint Cyprian, 28
Salicet, Guillaume de, 351
Salk, Dr. Jonas Edward, 363, 366, 367
Sanctorius, 104, 112
Schaudinn, Fritz Richard, 381
Schick, Bela, 357
Scott, Moncrief, Sir Colin, 279, 280
Semmelweis, Ignaz Philipp, 220, 223,
    224, 225, 226
Semple, 260
Seneca, 342
Servetus, Michael, 80, 105
Shattuck, Lemuel, 277
Siebold, Karl Theodor Ernest Von, 291
Simmonds, 379
Simon, Dr. John, 276, 277
Simond, P. L., 298, 299
Simpson, James, 277
Sloane, Sir Hans, 108, 163, 176, 177
Smith, Dr. Southwood, 275, 277
Smith, Dr. Theobald, 258, 294, 295,
    357
Smith, Dr. Wilson, 384
Snow, Dr. John, 265, 266, 267
Sonnerat, 281
Soper, George A., 288
Soxhlet, Franz Von, 254, 255
Spallanzani, 205, 206, 207
Steenbock, 374
Stenson, Neils, 111
Sternberg, Surgeon General, 318
Stokes, Dr. Adrian, 322
Straus, Nathan, 255
Sutton, Robert, 177, 178
Swieten, Gerhard Van, 147, 150
Swift, Jonathan, 291
Sydenham, Thomas, 67, 107, 108, 109,
    110, 113, 146, 184, 325, 345
Sydenstricker, 378
Sylvius, Franciscus, 111, 112, 325
Szent-Gyorgyi Albert, 371, 372

Tabor, Robert, 311
Takaki, Kanehiro, 375
Taylor, Dr. Michael, 252
Thacker, Thomas, 183
Theiler, Dr. Max, 322
Thompson, 350
Thullier, 237
Timoni, Emmanuel, 174
Todd, 296, 306
Topley, W. W. C., 384
Torti, 309
Traube, Frantz, 245
Traum, Jacob, 260
Trotula, 42
Trousseau, 354
Trudeau, Dr. Edward Livingston, 333,
    334, 335
Tulp, Nicolaas, 111, 375
Typhoid Mary, 287, 288, 289

Underwood, Michael, 359
Ulsenius, Theodore, 89

Valdes, Gonzalo Fernandez de
    Oviedo -y, 88
Valens, Ezio, 343
Valsalva, 149
Van Slyke, 351
Variot, Gaston, 255
Varro, 96
Vesalius, Andreas, 79, 80, 81, 82, 85,
    98, 104, 105, 149
Vespasius, Emperor Flavius, 26, 273
Villemin, Jean Antoine, 329
Vinci, Leonardo da, 79
Virchow, 354
Vitry, Jacques de, 196
Vitruvius, 25
Von Behring, *see* Behring von

Waksman, Selman A., 338, 339
Wasserman, August Paul von, 381
Waterhouse, Dr. Benjamin, 142, 194
Waugh, 371
Weigart, Carl, 245, 246
Weisner, von, 360

Welch, William H., 248, 319
Weller, Dr. Thomas H., 362
Wesley, John, 145, 146
Wharton, Thomas, 110
Wheeler, G. A., 370, 378
Wherry, 299
Whistler, Daniel, 372
White, Dr. Charles, 221
Wickman, 360
Widal, Georges Fernand Isidore, 286
Wiener, Alexander S., 387
Williams, Robert Runnel, 369, 370, 376
Willis, Thomas, 111, 284
Windaus, 376
Wiseman, Richard, 325

Withering, William, 159, 161, 162
Wolbach, 306
Woods, Surgeon Major W. W., 305
Woolf, 390
Wren, Sir Christopher, 128, 129
Wright, Sir A. E., 287

Yersin, Alexandre-Emil-Jean, 297, 356
York, John, 266
Young, Dr. William A., 322

Zeidler, Othmar, 307
Zink, 238
Zinsser, Hans, 304, 305

SUBJECT INDEX

A

Alcoholism, 141
Amoebic dysentery, 271
Amonites, 238
Anatomy, 79, 80, 81, 85, 104, 106,
    110, 111, 112, 147, 149, 152,
    153, 154
Antiseptic surgery, 234, 235
Antivaccinationist, 193
Anthrax, 37, 235, 236, 237, 244, 245
Aqueducts, 24
Arabian medicine, 33, 34, 40, 42
Arthropod-Borne diseases, 290-301,
    306
Ascorbic acid, see Vitamin C
Asiatic cholera, see Cholera
Assyrians, 3
Auscultation, 326, 327

B

Baal-Zebub, 4
Babylonians, 3, 4, 5
Bacillus pestis, 247
Bacteriology, 95, 117, 118, 227-252
Baths, 26, 27, 29, 77, 131
BCG, 336, 337, 340
Beriberi, 369, 370, 374, 375, 376
Bible (biblical medicine), 6-11, 49-51,
    54, 272, 324, 341, 353, 368
Bills of mortality, 121, 122, 128, 170
Black Death, see Plague
Blood pressure, 155, 156
Botany, 159-161
Brill's disease, 304, 305
Broad Street well, see Cholera
Brucellosis, 259-261
Bubonic plague, see Plague

C

Cancer, 390, 391
Canning, 206, 207

Certified milk, see Milk
Chaldeans, 3
Charlatan, see Quacks
Chemistry, 113, 159
Chemotherapy, 85, 339, 340
Chicago drainage canal, 270, 271
Chlorination, 264, 278
Childbed fever, see Puerperal sepsis
Child care, 130, 138, 139, 142
Chinchona, 113, 310
Cholera, 236, 247, 264-270, 281-289
Cholera infantum, 255, 262
Chorea, 66
Christian charity, 31, 32, 52, 53
Circulation, 105, 106, 111, 119
Circumcision, 6
Clap, see Gonorrhea
Cleanliness, 6, 145, 146
Cloaca Maxima, 23, 273
Condensed milk, see Milk
Condom, 351, 352
Consumption, see Tuberculosis
Contagion, 95, 96, 148
"Corpus Hippocraticum," 14, 15
Cowpox, 188, 189, 190, 191, 192, 193
Crusades, 35-40, 44, 50, 168

D

Dancing mania, 64-68
Dark Ages, 29, 31-36, 40
DDT, 307
De Contagione, 95, 169, 173
Deficiency diseases, 368-380
De Medicina, 18
Dengue, 296
Dental health, 385, 386, 387
Devonshire colic, 207
Diabetes, 111
Diet, 10, 11, 13, 14
Digitalis, 161, 162
Diphtheria, 39, 110, 252, 353-358
    antitoxin, 356, 357
    toxoid, 357

Drunkenness, *see* Alcoholism
Dysentery, 109

E

Ebers Papyrus, 6, 342, 351
Egyptian medicine, 5-7
Eighteenth century, 132-166
English sweat, *see* Sweating sickness
Enlightenment, age of, 132
Ergot-ergotism, 68, 69
Eye of Horus, 5

F

Fecal discharge diseases, 264-280
Filaria, 292, 293, 313
Fleas, 297, 298, 299, 301-307
Flouridation, 385, 386, 387
Food preservation, 206, 207

G

German measles, 388
Gibralter fever, *see* Brucellosis
Gin acts—Gin drinking, 140
Glauber's salt, 113, 114
Gonorrhea, 10, 341-352
Gonorrheal opthalmia, 346-350
Grecian health and medicine, 12-17
Guaiacum, 92

H

Hamburg, cholera epidemic, 268-270, 283
Hammurabi, Code of, 4
Hanging drop, 244, 245
Hebraic health code, 7-11
Hydrophobia, *see* Rabies
Hygiene, 15, 145

I

Indians, 179-183
Industrial awakening, 135, 136
Industrial diseases, 133, 134
Industrial medicine, 133, 134, 136, 137
Industrial Revolution, 212

Infant care, 137-139, 253
Infant feeding, 139, 253-255
Infant feeding stations, 255, 256, 257
Infantile paralysis, *see* Polio
Influenza, 73, 109, 382-385
Inoculation, 173-179, 184-186, 189
Isoniazid, 339

J

Jail fever, *see* Typhus
Jews, 6, 60, 62, 342

K

Kings evil, 163, 164, 325
Knights Hospitalers, 39
Kosher, 11

L

Latrines, 3, 25, 26
Lausen, typhoid epidemic, 267, 268
Lazarettos, 52, 53
Lepers, leprosy, 9, 40, 49-53, 94
Lice, 301-307
Life table, 122, 124

M

Madstones, 238
Magnetism, 102
Malaria, 16, 308,-323
Malta fever, *see* Brucellosis
Measles, 33, 96, 109, 385, 388
Mediterranean fever, *see* Brucellosis
Mercury, 89, 91
Miasma, 110
Microscopists, 104, 115-120
Military hygiene and medicine, 21, 203, 204
Milk
  adulteration, 252
  -borne diseases, 250-263
  certified, 257, 258
  condensed, 257
  depots, 255, 256
  sickness, 250, 251
Monastic medicine, 31, 32
Mosquitoes, 293, 308, 311-322

N

National Foundation for Infantile Paralysis, 361, 363, 364
National Tuberculosis Association, 335
Naval hygiene, 196-203
Negroes, 181
Nurses, nursing, 213-219

O

Occupational diseases, 133, 134
Occupational medicine, 133, 134
Ophthalmia neonatorum, 346-350
Orthopedics, 139, 140
Oxygen, 157, 158

P

Pap smears, 391
Parasitism, 291
PAS, 339
Pasteurella pestis, 298, 299
Pasteurization, 232, 253, 256, 259, 261-263
Pediatrics, 253, 254
Pellagra, 376-379
Penicillin, 350, 381, 385
Percussion, 150, 151, 326
Pharmacology, 159
Physiology, 112, 147, 155, 156
Pilgrims, 35-40
PKU, 388-390
Plague, 20, 27, 28, 37, 39, 48, 53-64, 74, 109, 110, 148, 296-298
Pneumothorax, 332
Polio, 359-367
Polio vaccine field trials, 365
Pocks, *see* Smallpox
Postulates of Koch, 246, 247
Pox, *see* Smallpox
Preventive medicine, 227
Prisons, 143, 144, 207
Prostitution, 211
Public baths, *see* Baths
Public health, 22, 78, 110, 129, 130, 208, 209, 211, 275
Puerperal fever and sepsis, 220-226

Q

Quacks, quackery, 162-166
Quarantine, 61, 62, 127, 315
Q fever, 306
Quinine, 310, 311

R

Ra, 5
Rabies, 96, 237-241
Rats, 128, 297, 298, 299
Red Cross, 218, 219
Regimen Sanitatis Salernitum, 45, 46, 47
Relapsing fever, 296
Renaissance, 74-85, 92, 96, 97, 99
Rheumatic fever, 110
RH factor, 387, 388
Rickets, 110, 139, 372, 373, 374
Rickettsia, 305
Rocky Mountain spotted fever, 305
Rodents, *see* Rats
Roman medicine, 17-28
Roman sanitation, 17-28
Royal College of Physicians, 85, 107, 127
Royal touch, 325

S

Salerno, School of, 40-48
Sanatoria, 333, 334, 336, 340
Sand filtration, 278, 279, 280, 283
Sanitary awakening, 274, 275
Sanitary food practices, 10, 11
Sanitation, early, 3, 8, 9, 15, 22, 30
Saint Anthony's Fire, 68, 69
Saint Vitus Dance, 66, 68
Scarlet fever, 39, 109, 252
Schick test, 357
Scrofula, 163
Scurvy, 37, 196-203, 371, 372
Septicemia, 220, 221
Septic tanks, 279
Seventeenth century, 100-115, 126
Sewage systems, 22, 23, 270-272, 280
Sewers, 3, 22-25
Sexual hygiene, 6
Shattuck Report, 277

Sleeping sickness, 295
Smallpox, 27, 28, 33, 39, 92, 94, 96,
    109, 142, 167-195
Spontaneous generation, 205, 206,
    230, 231
Statistics, 121-125
Stethoscope, 327, 328
Stream pollution, 279
Streptomycin, 338, 339
Sumerians, 3
Surgery, 80, 81, 82, 151, 152, 153, 154
Suttonian inoculation, *see* Inoculation
Sweating sickness, 70-73, 85
Syphilis, 85-99, 344, 345, 381, 382

T

Tetanus, 247, 356
Texas cattle fever, 294
Thoth, 5
Trembles, *see* Milk sickness
Trypanosomiasis, 295, 296
Tubercle bacillus, 259, 329-332, 334
Tuberculin, 248, 331, 336
Tuberculosis, 20, 96, 111, 163, 246,
    248, 258, 324-340
  bovine, 258, 259
  chemoprophylaxis, 339, 340
Tularemia, 300
Typhoid carriers, 288, 289
Typhoid fever, 252, 264, 267, 268,
    281-289
Typhus, 96, 98, 143, 145, 284, 301-307

U

Undulant fever, *see* Brucellosis

V

Vaccination, 142, 178, 189, 191-194
Variola, *see* Smallpox
Venereal disease, 9, 10, 92, 211, 341;
    see also Syphilis and Gonorrhea
Vital statistics, 121-125
Vitamins, 368-380

W

Water, 264-280
  -borne diseases, 264-280
  supplies, 3, 6, 24, 25, 27, 248, 277
  closet, 272, 274
Whooping cough, 110
Widal test, 286

X

X-ray, 326, 332
Xerophthalmia, 368, 379

Y

Yaws, 94
Yellow fever, 308, 315-323